PSYCHOACOUSTICS

Auditory Perception of Listeners With Normal Hearing and Hearing Loss

Second Edition

Editor-in-Chief for Audiology
Brad A. Stach, PhD

PSYCHOACOUSTICS

Auditory Perception of Listeners With Normal Hearing and Hearing Loss

Second Edition

Jennifer J. Lentz, PhD

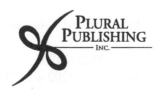

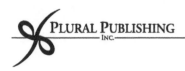

9177 Aero Drive, Suite B
San Diego, CA 92123

email: information@pluralpublishing.com
website: https://www.pluralpublishing.com

Typeset in11/13 Adobe Garamond by Flanagan's Publishing Services, Inc.
Printed in the United States of America by Integrated Books International

Library of Congress Cataloging-in-Publication Data:
Names: Lentz, Jennifer J., author.
Title: Psychoacoustics : auditory perception of listeners with normal
  hearing and hearing loss / Jennifer J. Lentz.
Description: Second edition. | San Diego, CA : Plural Publishing, Inc.,
  [2025] | Includes bibliographical references and index.
Identifiers: LCCN 2023024932 (print) | LCCN 2023024933 (ebook) | ISBN
  9781635505252 (paperback) | ISBN 9781635504392 (ebook)
Subjects: MESH: Auditory Perception--physiology | Psychoacoustics | Hearing
  Loss, Sensorineural
Classification: LCC QP461 (print) | LCC QP461 (ebook) | NLM WV 268 | DDC
  612.8/5--dc23/eng/20230911
LC record available at https://lccn.loc.gov/2023024932
LC ebook record available at https://lccn.loc.gov/2023024933

Contents

Introduction

The second edition of *Psychoacoustics* retains the modular organization, with each chapter including relevant information around a specific topic. Within each chapter, acoustics, physiology, and perception by adult listeners with normal hearing and those with hearing loss, as they relate to that topic, are presented. The book retains its focus on applications of psychoacoustics to clinical audiology. The many changes and updates are as follows:

- Chapters 2 through 7 remain similar to the first edition, but I have added a section on the perceptual consequences of SNHL on everyday listening to each chapter. Other changes include:
  - in Chapter 2, a reorganization to be more modular, additional content related to acoustics, ROC analysis, and the effects of hearing loss on the long-term average spectrum of speech (LTASS),
  - a section on the LTASS and treating hearing loss as a filter in Chapter 3,
  - review of auditory neuropathy spectrum disorders in Chapter 5,
  - more figures and additional text throughout, to clarify some points.
- Chapter 8 (Psychoacoustics and Advanced Clinical Auditory Assessment) has been revamped. This chapter now exclusively addresses elements within diagnostic audiology that are based on psychoacoustics, with added content on tinnitus assessment, automated (Békésy) audiometry, retrocochlear and pseudohypacusis evaluation, and the identification of dead regions.
- Chapter 9 (Improving Auditory Perception for Listeners with Hearing Loss) is a new chapter that exclusively focuses on the perception by individuals wearing hearing aids and cochlear implants. The content related to conventional hearing aids has been expanded, focusing on compression, digital noise reduction, and directional microphones. A section on cochlear implants has been added.
- More demonstrations, general exercises, and laboratory exercises have been added to the text and companion website. Icons new to the text remind the reader of the resources available on the website. I hope that these icons will allow these resources to be more accessible to users of this textbook, particularly students.
- With the idea of being more inclusive, person-first language is now used (including a change to the subtitle of the text), and I have added versions of some demonstrations to be more accessible to individuals with hearing loss. Chapter 1 includes a new section on the contributions of women and BIPOC scientists to the field of psychoacoustics.
- A few corrections to the text and figures have also been made, thanks to the feedback provided to me by colleagues and students.

Acknowledgments

This textbook has been strongly influenced by the many audiology and PhD students that I have taught while at Indiana University (IU). I would personally like to thank all those students at IU who took my course on psychoacoustics and taught me as much as I taught them (I hope). Some of those years were harder than others, but there is no doubt that working with audiology students over the years showed me how to better communicate psychoacoustics material. Specifically, I would like to mention the invaluable assistance of Yuan (Kim) He, who made many of the figures in this text and reviewed some of the content in the first edition. I also thank my clinical colleagues at IU for their years of discussion on the connection between psychoacoustics and audiology, particularly Nancy Nelson, Carolyn Garner, and Lisa Goerner. Those conversations have allowed me to better discuss the principles of psychoacoustics applied to clinical practice. I am also grateful to Larry Humes, Robert Withnell, and William Shofner for numerous fruitful conversations regarding the connection between physiology and psychoacoustics.

I can only begin to thank my PhD mentor, Virginia Richards, for taking a chance 30 years ago on an engineering student who knew nothing about experimental psychology and for giving me the foundation for the content of this text. The contributions of my postdoctoral advisor, Marjorie Leek, who taught me the value of scholarship and the impact of hearing loss on auditory perception, are also evident throughout this book. I am fortunate to have had two outstanding women mentors, and I thank them for their ongoing advice and mentorship over the years. Last, but most definitely not least, I would like to thank my family and loved ones for their tireless support and patience. I dedicate this edition to my father, who passed away in 2020, for his willingness to foster my interest in science as a child.

Reviewers of the Second Edition

Plural Publishing and the author would like to thank the following reviewers for taking the time to provide their valuable feedback during the manuscript development process. Additional anonymous feedback was provided by other expert reviewers.

Richard J. Baker, BSc, PhD
Reader in Audiology
Manchester Centre for Audiology and
    Deafness
The University of Manchester
Manchester, United Kingdom

Kathryn Bright, PhD
Professor Emeritus
University of Northern Colorado
Greeley, Colorado

Deborah Culbertson, PhD
Clinical Professor
East Carolina University
Greenville, North Carolina

Lilian Felipe, PhD
Professor
Lamar University
Beaumont, Texas

Scott A. Hansson, AuD
Western Michigan University
Kalamazoo, Michigan

Miwako Hisagi, PhD, AuD, CCC-A, ABA Certified
California State University, Los Angeles
Los Angeles, California

Mary Kassa, AuD
Henry Ford Health—Division of Audiology
Wayne State University
Detroit, Michigan

Adrian KC Lee, ScD
Professor and Chair
University of Washington
Seattle, Washington

Janet R. Schoepflin, PhD
Professor
Adelphi University
Long Island AuD Consortium
Garden City, New York

Kimberly Skinner, AuD, PhD
Assistant Professor
A.T. Still University
Mesa, Arizona

Nirmal Srinivasan, PhD
Assistant Professor
Towson University
Towson, Maryland

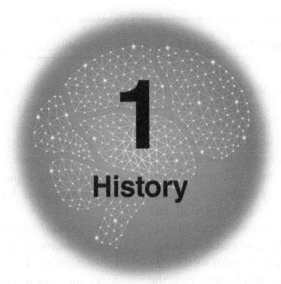

1

History

LEARNING OBJECTIVES

Upon completing this chapter, students will be able to:

- List the main pioneers in psychoacoustics
- Describe how the history of psychoacoustics has influenced the field of audiology
- Explain the history of audiometric threshold measurement

INTRODUCTION

Humans have been curious about music, hearing, perception, and communication throughout much of the history of our species. Yet, the primary roots of psychoacoustics date back to the early 1700s, when the philosophers of the time began to lay the foundation for the field of experimental psychology, which studied human behavior. This chapter provides a historical perspective of psychoacoustics by first presenting a history of experimental psychology and then discussing how those developments led to the fields of psychoacoustics and audiology, which were, in some ways, developed together. For this chapter, I have particularly relied on the publications by Boring (1961) on the history of experimental psychology, Schick's (2004), and Yost's (2015) articles on the history of psychoacoustics, and Jerger's (2009) book on the history of audiology.

This chapter reviews the origins of modern psychoacoustics by covering:

- The roots of psychophysical measurement
- The development of psychoacoustics
- The role of Bell labs
- Connecting psychoacoustics, Bell labs, and audiology
- The history of the audiogram
- Women and BIPOC pioneers in psychoacoustics

EARLY INVESTIGATION OF PERCEPTION

The connection between sound and auditory perception and has been around for millenia: In Europe, archaeologists have discovered prehistoric flutes dating from at least 35,000 years ago (Conard et al., 2009). Ancient flutes have also been uncovered in Asia, North and South America, Africa, and Australia. Early cultures developed a variety of instruments that were blown (e.g., trumpets in Egypt), struck (e.g., bell chimes in China; stones, or lithophones, from India and Vietnam), and rotated (e.g., the bullroarer found across the world). Creating these instruments required skill and craftmanship but also knowledge of how to generate sound with different perceptual characteristics. Although the Western world may consider the advent of *psychoacoustics*, the study of the relationship between sound and its perception, to have begun in the 1800s, we should credit prehistoric and ancient cultures, including those that are non-European, for their groundbreaking developments in our understanding of auditory perception. Without the development of musical instruments that could generate different types of sounds and the curiosity of prehistoric and ancient humans, Western science would not have achieved the advances of the 19th and 20th centuries.

The application of rigorous and systematic tools to the assessment of perception and its relationship to the physical world began in the early 1800s, and the field of *psychophysics* was born. At this time, scientists were interested in the sense of hearing, but they also evaluated the senses of touch and vision. Many of the techniques used to study auditory perception were originally developed for the purposes of evaluating other sensory modalities. Some techniques, particularly the scientific instruments but also the measurement methods, were designed specifically for the assessment of hearing. In a reciprocal relationship, those other disciplines adopted and modified the tools that were originally created for the hearing sciences. The purpose of this chapter is to give the reader a brief overview of principles of psychoacoustics from a historic perceptive and to illustrate how these discoveries have impacted modern audiology.

As we travel back in time to the early 1800s, we observe the development of the field of psychophysics and more specifically, psychoacoustics, which involved the evaluation of the perception of sound. These early investigators asked questions such as "under what parameters can humans:

- *detect stimuli?* Measurements in this vein usually involve manipulating various stimulus parameters (like frequency and amplitude) and measuring the *absolute threshold*, the lowest stimulus level that evokes a sensation.
- *differentiate between two stimuli?"* These experiments measure the *just noticeable difference (JND)*, also known as the *difference limen*, defined as the amount a stimulus must be changed on a particular dimension before the change is detectable.
- *describe the magnitude of the stimulus or the difference between stimuli?"* In these experiments, the *loudness*, the *pitch*, or the *quality* of sounds is measured.
- *recognize sounds?"* Here, experiments adopt meaningful stimuli, and we measure the ability to identify musical instruments, words in speech, and even environmental sounds.

Our discussion of the origin of psychological measurement begins with Ernst Heinrich Weber (pronounced Vay-burr; 1795–1878), although he was not the first to connect observation of perception with a physical stimulus. Weber, however, was the first to develop a systematic method of inquiry evaluating the relationship between the magnitude of physical stimuli and their associated sensation or perception. Although his work was conducted primarily in the areas of touch and vision, in 1834 he discovered what is now known as *Weber's law* (see Chapter 4). He noticed that, for pressure on the skin, the JND in weight could be described as a proportion of the weight (in this case, the JND was about 1/30th of the weight).

Further evaluation has demonstrated that this principle has evidence from many other sensory modalities, including hearing and vision.

One of Weber's students, Gustav Fechner (1801–1887), formalized Weber's work with mathematics. He noted that there was a way to measure the magnitude of sensation. Fechner's work was revolutionary: His claim was that the conscious perception of a stimulus is related to size of the stimulus in the physical world and that there is a relationship between perception and physical stimuli. Although this idea may seem obvious through contemporary eyes, this claim formed the foundation for all modern psychophysics and opened the door to the measurement of perception. Because of his visionary work, he is now known as the *father of psychophysics*. Perhaps not surprisingly, he coined the term *psychophysics* and published his experiments on sensory measurements in his 1860 book *Elements of psychophysics*, where he described psychophysical methods and psychophysical relationships. His book marked the beginning of experimental psychology because it brought sensation and perception, otherwise thought to be unmeasurable, under the requirements of measurement. His three methods of measuring absolute thresholds and differential thresholds are still fundamental to psychoacoustic measurement. He developed the **method of limits** (which, in modified form, is the method used to measure an audiogram), the **method of adjustment**, and the **method of constant stimuli**, techniques discussed in Chapter 2. Variants of these methods have yielded efficient measurements of perception, many of which are in use today. His view that perception and physics are connected is a foundation of our current practice: In the fields of psychoacoustics and audiology, we manipulate sound and measure the perceptual consequences. Without his seminal contributions to the study of perception, diagnostic audiology and psychoacoustics would be very different fields.

THE ORIGINS OF PSYCHOACOUSTICS

Despite the impact that Fechner and Weber have had on the field, neither conducted experiments in hearing. Rather, Hermann von Helmholtz (1821–1894), made some of the first psychoacoustic observations in the auditory modality. His book, *On the Sensations of Tone*, published in 1863, served as the foundational text on auditory perception for decades. This book, along with Fechner's, allowed the evaluation of hearing to be more than scientific observation. Rather, experimentation allowed auditory perception to be quantified under systematic evaluation. We could now connect physical acoustics with the perception of the physical dimensions.

One important aspect of Helmholtz's view of sensory systems was the idea that physiology was the basis of perception. His views have greatly influenced contemporary psychoacoustics, which commonly strives to determine the limits of auditory perception, as well as to discern the physiological mechanisms responsible for auditory perception. Helmholtz's view laid the groundwork for physiological models, some of which were proposed in the mid-1800s. For example, Helmholtz's theory of pitch was based on the "acoustic law" developed by Georg Ohm (1789–1854) and applied the principles of **Fourier analysis** developed by Joseph Fourier (1768–1830). Helmholtz's theory stated that the ear conducts a form of Fourier analysis, which allows complex sounds to be divided into sinusoidal components. To test this spectral theory of pitch, Helmholtz developed the innovative *Helmholtz resonator* (shown in Figure 1–1). By varying the size of the neck opening and the volume of the cavity, the Helmholtz resonator could produce sounds of different frequencies.

Yet, August Seebeck (1805–1849) devised a clever experiment using a rotary siren (one of which is illustrated in Figure 1–2) that

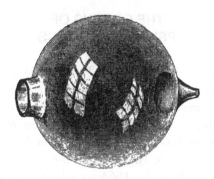

FIGURE 1–1. A Helmholtz resonator. From Helmholtz (1863).

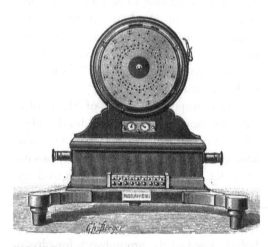

FIGURE 1–2. One of Seebeck's sirens. From Koenig (1889).

demonstrated inconsistencies in Helmholtz's spectral theory of pitch. Seebeck's results posed substantial problems for Helmholtz's theories and were bitterly disputed at the time (Turner, 1977). Unfortunately, Seebeck passed away almost a century before his experimental results were reconsidered and formalized into a theory by J. F. Schouten (1940). In contrast to the spectral representation proposed by Helmholtz, Schouten's residue theory suggested pitch perception could also be based on a temporal representation of sound. Variants of Helmholtz's and Schouten's theories are still discussed today, and both form the founda-

tion of modern models of pitch perception (see Chapter 6).

Lord Rayleigh (James William Strutt, 1843–1919) was strongly influenced by the work of Helmholtz. He discussed acoustic problems using mathematics in his book *The Theory of Sound* (1877). This work laid the groundwork for future study linking acoustics with perception. Rayleigh was also keenly interested in the ability to localize sounds in space. He proposed that two acoustic cues are used for sound localization: intensity differences and time differences across the ears. The intensity differences were produced by the presence of the head in the sound field, which can effectively block sound transmission. The time differences were produced by the different travel times of sound across the ears. This theory, called the **duplex theory of sound localization**, has been validated numerous times (see Chapter 7).

Although the investigations presented above are not exhaustive, these representative studies illustrate that the earliest psychoacoustic work was conducted on the perception of pitch and space. Little evaluation of loudness and its relationship to sound was conducted. If we pause to consider the environment that these pioneers were working in, we can gain a better understanding of why the early work was conducted in these primary areas. Technology such as sound level meters and earphones had not been engineered at that time. Although Fechner developed techniques to measure perception in the mid-1800s, the devices to manipulate and measure sound levels were not built until the 1920s. Controlling and characterizing the intensity of a sound was even more difficult than manipulating frequency or spatial location. For example, changing the length of strings, altering the properties of materials, or changing size of a tuning fork could manipulate frequency. A Helmholtz resonator or a siren, similar to that developed by Seebeck, could also be used to generate sounds with specific frequencies. On the other hand, techniques at that time did not allow manipulation of intensity without also varying the frequency of a sound.

Measurements of the auditory perception of intensity were therefore somewhat restricted and were extremely imprecise. Otologists quantified hearing loss by using tuning forks and made measurements of how long a patient could hear a sound or how far away an examiner could be before a patient could not hear a sound. Due to the limitations in achieving both accurate and precise intensity levels, early scientists focused their endeavors more on pitch and sound localization than other acoustic quantities.

Yet, one of Helmholtz's students, Wilhelm Wundt (1832–1920), did not let these limitations stymie his interest in sound perception and the perception of sound intensity. Notably, Wundt developed many instruments that allowed him to measure the perception of sound in a controlled way. His sound pendulum and falling phonometer allowed him to alter sound intensity without changing the frequency characteristics of a sound (Schick, 2004). Examples of these devices are shown in Figures 1–3 and 1–4. Both devices functioned by dropping an object that struck a panel. The height of the object would determine the intensity of the sound generated when the object struck the panel. He also developed a sound hammer and a sound interrupter, which allowed the quantification of intensity and time, among a variety of other devices.

Wundt performed some of the earliest quantitative experiments evaluating the perception of tones at different levels and why some combinations of musical notes are appealing to the ear and some are not. His work, published in his writings *Principles of Physiological Psychology* (1902) came to be one of the more important texts in psychology, and he founded

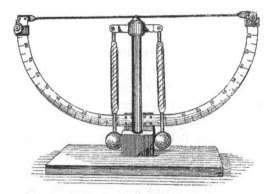

FIGURE 1–3. A sound pendulum used by Wundt. From Spindler and Hoyer (1908).

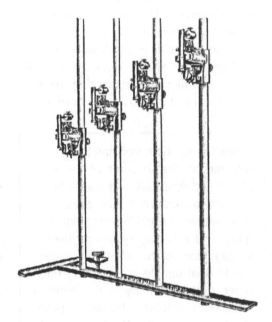

FIGURE 1–4. A falling phonometer used by Wundt. From Zimmerman (1903).

the first formal laboratory for psychological research in 1879 at the University of Leipzig. Wundt is considered the *father of experimental psychology*, as he treated psychology as separate from biology or philosophy and was the first to call himself a psychologist. His influence was far reaching and has had an impact on all areas of experimental psychology.

THE ADVENT OF THE TELEPHONE

Although Wundt was able to control the sound intensity in his experiments, the introduction of telephone receivers and sound level meters made measurements of the perception of sound intensity far more feasible. Alexander Graham Bell's (1847–1922) invention formed the basis of the technology that allows us to control and manipulate sound precisely and accurately. Along with Western Electric, its precursor company, Bell Telephone Labs (commonly called Bell Labs), focused on the research and development of telephone-associated equipment. The contributions of Bell Labs after its formation in 1925 have been integral to the fields of psychoacoustics and audiology. Much of their work involved the development of technologies that are now used to assess and to characterize hearing.

> Alexander Graham Bell has been both admired as the inventor of the telephone and despised as a leader in the oralism movement, which pressured deaf people to avoid learning sign language. He was also loosely connected to eugenics, as he attempted to persuade deaf people not to marry each other. Although many in the hearing community celebrate his accomplishments, many in the Deaf community feel very differently.

During this time frame, we also saw the development of the decibel as a unit to describe sound level. The unit, of course, was named to honor A. G. Bell, who passed away in 1922. Development of the decibel has had a profound impact on our ability to characterize hearing, including the use of suffixes such as dB SPL (sound pressure level), dB A (A weighted), and dB HL (hearing level), all of which are used to describe the level of sound in various ways. Some of the most seminal work in the field of psychoacoustics originated at Bell Labs. Examples include:

- Wegel and Lane (1924), who made the first quantitative measurements on masking, the process by which one sound influences the ability to detect another sound (see Chapter 3)
- Sivian and White (1933) measured some of the first calibrated auditory detection thresholds and compared measurements made over headphones with those obtained in the free field (see Chapter 2)
- Fletcher and Munson (1933), who, along with Steinberg, made the earliest measurements of equal loudness contours (see Chapter 4)
- Steinberg et al. (1940) conducted large-scale measurements of auditory detection abilities across a representative group of people living in the United States.
- Fletcher (1940) formalized theories of masking (see Chapter 3).

The investigations mentioned here represent some of the more important studies conducted at the time. Their work was innovative, inventive, and impactful. Their investigations have proven to be foundational on the topics of threshold, loudness, and masking. Interestingly, however, unlike in the previous century, the investigations at that time did not involve other auditory percepts, such as pitch and spatial hearing. Such experiments were not as relevant to the development of the telephone, where engineers were evaluating the limits of hearing to establish the constraints necessary for telephone receivers and associated equipment.

Although all of the investigators listed above deserve credit and recognition, it is worth pointing out the contributions of Harvey Fletcher (1884–1981), a research engineer at Western Electric and later Bell Labs from 1916 to 1949. Fletcher made some of the greatest contributions to both psychoacoustics and audiology during his tenure there and was also a founding member of the Acoustical Society of America, one of the premier organizations in support of acoustics. His contributions to the field were widespread and influential. Remarkably, he, along with R. L. Wegel (birth and death dates unknown), developed the first commercial audiometer, the Western Electric Model 1–A audiometer (Fletcher, 1992), which was the size of a large cabinet and therefore was not practical. Yet, none of the other audiometers in use at the time were practical either. For example, Cordia Bunch (birth and death dates unknown), a psychologist at the University of Iowa, built the first audiometer in the United States, but he and his colleagues were the only ones to use it. Fletcher and Wegel's audiometer, on the other hand, was a commercial audiometer that could test hearing up to 16,000 Hz. However, it was expensive and sold for roughly $1500, about 4 times the price of a car (a model-T Ford sold for about $400) and just slightly less than a house, at the time. Because of the steep price tag and the lack of portability, Fletcher and Wegel developed the first commercial and portable audiometer, the Western Electric Model 2–A (with test frequencies up to 8000 Hz) soon afterward.

Developing the audiometer was only one of Fletcher's many achievements. As Allen (1996) describes, Fletcher was the first to accurately measure auditory threshold, the first to measure the relationship between loudness and intensity and loudness and frequency (see Chapter 4). Further, he developed the model of masking in application still today (see Chapter 3). His two books *Speech and Hearing*, published in 1929, and *Speech and Hear-*

ing in Communication, published in 1953, were considered authoritative at the time and, in many cases, remain so today. Fletcher also coined the term *audiogram* and developed the unit of dB hearing level (dB HL), the decibel metric in use today to describe hearing abilities (Jerger, 2009). If that were not enough, he also made substantial contributions to our knowledge of speech perception and developed the Articulation Index, now revised to the Speech Intelligibility Index (SII), that allows one to calculate the amount of speech information available in different frequency bands. The SII is able to robustly predict intelligibility scores for certain speech materials and acoustic environments (ANSI S3.5, 2017) and is now used in industrial applications and to assess the impact of hearing loss on speech perception.

Of course, research on auditory perception did not end with the development of the telephone. In fact, the 1940s really marked the beginning of a new era, as the tools to assess auditory perception were now readily available. The accomplishments of these more recently investigators are discussed throughout this text.

CLINICAL AUDITORY ASSESSMENT

During the early-mid 1900s, we saw a revolution in the way that hearing was tested. Fletcher, along with his colleague Wegel, collaborated with an otologist, Edmund Prince Fowler (1872–1966), and began their work in measuring hearing thresholds. Regarding assessing hearing, these scientists evaluated absolute threshold (the lowest detectable sound level) and quantified the upper limit of loudness in terms of the *threshold of feeling*, which they called *maximum audibility*. Along the way, they also developed the tools and units with which to quantify the threshold and developed the graphical depictions we use today.

Developing the Audiogram

Fowler and Wegel created what we now call the ***audiogram***, a graph depicting absolute thresholds measured at specific octave and inter-octave frequencies. At the time, it was standard to quantify frequency in cycles per second (note: the unit *hertz* was established in the 1930s), and in the 1920s, Wegel had been plotting frequency in octaves, rather than using a linear scale. However, there was no standard for depicting the level (*y*) axis, and this was a topic hot for discussion. Two issues were of interest: what units to use and what scale would be best. At the time, auditory thresholds (as well as other auditory measurements, such as the maximum audibility) were plotted in sound pressure units, such as dynes/cm². It was common to use a logarithmic axis at the time, based on the works of Weber and Fechner, and was consistent with engineering tradition. Although the decibel was not in use yet, plotting auditory thresholds on a logarithmic scale was very similar to the modern practice of plotting thresholds in decibels.

An illustration of Wegel's representation is shown in Figure 1–5, which plots both auditory threshold (*minimum audibility*) and the threshold of feeling (*maximum audibility*), measured in more than 40 people. Wegel defined the range between the minimum audibility and maximum audibility curves as the *sensation area*. Wegel's sensation area had an elliptical shape because both the minimum and maximum audibility curves were frequency dependent. Today, we would call the difference between maximum and minimum audibility the ***dynamic range of hearing***. From Wegel's data, we see that the dynamic range of hearing was frequency dependent and was the largest in the mid-frequency range (e.g., about 500 to 4000 Hz).

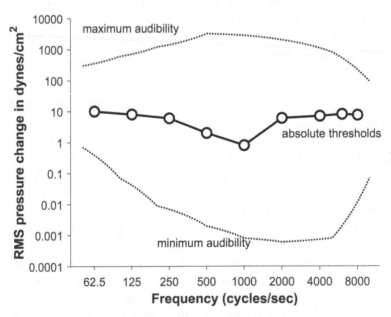

FIGURE 1–5. Illustration of early measurements of auditory abilities. The maximum audibility represents the threshold of feeling, and the minimum audibility curve represents auditory threshold in listeners with normal hearing. Thresholds obtained from an individual with hearing loss are also shown. Adapted from Wegel (1922).

At that time, Wegel and Fowler also conducted measurements of hearing in listeners with hearing loss. The absolute auditory thresholds of a listener with hearing loss, reported by Wegel (1922), are also plotted in Figure 1–5. We observe that this patient's thresholds were higher than the minimum audibility curve and fell in the middle of the sensation range. Using data such as these, Wegel and Fowler thought that there might be an easier way to depict the amount of hearing loss in which the dynamic range of hearing was considered. Wegel and Fowler observed that hearing thresholds could be quantified as a percentage of the dynamic range at each frequency. They counted the number of logarithmic steps between the minimum and maximum audibility curves and then counted the number of steps between minimum audibility and the patient's threshold. Dividing these two values and subtracting from 100% provided a *percent of normal hearing*. To illustrate this method, Figure 1–6 shows data from the same patient in Figure 1–5. Wegel and Fowler felt that plotting the data in this way better quantified how much dynamic range was left for a listener with hearing loss.

Fletcher, however, did not agree with the percent of hearing loss approach, and strongly argued against it. He renamed the *y*-axis to sensation units and changed the line at the top of the graph to *0 sensation loss*. Essentially, Fletcher's rearrangement put zero at the top, rather than at the bottom, of the figure and did not represent hearing loss in terms of the range of hearing, but rather the amount of sensation loss with respect to the minimum audibility curve. Over the years, as the dB became more widely used, it became common to plot the *y*-axis of an audiogram using dB hearing level, rather than sensation loss. The line at the top, however, remained at 0 dB HL, the value used in audiograms today (see Chapter 2).

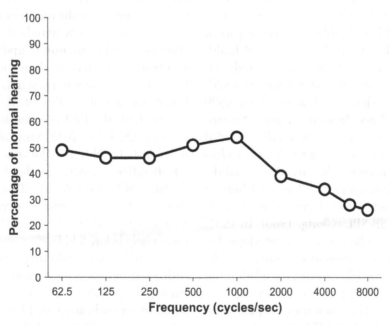

FIGURE 1–6. Early audiometric report in which the hearing threshold is converted into a percentage of normal hearing. Based on the patient's threshold from Figure 1–5.

> Fowler conducted numerous studies on measuring absolute thresholds in listeners with hearing loss. He was the first to report that listeners with sensorineural hearing loss experience a smaller dynamic range but a similar range of loudness as listeners with normal hearing. He called this phenomenon *loudness recruitment* (Fowler, 1928), a term we still adopt today (see Ch. 4).

Hearing Surveys

As the audiogram and audiometers became more widespread in their use, measurements of hearing abilities in listeners with good and poor hearing were conducted on both large and small scales. Such work was necessary to quantify hearing loss and to establish normative data in the healthy population. Due to the necessity of normative measures, Willis Beasley carried out a large survey to establish the thresholds of healthy listeners as part of a U.S. Public Health Service general health survey in 1935 and 1936. Beasley's study was designed to obtain the audiometric thresholds for people who had good hearing (about 4,500 people), and people with presumed or suspected hearing loss were specifically excluded from data analysis. Using the Western Electric 2–A audiometer, the survey provided the first large-scale estimates of normal hearing in the frequency range from 64 to 8192 Hz reported in dB SPL (Glorig, 1966). In 1951, results from the *Beasley survey* were adopted as the basis for calibration of audiometers in the United States and determined the relationship between dB SPL, which uses a physical reference, and dB HL, which uses the perceptual reference, in the ASA-1951 standard.

Beasley's survey results were problematic, however. In 1952, Dadson and King conducted

a similar survey in England and found thresholds to be approximately 10 dB better than those reported in the United States. Studies were then conducted in several other countries, all of which conformed to the English measurements and not those made in the United States. In an effort to determine the source of this discrepancy, Aram Glorig conducted another survey at the Wisconsin State Fair in 1954, in which the exact procedures used by Beasley were adopted. These data essentially replicated the results of Beasley, leading Glorig to return to the Wisconsin State Fair in 1955 and use a different method to estimate threshold, which adopted an ascending and descending method of limits. Using this procedure, Glorig found measurements to agree with those obtained in the United Kingdom and Japan. Glorig was able to conclude that by using better threshold estimation techniques than those adopted by Beasley, lower threshold estimates were achievable. His work illustrated that both the auditory sensitivity of the listener and the method used to estimate that sensitivity influence the measurement.

In 1964, a new standard was issued (ISO-64). Although minor updates to the standard have been made throughout the past 50 years, the audiometric standard remains largely unchanged. To illustrate this, the ASA-51 standard, the ISO-64 standard, and the modern ANSI 3.6 (2018) standard are listed in Table 1–1. Table 1–1 illustrates a roughly 10-dB difference between the ASA-51 and the later ISO-64 and ANSI (2018) standards. Note the drastic similarity between the ISO-64 standard and the ANSI-2018 standard, particularly below 6 kHz.

In addition to collecting data on people with good hearing, investigators were interested in the prevalence of hearing loss and the effects of age on hearing. Bell Labs conducted another survey of hearing designed to sample the range of auditory thresholds in the population. These measurements at the San Fran-

TABLE 1–1. Reference Threshold Levels in dB SPL (RETSPL) for Standards ASA-51 (First Column), ISO-64 (Second Column), and ANSI-2018 (Third Column)

Frequency (Hz)	Reference Threshold Levels in dB SPL		
	1951 ASA	1964 ISO	2018 ANSI
125	54.5	45.5	45
250	39.5	24.5	25.5
500	25	11	11.5
1000	16.5	6.5	7
1500	16.5	6.5	6.5
2000	17	8.5	9
3000	16	7.5	10
4000	15	9	9.5
6000	17.5	8	15.5
8000	21	9.5	13

Note: ASA-51 and ISO-64 adopted a Western Electric 705-A earphone, and ANSI-2018 uses a TDH-39 supra-aural earphone.

cisco and New York world fairs in 1939, therefore, did not exclude listeners with suspected auditory problems. Steinberg et al. (1940) reported their data on the hearing abilities of over 15,000 people with ages ranging from 10 to 59 years. Although these measurements were not made with robust threshold estimation procedures, the measurements largely characterized the hearing of the population of average Americans. They noted that hearing was best for their participants between the ages of 10 and 19 and slowly worsened with age. They also documented that these declines predominantly occurred in the high frequencies and that thresholds were better for women than for men, even in the same age group.

Clearly, the contributions of these investigators to the fields of psychoacoustics and audiology have had great impact. As we have seen, work in auditory perception prior to the 1900s predominantly focused on pitch and spatial perception, whereas the work between

1920 and 1940 focused on threshold testing, loudness, and masking. The work conducted by Bell Labs, of course, was directed toward developing technologies for the telephone and focused on knowledge that was important for advancing that technology. Consequently, the study of auditory perception was strongly influenced by the goals of the day. Now, modern psychoacoustics evaluates a variety of auditory perceptual abilities and considers physiological mechanisms responsible for those abilities. Since the time of Bell labs, we have greatly advanced our knowledge of hearing loss beyond that provided by the audiogram.

The audiogram, as a representation of hearing abilities, has a great deal of historical impact, and it has essentially been used in the same form for almost a century now. We should recognize, however, that the audiogram is grossly limited in its ability to characterize how well a particular patient might understand speech in a noisy or complex situation. Because it can only characterize perceptual abilities at the detection level, it is not a terribly useful tool for assessing perception at other levels. I would suggest that a focus of the next century could be the development of better tools and metrics that identify the specific deficits experienced by listeners, with thought toward using that information to determine which rehabilitation options may be the most beneficial to individual patients.

PIONEERS IN AUDITORY PERCEPTION: WOMEN AND SCIENTISTS OF COLOR

I close this chapter with an observation: Up until the 1960s and 1970s, research in psychoacoustics and audiology had limited, and maybe no, representation from female investigators or from BIPOC (Black, Indigenous, and people of color) scientists. As of 2023, the field has far greater representation of female and BIPOC investigators, but many barriers to their engagement still exist. Although more work is needed to attract and encourage scientists from these groups, I would like to highlight some of the pioneers who began to bridge these gaps prior to the 1990s. These exceptional investigators have provided examples and mentorship to younger scientists who are now following in their footsteps. Despite the lack of representation of women and BIPOC scientists in the preceding sections of this chapter, the work of many of these individuals is noted throughout this textbook. Here I point out some of these pioneers who have made significant contributions to the field of auditory perception in the 20th century. For those who are cited in this text, I have indicated the associated chapters in parentheses.

- *1960s*—Laura Ann Wilber's contributions spanned the fields of audiology, auditory perception, and acoustics. Some of her seminal work focused on measuring auditory detection abilities for bone (via a bone oscillator) and air (via headphones) conduction. Her work has influenced the standardization of procedures and established reference values used in audiometric testing. Rhona Hellman (Ch. 4) studied loudness perception in listeners with normal hearing, and her research has been fundamental to the development of current loudness standards and hearing aid algorithms. Marion Cohen also started a multiple-decade career that focused on temporal processing, and Anna Nábělek (Ch. 2) applied psychoacoustic principles to evaluate speech perception and hearing aid acceptance.

- *1970s*—Mary Florentine (Chs. 3, 4, and 5) has studied masking, temporal processing, and loudness perception of listeners with normal hearing and hearing loss. Of note is her theory called *softness imperception,* which posits that sounds at and near threshold may be louder for listeners with sensorineural hearing loss than for those with normal hearing. Glenis Long also started a storied career in auditory perception and physiology. Her work evaluated perception in humans and animals (such as the chinchilla and bat) and used both physiological and behavioral measures to investigate the mechanisms responsible for perception. Diana Deutsch is well-known for groundbreaking work on auditory illusions and the relationship between experience and beliefs on auditory perceptions. Diane Kewley-Port (Ch. 2), the only female engineering student in her graduating class, connected psychoacoustics with speech perception, focusing on the perception of vowels. Around the same time, MJ (Lynn) Penner (Ch. 8) started research in auditory perception and later applied psychoacoustic techniques to better understand the perception of tinnitus while Sharon Abel began studying temporal processing and the impact of hearing loss.

- *1980s*—Some of the women and BIPOC investigators who began their careers in the 1980s are still active in the field today. Collectively they have made contributions to our understanding of a variety of auditory perceptual processes. Specific examples include the assessment and development of measurement techniques (Lynne Marshall —Ch. 2), masking under uncertain conditions (Donna Neff, Chris Mason—Ch. 4), spectro-temporal processing in listeners with normal hearing (Virginia Richards —Chs. 3 and 5) and those with hearing loss (Marjorie Leek—Chs. 3, 6; Blas Espinoza-Varas), multi-sensory temporal processing (Charlotte Reed), and temporal processing in older listeners (Sandra Gordon-Salant—Ch. 5). Lynne Werner's work on auditory perception in infants has resulted in methodological advancements and an understanding of auditory perceptual development, and Judy Dubno (Ch. 3) has had a significant career studying the influence of aging and sensorineural hearing loss on auditory and speech perception. In 2020, Judy became the third woman to receive the Acoustical Society of America's gold medal, the ASAs highest award (the other two winning for speech communication—Kathy Harris in 2007 and Patricia Kuhl in 2008).
- Late *1980s* and early *1990s*—This era has much better representation from women in the field, and contributions from people of color really began around this time. Here are a few highlights: Ruth Litovsky's (Chs. 7 and 9) work evaluating the auditory mechanisms responsible for listening in complex environments for adults and children has been particularly influential. Her studies evaluating the benefits of bilateral cochlear implantation have informed modern medical recommendations. She was the first woman to receive an ASA prestigious silver medal in the area of Psychological and Physiological Acoustics for her contributions in

the area of cochlear implants. Toshio Irino's developments (Ch. 3) in auditory modeling and signal processing are now used in modern perceptual models, whereas Fan-Gang Zeng (Chs. 5 and 9), and Qianje Fu (Ch. 9) have informed our understanding auditory perception by cochlear implant users. Fan-Gang Zeng also has studied perception by individuals with tinnitus and auditory neuropathy. Beverly Wright's work (Ch. 3) has advanced our understanding of auditory learning and plasticity and the connection between masking and speech perception.

Although this list of scientists is not exhaustive, I note that the contributions of women and BIPOC scientists really did not begin until the latter part of the 20th century. We can't change the past, but we can acknowledge the importance of change. We can all take steps to encourage the work of investigators from different backgrounds to the benefit of the field and ourselves as scientists. Even today, more work needs to be done to celebrate the work of these investigators: A colleague estimated that as of 2023, roughly 10% of fellows of the ASA are BIPOC and about 23% to 24% are female, suggesting as such.

Yet, the demographics of the field are changing, and the field is becoming more diverse. Today, both women and BIPOC individuals hold leadership roles within local and professional institutions, providing examples for a younger generation. In the past 10 years, three women with expertise in psychoacoustics have served as president of the ASA, an institution historically dominated by men: Judy Dubno (2014–2015), Diane Kewley-Port (2020–2021), and Peggy Nelson (2022–2023). All three previously served as vice president, along with Donna Neff (2005–2006) and Barbara Shinn-Cunningham (2014–2015). Many people of color with backgrounds in psychoacoustics have also achieved leadership roles or the rank (or its equivalent) of full professor (e.g., Denis

Başkent, Monita Chatterjee, Lei Feng, Shuman He, Sridhar Kalluri, Adrian K.C. Lee, and Vishakha Rawool). However, there still is significant underrepresentation from individuals of minoritized groups, and barriers to engagement remain. Lack of representation is only one of those barriers. I encourage us all, myself included, to consider how the field of psychoacoustics can continue the trajectory of becoming a more inclusive space and work actively to reduce these hurdles.

REFERENCES

Allen, J. B. (1996). Harvey Fletcher's role in the creation of communication acoustics. *Journal of the Acoustical Society of America, 99*(4), 1825–1839.

ANSI/ASA S3.5 (1997; R2017). *American National Standard methods for calculation of the speech intelligibility index.* American National Standards Institute.

ANSI/ASA S3.6 (2018). *American National Standard specification for audiometers.* American National Standards Institute.

Boring, E. G. (1961). The beginning and growth of measurement in psychology. *Isis, 52*(2), 238–257.

Conard, N. J., Malina, M., & Münzel, S. C. (2009). New flutes document the earliest musical tradition in southwestern Germany. *Nature, 460*(7256), 737–740.

Dadson, R. S., & King, J. H. (1952). A determination of the normal threshold of hearing and its relation to the standardization of audiometers. *Journal of Laryngology and Otology, 66*(8), 366–378.

Fechner, G. (1966). *Elements of psychophysics* (Vol. 1). Holt, Rinehart and Winston.

Fletcher, H. (1929). *Speech and Hearing.* Van Nostrand.

Fletcher, H. (1940). Auditory patterns. *Reviews of Modern Physics, 12*(1), 47.

Fletcher, H. (1953). *Speech and Hearing in Communication.* Krieger.

Fletcher, H. (1992). *Harvey Fletcher 1884–1981.* NAS Online. National Academy of Sciences. https://www.nap.edu/read/2037/chapter/10#180

Fletcher, H., & Munson, W. A. (1933). Loudness, its definition, measurement and calculation. *Bell Labs Technical Journal, 12*(4), 377–430.

Fowler, E. P. (1928). Marked deafened areas in normal ears. *Archives of Otolaryngology, 8*(2), 151–155.

Glorig, A. (1966). Audiometric reference levels. *Laryngoscope, 76*(5), 842–849.

Helmholtz, H. (1863/1954). *On the sensation of tone.* English translation published in 1954 by Dover Publications. (First German edition, On the sensation of tone as a physiological basis for the theory of music, published in 1863.)

Jerger, J. (2009). *Audiology in the USA.* Plural Publishing.

Koenig, R. (1889). *Catalogue des appareils d'acoustique construits par Rudolph Koenig.* s.n.

Schick, A. (2004). History of psychoacoustics. *Proceedings of 18th International Congress on Acoustics (ICA)* (Vol. 5, pp. 3759–3762), Kyoto Acoustical Science and Technology for Quality of Life.

Schouten, J. F. (1940). The residue and the mechanism of hearing. *Proceedings of Koninklijke Nederlandse Akademie Van Wetenschappen, 43,* 991–999.

Seebeck, A. (1843). Ueber die Sirene. *Annals of Physics and Chemistry, 60,* 449–481.

Sivian, L. J., & White, S. D. (1933). On minimum audible sound fields. *Journal of the Acoustical Society of America, 4*(4), 288–321.

Spindler, & Hoyer (1908). *Apparate für psychologische untersuchungen.* Preisliste XXI.

Steinberg, J. C., Montgomery, H. C., & Gardner, M. B. (1940). Results of the World's Fair hearing tests. *Bell Labs Technical Journal, 19*(4), 533–562.

Strutt, J. W. (Lord Rayleigh; 1877). *The theory of sound: Volume I.* Macmillan.

Turner, R. S. (1977). The Ohm–Seebeck dispute, Hermann von Helmholtz, and the origins of physiological acoustics. *The British Journal for the History of Science, 10*(1), 1–24.

Wegel, R. (1922). Physical examination of hearing and binaural aids for the deaf. *Proceedings of the National Academy of Sciences, 8,* 155–160.

Wegel, R., & Lane, C. E. (1924). The auditory masking of one pure tone by another and its probable relation to the dynamics of the inner ear. *Physical Review, 23*(2), 266–285.

Wundt, M. (1902). *Principles of physiological psychology* (5th ed., English translation published in 1904). Swan Sonnenschein and Co.

Yost, W. A. (2015). Psychoacoustics: A brief historical overview. *Acoustics Today, 11,* 46–53.

Zimmermann, E. (1903). XVIII. *Preis-Liste über psychologische und physiologische Apparate* (p. 29). Eduard Zimmermann.

2

Estimating Threshold in Quiet

INTRODUCTION

Psychophysics is the systematic assessment of perception and its relationship to the physical world, and *psychoacoustics*, a subset of psychophysics, specifically focuses on the connection between auditory perception and sound. One of the core psychoacoustic and audiological assessments is the measurement of *absolute threshold*, the minimum detectable level of a sound in the absence of external noise. The absolute threshold reflects *auditory sensitivity* at the detection level and provides a

measure of the lower limit of hearing. From a psychoacoustic standpoint, measurements of absolute threshold have greatly influenced the development of technologies (such as the telephone, stereo systems, and hearing aids) but also have contributed to our understanding of the relationship between sound and its perception. In clinical audiology, measuring absolute threshold is part of diagnostic assessment, useful for characterizing the hearing loss of a particular patient and in guiding hearing aid fittings. To obtain a full understanding of this important measurement, one must also possess an understanding of a variety of concepts underlying sound detection, including acoustics, measurement techniques, and psychophysical principles.

Although this chapter primarily focuses on the ability of the ear to detect sounds, we should also recognize that detection is an important precursor to the comprehension of complex sounds such as speech, music, and environmental sounds. Detection is often considered the lowest level of auditory behavior in the hierarchy of auditory skills, as described by Erber (1982). In this hierarchy, there are four levels of auditory perception:

- *Detection:* Detection of sound simply implies that one is able to perceive the presence of a sound stimulus. Detection is often quantified in terms of the lowest *sound level* necessary for a stimulus to be detected.
- *Discrimination:* Discrimination is the ability to hear that two sounds are different from each other. A variety of different acoustic dimensions can be evaluated using discrimination tasks (such as frequency, intensity, or timing).
- *Recognition:* Recognition occurs when a sound is attached to an object, or a label. It is also sometimes referred to as *identification*, a term also used throughout this book.
- *Comprehension:* Comprehension is the process by which sounds are assigned meaning.

Psychoacoustics primarily focuses on the detection and discrimination levels, although some experiments also address identification abilities. Both detection and discrimination abilities are necessary precursors to recognize and comprehend complex sounds. Deficits in low-level abilities preclude good performance in higher-level abilities, although a listener could have a deficit in a higher-level ability and not a lower-level one. For example, problems with detecting sounds can have a large impact on the ability to recognize and comprehend speech. In contrast, a listener may have difficulty comprehending speech in the absence of deficits at the detection level.

This chapter specifically focuses on interpreting *absolute threshold* measured using *detection*. Other chapters cover a variety of auditory abilities at the discrimination level, with some discussion of identification. This chapter is divided into three sections: Foundations: Acoustics and physiology, Psychoacoustical measurement and signal detection theory, and the Threshold of human hearing. Students with sufficient background in acoustics and physiology may begin with the section on measurement techniques, but acoustics of pure tones and physiology are provided for those who would like a review.

This chapter covers the following topics:

- Foundations: Acoustics and physiology
  - Acoustics of pure tones (the spectrum, waveform, and the decibel)
  - Physiological representation of pure tones
- Psychoacoustic measurement and signal detection theory
  - The psychometric function
  - Research and clinical methods
  - Signal Detection Theory and applications within clinical audiology
- Threshold of human hearing
  - Absolute threshold measured in the free field and over headphones
  - The effects of hearing loss on threshold and dB HL
  - The relationship between the long-term average spectrum of speech (LTASS) and elevated thresholds

FOUNDATIONS OF ABSOLUTE THRESHOLD: ACOUSTICS AND PHYSIOLOGY

Psychoacoustics is the study of the relationship between perception (the psychology) and sound (the acoustics). In order to understand perception, a general understanding of sound and auditory physiology is critical. The concept of sound is important so that we can interpret psychoacoustical data, whereas physiology is the basis of perception. Here, we review the components of sound—waveforms, spectra, and the decibel – that are necessary to understand and interpret perceptual measurements, focusing on detection and pure tones.

Acoustics: Pure Tones and the Decibel

This section provides a general overview of some of the important acoustic concepts used within psychoacoustics and audiology, but the interested reader is referred to Charles Speaks' book *An Introduction to Sound* (2018) for additional detail.

The Sinusoidal Pressure Wave

Very generally, **sound** is a pressure wave that results from oscillation of particles within a medium. Sound is generated when a source is set into vibration and that vibration is transmitted through a medium. For audiology, the medium is commonly air for audiology applications but can also be bone and liquid. The oscillations occur in the form of high- and low-pressure variations that occur over time and distance. To illustrate these oscillations, we can visualize sound by looking at the vibratory motion of a tuning fork.

Striking a tuning fork sets the tines into an oscillating motion, moving inward and then outward from their initial resting place. Figure 2–1 illustrates the motion of tuning fork, shown on the left side of the figure. The outward and inward movement of the tines cause regions of high and low pressure, respectively, in the air adjacent to the tuning fork. For reference, the various shapes of the tuning fork are illustrated in the bottom panel of Figure 2–1, with the main panel showing the associated regions of high and low pressure resulting from the different portions of tuning fork vibration. When the tines move outward, the air molecules immediately adjacent to the tuning fork are compressed, yielding a region of *high pressure* (illustrated by the regions of crowded air molecules in Figure 2–1), also referred to as the *compression* portion of the wave. The tines then pass through their equilibrium state and move inward, producing a region of *low pressure* (illustrated by the regions in which the air molecules are far apart in the middle panel), called the *rarefaction* portion. The pressure wave then *propagates* away from the tuning fork, although the air molecules

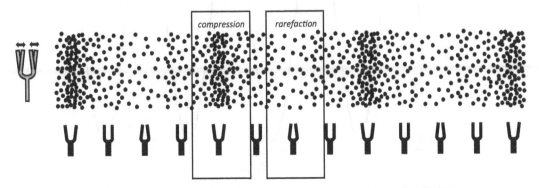

FIGURE 2–1. An illustration of sinusoidal vibration of a tuning fork. The main panel illustrates the air molecules with regions of high (compression) and low (rarefaction) pressure that result from the various phases of the tuning fork, illustrated in the bottom panel.

themselves do not move from their local positions. High- and low-pressure oscillations also occur *over time* at a single point in space.

The form of sound produced by a tuning fork is commonly called a ***pure tone***. A pure tone is a sound, or signal, with pressure variations occurring over time that follow a *sinusoidal* pattern. That is, the variations in pressure over time can be described by a sinusoidal function, as illustrated in Figure 2–2, which shows the instantaneous amplitude versus time. One *cycle* of a sine wave is one repetition of the sinusoidal repeating pattern and includes one compression phase and one rarefaction phase. Because a sine wave repeats over time, it is a *periodic* sound. On Figure 2–2, the deflections above zero refer to regions of high pressure, and the deflections below zero refer to regions of low pressure. The ***amplitude***, which describes the *size* of the stimulus, reflects the amount of pressure variation. Notably, a pure tone always reaches the same maximum and minimum amplitude each cycle, as illustrated in Figure 2–2, labelled as *a* and *-a*. A pure tone also has a single ***frequency***, or the rate of oscillation, defined as the number of cycles

that the sound completes in one second. For a pure tone, there is only one rate of oscillation—it does not change over time. We can observe this in Figure 2–2, as the time it takes for one cycle to complete (the ***period***, *T*) is the same for every cycle.

Because of the simple and regular characteristics of this sound, the pure tone is a foundational stimulus for audiometric assessment and psychoacoustics. Pure tones are particularly useful for the ***audiogram***, a report of the ability to detect pure tones as a function of frequency. They are preferred for standard audiometric testing over other sounds as they are characterized by only one frequency and therefore are the most ***frequency-specific*** sounds available. Of all potential stimuli, the pure tone is acoustically very simple and produces a relatively simple response in the auditory system.

Representations: Waveforms and Spectra

As described previously, pure tones follow a pattern of vibration that is sinusoidal, char-

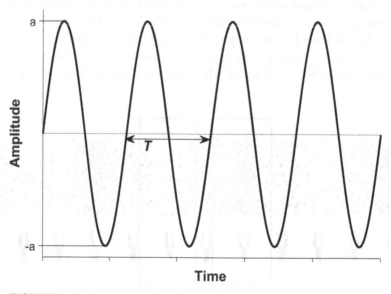

FIGURE 2–2. A pure-tone stimulus waveform. The maximum amplitude, a, and the period, T, are labelled.

acterized by the following equation that describes the ***waveform***, which is a plot of instantaneous amplitude (y) versus time (t), also illustrated in Figure 2–2:

$$y = a \ sin(2\pi f t + \theta), \qquad \text{Eq. 2–1}$$

where a = maximum amplitude, f = frequency, and θ = phase. When referring to actual physical stimuli and their representation in the environment, we describe the amplitude of sound in terms of sound pressure in pascals (Pa), a metric unit named after Blaise Pascal, which is defined as a force per unit area (newtons per square meter; N/m^2). The frequency of a stimulus is quantified in cycles per second (hertz; Hz), or the number of times a stimulus repeats itself over one second. The starting phase, θ, is quantified in degrees or radians (0° – 360° or 0 – 2π radians) and describes how much a wave is shifted compared to its reference starting phase at t = 0 seconds.

To fully represent a pure tone, then, one needs to specify the *maximum amplitude*, the *frequency*, and the *phase*. For the purposes of this chapter, we consider the starting phase of the pure tone to be zero degrees, as the ear cannot sense the starting phase of a single pure tone. However, the ear can sense phase differences between tones and across the two ears (see Chapter 7 on Hearing with Two Ears), and so we should not always neglect the phase of pure tones.

The waveform is used to represent temporal properties of sound, or how sound varies over time. The waveform of a pure tone follows a simple sinusoidal pattern in which the maximum amplitude is equal to the minimum amplitude but with the opposite sign. We can refer back to Figure 2–2, which shows how the maximum amplitude (a) manifests on the waveform. The maximum amplitude, often also referred to as the *peak amplitude*, is rather straightforward to visualize and label, as it is the highest amplitude reached by the sinu-

soidal waveform. Because sound is a pressure wave, the peak amplitude is a term often interchanged with the term ***peak pressure***, or the highest pressure achieved by the sound stimulus. The waveform illustrates variations over time and allows visualization of the period (denoted T; see also Figure 2–2). Although the period is easily noted on the waveform, the frequency (the number of cycles completed in one second), is not so obvious. Thus, we usually plot the waveform over a time interval that allows us to observe the period, and we then calculate the frequency from the period using the formula, $f = 1/T$, with T specified in seconds.

Figure 2–3 illustrates a more specific example and shows 10 cycles of a waveform with an amplitude of 1 and a period of 0.001 seconds, or 1 millisecond (ms). The period can be converted into frequency (hertz) by the formula $f = 1/T$ (1/0.001 s = 1000 Hz).

The waveform is related to the ***spectrum***, a plot of amplitude versus frequency through a process called ***Fourier analysis***, which allows any stimulus waveform to be represented by a series of pure tones. A line at a single frequency illustrates the spectrum of a pure-tone stimulus, as observed in Figure 2–4 for the 1000-Hz tone plotted in Figure 2–3. A complex stimulus, on the other hand, can be represented as a series of lines, with each line representing the amplitude and frequency of a constituent tone. This representation of the spectrum can be referred to as a line spectrum.

Figure 2–4, which plots the spectrum in terms of amplitude versus frequency, illustrates that the pure tone contains only a single frequency, making it quite straightforward to determine that the frequency of this particular pure tone is 1000 Hz. Notably, the spectrum does not represent the temporal characteristics of sound like the waveform, and the waveform does not represent the frequency characteristics like the spectrum. Both representations have their advantages, and students should

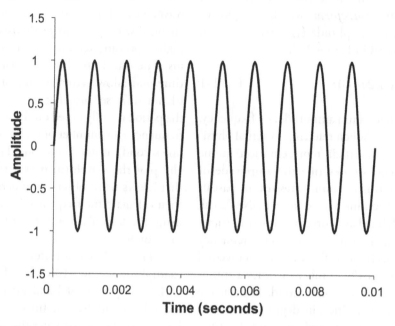

FIGURE 2–3. A waveform of a 1000-Hz tone with an amplitude of 1 and 0° starting phase.

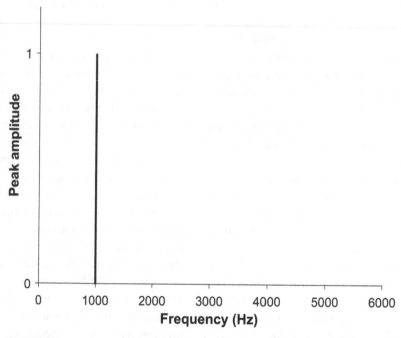

FIGURE 2–4. The spectrum of the 1000-Hz tone illustrated in Figure 2–3.

be comfortable with both representations in order to fully understand the range of auditory abilities covered in psychoacoustics.

A common question is when to use a waveform to represent sound and when to use a spectrum to represent sound. For some types of sounds, either representation is equally effective. A pure tone is a good example of this—the frequency and amplitude of the sound can be determined from both the waveform and the spectrum. On the other hand, the waveform is most useful if one is interested in evaluating the temporal characteristics of a stimulus, such as how the amplitude of speech changes over time. The spectrum is more valuable when one wants to evaluate the frequency content of sounds, such as the spectral prominences, or formants, in a vowel stimulus.

Duration Effects

Acoustic Considerations. The spectrum illustrated in Figure 2–4 represents a pure tone of infinite duration. However, it is physically impossible to generate a sound of infinite duration. Therefore, we must also consider the effect that the duration of a sound stimulus has on the representation of that sound. The longer the duration of a pure tone, the more *frequency specific* that pure tone will be. The ***time-frequency tradeoff*** governs this relationship in the following way: a short-duration sound must have a broad bandwidth spectrum. The only way to achieve a narrow bandwidth spectrum is to provide a long duration. However, long-duration sounds can, and often do, have broad spectra, such as white noise. More detail is provided about noise stimuli in Chapter 3.

In sum, a long-duration tone has only one frequency: It is very frequency specific. A short-duration tone can never be frequency specific. The duration of a tone has a drastic influence on the frequencies present in the stimulus and has a primary effect of broadening the spectral peak of the stimulus. The increase in the frequencies present in the stimulus is called ***spectral splatter***, which is characterized by the ***bandwidth***, or the range of frequencies contained within the stimulus. Figure 2–5, which shows the spectrum of a short-duration pure tone, illustrates this effect and shows a stimulus with a much broader bandwidth than the infinitely long pure tone illustrated in Figure 2–4. The duration of the pure tone determines the frequencies of the *nulls*, which are frequencies at which there is no energy. We can calculate the high-frequency and low-frequency nulls of the primary spectral peak for a tone with center frequency, f_c, as

$$hf_{n1} = f_c + 1/d, \text{ and}$$
$$lf_{n1} = f_c - 1/d.$$

Eq. 2–2

where d = the duration of the stimulus; hf_{n1} is the high-frequency null of the primary lobe, and lf_{n1} is the low-frequency null of the primary lobe. Additional nulls, both higher and lower than the frequency of the pure tone, occur. Their frequencies are also related to the duration of the stimulus. As we observe in Figure 2–5, the spectrum is no longer a line at a single frequency at f_c, the frequency of the tone. Rather, additional frequencies are now present in the spectrum, which shows a broadening of the spectral peak and a small number of *side lobes*, small *bumps* in the spectrum at frequencies higher and lower than the center frequency. The duration of the stimulus determines the bandwidth (BW) of the primary lobe and the bandwidth of the side lobes. Because the location of the nulls can be calculated directly from the duration, reducing the duration of the tone increases the

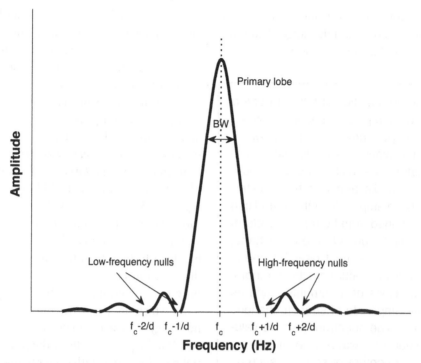

FIGURE 2–5. Spectrum of a short-duration pure tone. The frequency of the pure tone is indicated by f_c, which is the center frequency of the spectral representation. Nulls are shown to occur at $f_c \pm n$/duration (d), where n is the nth null.

breadth of the spectral peak and increases the distance between the side lobes.

From Eq. 2–2 we can calculate the amount of spectral splatter generated by decreasing the duration. One way to define the bandwidth of the spectral peak is the distance between the nulls, or $BW = hf_{n1} - lf_{n1} = 2/d$. For example, a tone with a 2-sec duration has a bandwidth of the main lobe of 1 Hz:

$$BW = 2/2s = 1 \text{ Hz}.$$

A tone with a 2-ms duration has a bandwidth of the main lobe of 1000 Hz:

$$BW = 2/.002s = 1000 \text{ Hz},$$

and a tone that is 10 microseconds (μs) in duration has a bandwidth of 20000 Hz:

$$BW = 2/0.000010s = 20000 \text{ Hz}.$$

Thus, a very brief tone is not frequency specific and may contain unwanted frequencies. Extremely short tones, like those that are 10 μs or 1 μs in duration, are considered broadband within the scope of audiology and psychoacoustics. On the other hand, a 2-second tone, like the one used for audiometric testing is very frequency specific, with a bandwidth of 1 Hz. Thus, it is very important to consider the duration of a sound and its relationship to the frequency content of sounds. We must always be cognizant of the consequences of stimulus manipulations when determining the sounds and their durations for psychoacoustic and audiologic considerations.

Tone Duration in Assessment of Auditory Threshold. With respect to measuring absolute threshold, we should ensure that we are using frequency-specific stimuli. For audiometric measurements, the American Speech-

Language-Hearing Association (ASHA) has developed a set of specific recommendations for the durations of the pure tones used in audiometric testing. These recommendations are specific to audiometry, and different stimulus durations may be used for psychoacoustic testing. Here, we will evaluate the relationship between the ASHA recommended pure-tone durations and the frequency specificity of the stimuli used in audiometric testing. When measuring the audiogram, ASHA recommends using a pure-tone duration of 1 to 2 seconds for testing with steady tones and three, 200-ms presentations when testing with pulsed tones (ASHA, 2005). Because audiometric testing is most commonly conducted at the octave and inter-octave frequencies ranging from 250 to 8000 Hz, we will evaluate the time-frequency tradeoff for the frequencies across this range. Consider two of the durations within ASHA's recommendations: 2 seconds for a steady tone and 200 ms for a pulsed tone.

According to our previous analysis of spectral splatter, the 2-second tone has a spectral-peak bandwidth of 1 Hz, whereas the spectral-peak bandwidth of the 200-ms tone is 10 Hz. For both of these durations, the majority of stimulus energy is contained within a fairly narrow frequency range around the signal frequency. Thus, ASHA's recommendations for the durations of pure tones yield very little spectral splatter. No matter the audiometric frequency tested (e.g., 250 Hz or 500 Hz), these durations will yield pure tones that have no frequencies in common with other frequencies tested during audiometry. We can then treat each frequency tested in the audiogram as being independent from the other frequencies from an acoustic standpoint.

In fact, from an acoustic standpoint, ASHA's guidelines are extremely conservative. Even 20-ms pure tone would have a spectral peak bandwidth of 100 Hz, and thus the spectral spread of a 20-ms, 250-Hz tone used in audiometry would still provide a frequency representation independent from a 500-Hz

tone. We can conclude, then, that ASHA's recommendations of pure-tone durations are not primarily driven by acoustic principles. Rather, as we will see in Chapter 4 of this text, the pure-tone duration requirements are driven by the perceptual principle of *temporal integration*.

There are times, however, when testing requires the use of brief tones. Consider the impact of using a 2-ms tone. A 2-ms, 500-Hz tone will contain frequencies from 0 to 1000 Hz, and a 2-ms, 1000-Hz tone will contain frequencies from 500 to 1500 Hz. In this case, both tones have frequencies between 500 and 1000 Hz in common. From an acoustics perspective, these two tones are not independent, and this duration would be a poor choice for audiometric testing, particularly for low audiometric frequencies. An audiological application of the use of short-duration stimuli is tone-burst auditory brainstem response (ABR), which is sometimes used as a physiological alternative to an audiogram. This tool uses durations between 2 and 10 ms. As a result, the technique yields less frequency-specific results than audiometry.

Decibels (dB)

We have seen previously that the peak amplitude is sufficient to characterize a pure tone. However, there is a drawback to using peak amplitude when describing sounds other than pure tones. Although the peak amplitude provides an unambiguous descriptor of the size of the sine wave, it is rarely appropriate for complex sounds because many of these sounds experience large amplitude changes with time. To demonstrate this point, the waveform of a complex sound is shown in Figure 2–6. In this stimulus, the peak (maximum) amplitude does not provide a strong depiction of the overall amplitude characteristics of that sound. Most amplitude in this sound is low relative to the peak amplitude. Consequently, we can also represent the amplitude of a sound using metrics other than the peak amplitude.

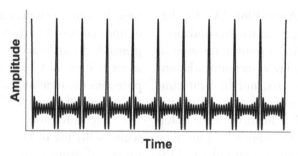

FIGURE 2–6. Waveform of a complex sound with large amplitude variation.

A common way to represent the overall amplitude, or pressure, of a complex sound is to use *root mean squared (rms) pressure*, which provides a characterization of the amplitude over *some time interval*. The rms pressure contrasts with the *instantaneous pressure*, which is the pressure of the wave at any moment in time, and the *peak pressure*, which is the maximum pressure achieved. For a pure tone, there is a fixed relationship between peak pressure and rms pressure, given by Eq. 2–3.

$$P_{rms}=0.707 p_{peak}, \qquad \text{Eq. 2–3}$$

where P_{rms} = rms pressure and p_{peak} = peak pressure. Note that the units for rms pressure and peak pressure are the same and are pascals (Pa; N/m^2).

Rather than being a simple average, which would be zero for any sine wave, rms pressure is calculated by

$$\sqrt{\sum \frac{(p_i)^2}{N}}.$$

In this equation, the pressure (p) at time i is calculated at each of N points that sample a single period. Essentially, the rms calculation squares the wave, takes the mean of those squared values across one period (for a periodic sound), and then takes the square root.

Visit the companion website for an example calculation of the rms pressure for a pure tone.

Although the rms calculation allows characterization of complex sounds by a single number, we do not use it when describing sound for perceptual applications. The smallest detectable pressure by the human ear is roughly 20 µPa (or 20×10^{-6} Pa) and the sound pressure associated with excessively loud sounds is about 0.2 or 2 Pa. Because the range of pressures represented by the ear is so large, we rarely use pressure in pascals in acoustics, psychoacoustics, or audiology. Rather, the decibel is almost ubiquitously utilized.

The decibel is based on the long-term rms pressure, rather than the peak pressure, and is always used in reference to a quantity. With respect to sound, a common decibel metric used to describe sound is *dB SPL*, or decibels in *sound pressure level*. dB SPL can be calculated by the following equation:

$$dB\ SPL = 20\ log(P_1/P_{ref}), \qquad \text{Eq. 2–4}$$

where P_1 is the rms pressure of the measured sound and P_{ref} is the reference pressure of 20 µPa. Using dB SPL is very specific, as it commonly implies the 20 µPa reference. The 20 µPa reference is quite handy, as using this reference allows us to characterize sound levels in our environment using numbers ranging between -10 dB SPL and 120 dB SPL or so. As an aside, we often see the term *sound level* used to describe how big a sound is. This term is purposely general, and it is similar to the term *amplitude*, in that it refers to the size of the sound but can be used without reference to the specific units of measurement.

> To illustrate the relationship between pascals and dB, we can use the stimulus in Figure 2–3 to determine the rms amplitude and dB SPL level. First, we treat the peak amplitude in the waveform of Figure 2–3 as represented in pascals, and is 1 Pa. From Eq. 2–3, we can calculate the rms pressure as 0.707 Pa. Substituting this value for P_1 in Eq. 2–4, we see that the dB SPL value of this tone is 91 dB SPL [20 log(0.707/20 × 10^{-6})].

> Visit the companion website for an illustration that shows a 10-fold increase in pressure translates to a 20-dB increase in dB SPL.

Summary

Because psychoacoustics is concerned with measuring the limits of auditory perception on various acoustic dimensions, understanding the waveform and spectral representation of sound is important. The waveform, which plots instantaneous amplitude versus time, contrasts with the spectrum, which plots amplitude versus frequency. The waveform can only be represented using instantaneous amplitude/pressure, but in audiology and psychoacoustics applications, the spectrum typically uses a decibel metric. However, the two representations are two sides of the same

coin, so shortening the duration of the stimulus will concomitantly lead to a broadening of the bandwidth of the stimulus.

Physiological Representation of Sound

We consider the auditory system to consist of the *periphery* (the outer, middle, and inner ear) and the *central* auditory system, connected by the *vestibulocochlear nerve*. Each of these components has a distinct role to play in the ability to hear, and changes to each of these systems can drastically affect perception. Consequently, a brief review of each component of the auditory system is provided here. A schematic of the main anatomical structures of the ear is shown in Figure 2–7.

Outer and Middle Ear

The outer ear primarily consists of the pinna and ear canal. The components of the pinna and ear canal, together, modify the amplitude of the incoming sound, and add gain predominantly for frequencies ranging between 2000 and 3500 Hz (Shaw, 1974). The tympanic membrane lies at the end of the ear canal and vibrates in response to the incoming, and now modified, sound. The middle ear transmits the vibrations of the tympanic membrane to the cochlea, via the ossicular chain, which consists of the malleus, incus, and stapes and serves to provide an impedance match between the air-filled communication medium and the fluid-filled cochlea. The ossicular chain provides a second source of gain, with an emphasis on frequencies between 600 and 1800 Hz (Kurokawa & Goode, 1995). The *frequency-gain functions*, also referred to as *transfer functions*, for the outer and middle ears are shown in Figure 2–8.

The transfer function of the outer ear shows only a small amount of gain below 1000 Hz, and the amount of gain increases

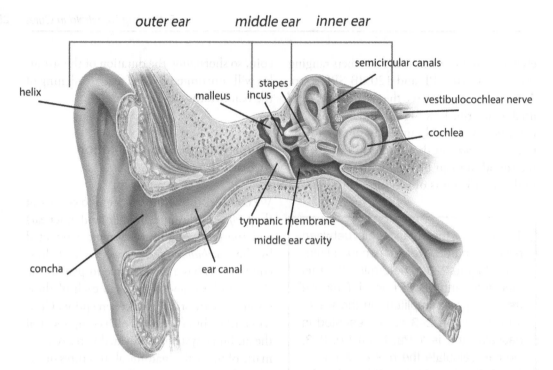

FIGURE 2–7. Depiction of the anatomical structures of the peripheral auditory system. Image adapted from Medical Art Inc/Shutterstock.com.

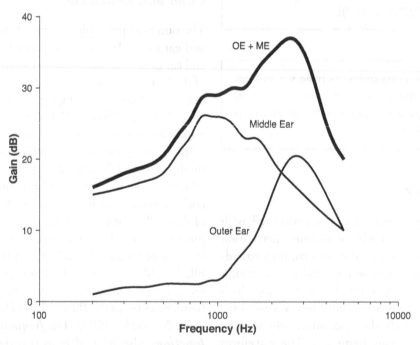

FIGURE 2–8. Schematics of transfer functions of outer ear (OE) and middle ear (ME), along with the total gain provided by the combined outer and middle ear. The combined function reflects amplification between 2000 to 3500 Hz from the outer ear and 600 to 1800 Hz from the middle ear. Based on data from Abiara et al. (2001) and Mehrgardt and Mellert (1977).

with increasing frequency until it peaks at approximately 2500 Hz. The middle ear shows a broader response, with the most gain around 800 Hz. The heavy, solid line illustrates the combined response of the outer and middle ears. The combined transfer function demonstrates that the outer and middle ear, together, provide gain over a wide range of frequencies, between 600 and 4000 Hz.

Changes to the outer and middle ear structures can have a direct influence on their transmission properties. Damage to these structures may result in a **conductive hearing loss**, which reduces the amount of vibration transmitted to the inner ear. Middle ear disorders such as otosclerosis and otitis media can affect the stiffness and the mass of the middle ear. Increasing the stiffness of the middle ear system primarily reduces the gain provided in the low frequencies, whereas increasing the mass mostly reduces the gain provided in the high frequencies.

Inner Ear

The auditory portion of the inner ear is responsible for transducing sound energy into neural signals that are interpretable by the central auditory system and higher brain centers. The inner ear consists of a vestibular portion and an auditory portion (the cochlea); only the auditory portion is reviewed here.

The form of the inner ear is that of a snail-shaped coil embedded in the dense temporal bone of the skull. Figure 2–9, a depiction of a cross section of the cochlea, illustrates that the basilar and Reissner's membrane divide the cochlea into three chambers along its length. The **organ of Corti**, the sensory organ for hearing, sits atop the basilar membrane. Vibrations from the stapes footplate, connected to the oval window, stimulate the cochlear fluids and cause the basilar membrane (BM) to move. Different areas of the BM vibrate in response to different frequencies because the *base* (the portion closest to the stapes footplate) of the basilar membrane is relatively narrow and stiff, whereas the *apex* (at the center of the coil) is relatively wide and less stiff. This is a process that we now refer to as **tonotopic organization**.

Helmholtz (1857) developed the first sophisticated theory of tonotopic organization, and von Békésy's (1960) Nobel prize-

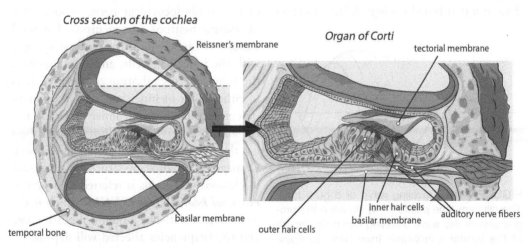

FIGURE 2–9. Anatomical drawing of the cochlea (cross section shown in the *left panel*) and the organ of corti (*right panel*). Image adapted from EreborMountain/Shutterstock.com.

winning experimental work directly supported this theory. From von Békésy's work, we now know the following:

- *Tonotopic organization occurs at the basilar membrane.* High-frequency sounds vibrate near the base of the basilar membrane while low frequencies peak near the apex of the basilar membrane. These results provided clear support for a frequency analysis mechanism being present in the ear.
- *Vibration occurs in the form of a traveling wave.* The **traveling wave** is a wave of basilar membrane vibration that travels through the basilar membrane until it reaches its place of maximum vibration. This movement is illustrated in Figure 2–10, which shows various time points of a wave as it moves down the length of the cochlea. We also observe that the traveling wave builds slowly as it travels down to the apical region of the basilar membrane and drops quickly after reaching its point of maximum vibration.

Von Békésy's studies used cadaver cochleae and high-level stimuli. As a result, he measured passive responses, reflecting purely mechanical properties of the BM. His measurements demonstrated broad tuning: A large portion of the BM was activated by a single sound. Modern in vivo measurements illustrate a much more narrowly tuned traveling wave, in that a pure tone vibrates many fewer basilar membrane locations (Rhode, 1971; Sellick et al., 1982). Thus, in vivo, the cochlea provides a more frequency-specific representation than originally thought. Although von Békésy was unable to measure BM responses to a variety of stimulus levels, modern measurements down to levels of 10 dB SPL indicate that cochlear tuning is much sharper at low versus high levels (Robles et al., 1986).

Referring back to Figure 2–9, the organ of corti has three rows of *outer hair cells* and one row of *inner hair cells* down the length of the cochlea. The outer hair cells are responsible for enhancing the vibration on the basilar membrane, particularly at low levels, sharpening the tuning of the vibration on the basilar membrane, and compressing the range of vibration represented by the basilar membrane. These hair cells lead to the mammalian ability to hear very low-level sounds, and loss of these hair cells can cause a reduction in hearing sensitivity up to about 60 dB (Sellick et al., 1982). The inner hair cells transduce the vibratory signal into neural activity and synapse with the **auditory nerve**, a portion of the vestibulocochlear nerve. About 95% of *afferent* neurons (the neurons that send signals to higher auditory centers) synapse with the inner hair cells, and they maintain the tonotopic organization of the BM. Loss of either outer or inner hair cells, the synaptic connections between inner hair cells and the auditory nerve, or auditory nerve fibers has the potential to cause complete deafness. Damage to any of these structures that leads to elevated thresholds is referred to as **sensorineural hearing loss (SNHL)**, which is the focus of this text. The amount of hearing loss and the frequencies affected will depend on the severity and location of the damage.

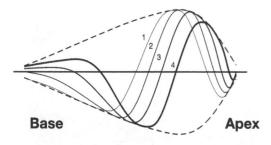

Base   **Apex**

FIGURE 2–10. Traveling wave of a pure tone. The different time points (1–4) illustrate the progression of the wave traveling down the length of the basilar membrane from base to apex. Adapted from von Békésy (1966).

Auditory Nerve: Amplitude Coding

The auditory nerve plays a critical component in transducing the amount of vibration on the basilar membrane. The type I fibers, afferent fibers that synapse with the inner hair cells and provide connections to higher levels in the auditory system, provide a neural representation, or code, of basilar membrane vibration. These fibers carry the information from the cochlea to the central auditory system in the form of action potentials, also known as spikes (Sachs & Abbas, 1974). Type I neurons code the amplitude of basilar membrane vibration via firing rate, defined as the number of spikes per second. Increasing stimulus level increases the firing rate of the fiber. Note that the size of an action potential does not vary with the frequency or amplitude of the stimulating sound stimulus (via the amount of BM vibra-

tion). Individual type I fibers typically have a spontaneous firing rate (SPR), in which they generate action potentials even in the absence of stimulation. Three different types of type I fibers are present in the auditory nerve fiber bundle, classified based on their spontaneous firing rates: high SPRs (about 18 to 250 spikes/ second), medium SPRs (about 0.5 to 18 spikes/ second), and low SPRs (<0.5 spikes/second).

As the amplitude of a stimulus is increased, the measured spike rate of a single auditory nerve fiber also tends to increase. To illustrate this, auditory nerve fiber behavior is often plotted using a ***rate-level function***, a plot of the neuron's output firing rate as a function of the input stimulus level. Figure 2–11 illustrates typical rate-level functions for auditory nerve fibers with different spontaneous rates, based on data collected by Winter

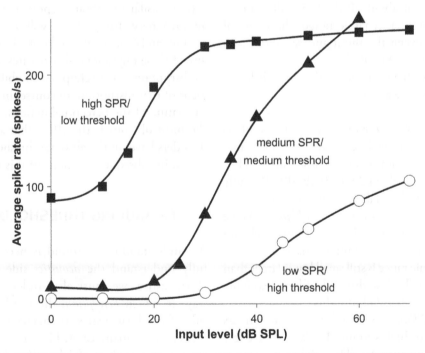

FIGURE 2–11. Auditory nerve rate-level functions for the three different Type I auditory nerve fibers, classified by their spontaneous firing rate (SPR). Based on data from Winter et al. (1990).

et al. (1990). We observe a strong relationship between the firing rate of a neuron and the stimulus level. Using Figure 2–11, we also note that the threshold and SPR of a neural fiber are related. The threshold of a neuron is defined as the lowest sound level that leads to a measurable increase in the driven spike rate. High spontaneous rate fibers have low thresholds, whereas low spontaneous fibers have high thresholds. Figure 2–11 shows that the high spontaneous rate fiber begins firing above its spontaneous rate at a very low input stimulus level (<5 dB SPL). On the other hand, the low spontaneous rate fiber does not fire above its spontaneous rate until an input level of roughly 25 dB SPL.

The neurons also demonstrate saturation, which occurs when increases in stimulus level no longer lead to increases in firing rate. For example, note the very low level at which saturation occurs for the high SPR/low threshold fiber in Figure 2–11, which begins at a level of about 30 dB SPL. All neurons demonstrate a dynamic range, the range of levels between threshold and saturation, on the order of 20 to 40 dB.

The characteristics of the three different fiber types are as follows:

- *high SPR/low threshold fibers.* These fibers respond at low levels, have high spontaneous rates, and small dynamic ranges. They saturate at about 25 to 30 dB SPL. Roughly 60% of fibers fall into this category.
- *medium SPR/medium threshold fibers.* These fibers code for moderate stimulus levels and have moderate spontaneous rates. Their dynamic range is still small but is larger than that of the low-threshold fibers. Roughly 25% of fibers fall into this category.
- *low SPR/high threshold fibers.* These fibers code for high stimulus levels and have low spontaneous rates. Their dynamic range is the largest of all fibers but rarely exceeds 60 dB (Palmer & Evans, 1979). Roughly 15% of fibers fall into this category.

Due to the saturation and limited dynamic ranges of individual fibers, an individual neuron cannot code the entire range of sound levels that are perceived by the human ear. The *dynamic range* of an individual neuron is on the order of 20 to 40 dB and rarely exceeds 60 dB. Note that the **dynamic range of human hearing**, the range of sound levels between absolute threshold and excessively loud, is considered to be approximately 100 to 120 dB, suggesting that all three fiber types must be used to represent the entire dynamic range of hearing. Consider, then, that the high SPR/low threshold fibers would be most involved in representing low-level stimuli, such as when auditory threshold is measured. On the other hand, high threshold/low SPR fibers are most involved in auditory detection when a background noise is present.

Our ability to hear sounds, then, is a consequence of outer and middle ear amplification, basilar membrane representation and auditory nerve firing. As we will see in other sections and chapters of this book, disorders of any of these physiological structures will lead to disruptions in psychophysical ability. The locus of that disruption, of course, influences the nature of the perceptual deficits. Perhaps the most obvious is the effect that auditory disorders have on the absolute threshold, discussed in subsequent sections of this chapter.

MEASURING THRESHOLDS

An understanding of sound is necessary to fully understand the *acoustics* side of psychoacoustics, we must also understand the ways in which *perception*, the psychological side of psychoacoustics, is characterized and measured. In many cases, like for audiology, we are interested in **absolute threshold**, the minimum detectable level of a sound in the absence of external noise. However, in other cases, we may be interested in other types of thresholds (such as a discrimination threshold). Regardless, an understanding of how psychoacoustical measurements are made is needed to interpret various aspects of auditory perception. This section of this chapter will review many of the methods used, with a focus on the measurement of absolute threshold.

The Psychometric Function and Classical Measurement Techniques

Measuring the ability of the ear to detect sounds is a core of both audiology and psychoacoustics. As noted, we are often interested in the absolute (or detection) *threshold*, particularly in the field of audiology. The term threshold is misleading, as it lends to an interpretation that stimulus levels above the threshold always yield detection and stimulus levels below the threshold are undetectable (or inaudible). It would be a mistake to think of

the threshold in this way. Rather, in auditory detection, the term threshold refers to a sound level associated with a somewhat arbitrarily chosen percentage of detections, like 50% or 75%, which means that at threshold, a listener could detect the sound 50% or 75% of the time. For any psychoacoustic task, there is a range of stimulus parameters for which performance is between 0% and 100%. For example, a range of stimulus levels (e.g., 0 to 25 dB SPL) might be associated with detection abilities ranging from 0 to 100%, as shown in Figure 2–12.

Figure 2–12 illustrates a *psychometric function*, which plots the percentage of sound detections as a function of signal level in dB SPL. In the example illustrated here, the method used to determine the response to a given stimulus was a *yes/no* task. In a yes/no detection task, a listener is given an *observation interval* in which the stimulus is either present or not. In many cases, the observa-

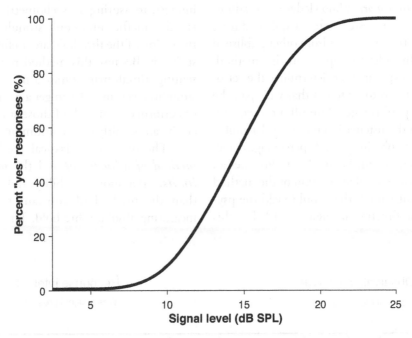

FIGURE 2–12. An example of a psychometric function for detecting a pure tone in quiet, which illustrates that performance increases with increasing signal level.

tion interval is *defined*, in which a subject is informed about when to listen. This is often done using a light that precedes, or is simultaneous with, the observation interval. The listener then responds either "yes, I heard a signal" or "no, I did not hear a signal." Figure 2–13 illustrates an experimental *trial* for a yes/no experiment. The trial is defined as the **observation interval** plus the **response interval**, the interval in which a listener is expected to respond.

> Visit the companion website for an auditory-visual demonstration of a yes/no detection experiment.

Measuring the psychometric function typically employs the **method of constant stimuli**, one of the three classical psychophysical procedures used to measure perceptual abilities. Implementation of this method requires some *a priori* knowledge of the stimulus levels to be tested, often acquired during pilot experimentation or from other published studies. In order to implement this method, then, the experimenter determines the set of stimulus levels to be tested that will span the range of performance. Stimuli are then presented to the listener in random order multiple times to obtain a reliable percentage detection measurement. Figure 2–14 illustrates an example of an implementation of the method of constant stimuli that would yield the psychometric function in Figure 2–12. For this

example, the stimulus levels of 7, 11, 15, 19, and 23 dB SPL were randomly selected and tones at those levels were presented six times each. Note that six stimulus presentations were chosen only for illustrative purposes—a robust psychometric function usually requires at least 25 to 30 presentations per stimulus level. The example in Figure 2–14 also includes no-signal trials, which allow an investigator to measure *false alarms*, responses in the absence of a stimulus. Figure 2–14 shows a "yes" response coded as a "+" whereas a "no" is coded as a "–." The psychometric function is generated by calculating the percent correct detections at each stimulus presentation level.

From this example, we see that increasing the sound level increases the percentage of stimulus detections. The threshold is then defined as some arbitrary level of performance, which is typically 50% or higher. If the threshold were defined as 50% detections, the threshold for this listener would be about 15 dB SPL. If only the threshold is of interest, measuring a psychometric function is rather inefficient, as only stimulus levels in the region of the threshold are useful for measuring it. Because this method requires presenting stimuli many times at many different stimulus levels in order to get a measurement of performance at each of those stimulus levels, it can be fairly time consuming.

The other two classical methods, the **method of adjustment** and the **method of limits**, offer more flexibility and efficiency than the method of constant stimuli for measuring absolute threshold. The *method of*

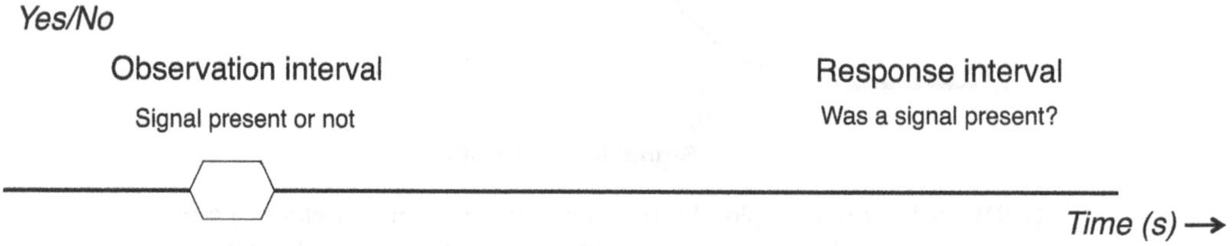

Yes/No

Observation interval

Signal present or not

Response interval

Was a signal present?

Time (s) →

FIGURE 2–13. Illustration of a single trial of a yes/no paradigm. This is a signal-present trial.

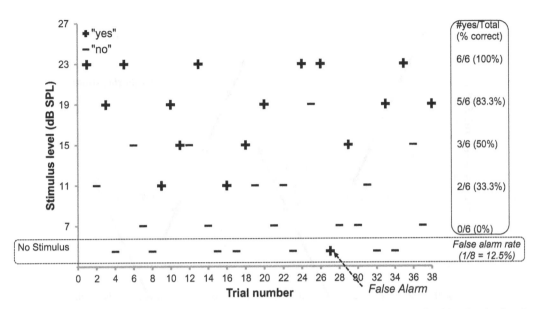

FIGURE 2–14. Illustration of an implementation of the method of constant stimuli, with stimulus level plotted versus the trial number. "Yes" responses are indicated as a "+", and no responses are indicated as a "–". Percent detections are calculated in the right of the panel for each stimulus level. A calculation of false alarms is also shown for no stimulus trials.

adjustment is unique in that it allows listeners to adjust the stimulus and find their threshold. Although this method is appealing and can yield a threshold in a matter of a few seconds, it has no fixed response percentage associated with threshold, and thresholds depend greatly on how individual listeners define their threshold. Due to the weaknesses of this method, we do not commonly use it for clinical purposes. However, it is becoming more widely accepted as an effective procedure for automated audiometry and screening, as recent evidence suggests that the technique rivals standard audiometry in terms of its validity and reliability for testing absolute thresholds of adults using earphones (Mahomed et al., 2013).

Regarding threshold estimation, however, a more widely adopted classical method is the *method of limits*. In the *descending* method of limits, the tester presents a stimulus at an audible level (selected randomly from a few pre-selected levels), and the experimenter gradually decreases the stimulus level until the listener cannot detect the stimulus. The tester averages the two final signal levels to obtain the threshold. In the *ascending* method of limits, the procedure starts at an inaudible stimulus level (also selected randomly) and the tester increases the stimulus level until the listener detects it. Again, the tester averages the two final signal levels to obtain the threshold. These procedures may be repeated a few times, and the average of all threshold estimates yields the final threshold. Figure 2–15 illustrates an example of the *ascending/descending* method of limits, in which a tester alternates between ascending and descending runs.

Experimentally, it was found that listeners can anticipate stimulus presentations or become accustomed to hearing a stimulus (habituation), and the ascending trials did not have this limitation. However, there was still room for more efficiency, which led to the development of adaptive procedures that are now commonly used in modern psychoacoustic applications. The procedure now adopted

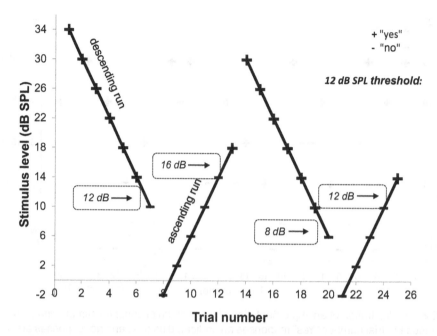

FIGURE 2–15. Illustration of an implementation of the ascending/descending method of limits. In this example, two descending and two ascending runs of the method of limits are shown, with signal level plotted versus the trial number. "Yes" responses are indicated as a "+" and no responses as a "–". A calculation of the threshold estimate is also demonstrated.

for clinical threshold measurement is a modified version of the method of limits and has similar characteristics to the adaptive procedures discussed next.

Adaptive Procedures

Adaptive procedures allow an experimenter or clinician to home in on the threshold level rather quickly. An adaptive procedure samples multiple points on the psychometric function, in an attempt to find a single point, such as the threshold. As long as the psychometric function governing the specific auditory behavior follows an increasing pattern like that shown in Figure 2–12, adaptive procedures can be used to estimate the threshold. In these cases, the percentage detection associated with the threshold is commonly defined by the adap-

tive procedure used. The parameters used for the adaptive procedures must be carefully considered in the context of the psychometric function. The adaptive procedure must sufficiently sample the psychometric function by testing stimulus levels that fall within the sloped portion. Because an adaptive procedure should obtain most of its measurements at signal levels within the sloped region of the psychometric function, it can be efficient by not presenting too many trials associated with 0% and 100% detections.

The Modified Hughson-Westlake Procedure

The *modified Hughson-Westlake method*, used to estimate auditory thresholds in the clinic (ASHA, 2005), is based on the method of limits and is rather similar to adaptive procedures. The modified Hughson-Westlake procedure provides an efficient measurement of the detection threshold and is the result of considerations of the following principles:

- limited effects of the patient anticipating a signal presentation
- familiarization
- sufficient sampling of the psychometric function, and
- efficient threshold estimation.

In this procedure, the tester (often the audiologist) presents a stimulus and waits briefly for a patient response (a "yes" or a "no"). This paradigm uses an *undefined observation interval*, that is, the patient (or listener) does not know when the stimulus will be presented. In this way, the method *prevents a patient from anticipating* when a stimulus is presented, ensuring that the method will not yield a threshold lower than the true threshold. The procedure begins testing with a stimulus presented at a level high enough to familiarize the patient with the test stimuli (usually 20–30 dB above the estimated threshold). *Familiarization* is needed so that a patient understands task requirements and what to listen for. Familiarization is achieved when the tester finds a stimulus level at which a patient responds reliably; this value is always above the patient's threshold.

After familiarization, the adaptive procedure begins. Upon a detection ("yes") response, the stimulus level is decreased by 10 dB. This change in level is the *step size* of the procedure. The sets of trials in which the stimulus level is decreasing are referred to as the *descending runs*, which continue until a listener does not detect the presence of the signal. At this point, the stimulus level is increased by 5 dB; these are the *ascending runs*, which will continue until the listener detects the signal. At that point, a descending run is again initiated. This procedure, commonly called the *10-dB down,*

5-dB up procedure or the *10-down, 5-up* procedure, is continued until the patient responds to at least two out of three stimulus presentations at the same level on the ascending runs. The final value is taken as the threshold, leading to a very *efficient* means of estimating threshold. This procedure yields a threshold that corresponds to <u>50% or higher</u> detections. Marshall and Jesteadt (1986) estimated that the clinical procedure converges at about 85 to 95% detections. An example of this procedure is illustrated in Figure 2–16, which shows a threshold estimate of 50 dB HL and a procedure that started at 30 dB HL. Familiarization occurred at the presentation level of 70 dB HL, even though the procedure began at 30 dB HL.

> Clinical audiology measurements use dB HL, which is a decibel measure that describes the amount of hearing loss with respect to normative data. We will discuss this metric in more detail in the section on Hearing Loss and Elevated Threshold.

The span of the psychometric function in dB drives the selection of the parameters of the modified Hughson-Westlake procedure. Without knowing the shape of the psychometric function, we could not determine the appropriate parameters for implementation of the procedure, and years of previous research support the implementation of the modified Hughson-Westlake procedure. Using the established parameters, the modified Hughson-Westlake procedure *sufficiently samples the psychometric function* to obtain a threshold. To see the reasons for this, we first look back to Figure 2–12, where we observe that the psychometric function for detecting a tone in quiet has a range of approximately 12 dB (the dB values that encompass about

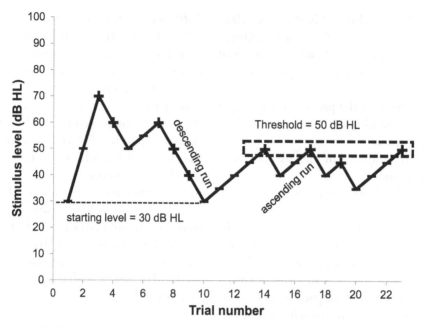

FIGURE 2–16. An example of the modified Hughson-Westlake procedure, estimating a threshold of 50 dB HL. The stimulus level in dB HL is plotted versus the trial number. A "+" sign indicates a positive response and a "–" sign indicates a no response.

5% to 95% detections). Although this psychometric function represents that of a listener with normal hearing detecting a pure tone in quiet, the range of a psychometric function for detection does not change in the presence of hearing loss (Marshall & Jesteadt, 1986).

Any adaptive procedure that samples the psychometric function for detection should use a step size smaller than the range encompassed by the psychometric function. This is the only way that a tester can ensure that an adaptive procedure will land on some of the stimulus levels that fall within the psychometric function. If the adaptive procedure selected presentation levels associated with 0% or 100% detections, the procedure could easily misestimate the threshold of the listener. Thus, an adaptive procedure must use a step size that, at some point, will test a presentation level that falls within the range of the psychometric function. By finding a signal level

associated with a no response and then using ascending runs with a 5-dB step size, the audiologist ensures that a presentation level will fall in the range of the psychometric function.

The 10-dB down and 5-dB up steps also allow for an efficient and relatively rapid

> Using a smaller step size can be appropriate for audiometric testing, as the ascending runs will sample the psychometric function using the smaller step size. Of course, this procedure will take longer to implement and may result in different test-retest reliability. Such modifications are usually only implemented in the clinic under uncommon circumstances, such as when a listener is suspected of feigning hearing loss, either intentionally or unintentionally.

assessment of threshold. Further enhancing the efficiency is the practice of stopping the threshold estimation procedure after at least two responses out of three stimulus presentations on the ascending runs. This allows an adept audiologist to collect a full audiogram in about 15 minutes, allowing time to conduct additional diagnostic assessments.

The Adaptive Staircase Procedure

Other forms of adaptive procedures are adopted for research purposes, as they can allow for better test-retest reliability, although they are typically more time consuming than the modified Hughson-Westlake procedure. The modified Hughson-Westlake procedure has a test-retest reliability of about ±5 dB, which can be sometimes too poor for psycho-acoustic testing. Furthermore, the modified Hughson-Westlake is only appropriate for estimating the absolute threshold and cannot be applied to other auditory abilities that involve discrimination or identification.

A common adaptive procedure used in psychophysical testing is the *adaptive staircase method*, an adaptive method in which the signal levels are determined by a listener's previous responses (Levitt, 1971). As with the clinical method, the staircase procedure makes the task easier (e.g., increases the stimulus level) when listeners make errors and makes the task more difficult (e.g., decreases the stimulus level) when listeners make correct detections or discriminations. The staircase

procedure is commonly paired with a forced-choice paradigm, illustrated in Figure 2–17. In a *forced-choice* paradigm, at least two, but sometimes more, observation intervals are presented. Only one randomly chosen interval contains the signal (the signal-present interval); all other intervals do not (the signal-absent intervals). The observation intervals are usually *defined* for the listener in some way (e.g., lights). Listeners select which interval contains the signal, and they will be either correct or incorrect. Figure 2–17 illustrates two-interval, two-alternative forced choice (2I-2AFC), which is a very common forced-choice paradigm. 3I-3AFC, three intervals and three choices (only one being correct), is also commonly adopted in psychoacoustics.

> Visit the companion website for an auditory-visual demonstration of a 2I-2AFC detection experiment.

> Most students are familiar with forced-choice procedures, as they are the basis of multiple-choice exams. A multiple-choice exam, in which each question has four answers and only one correct answer, would be the equivalent of four-alternative forced choice.

Implementing the staircase method requires selection of parameters that are already

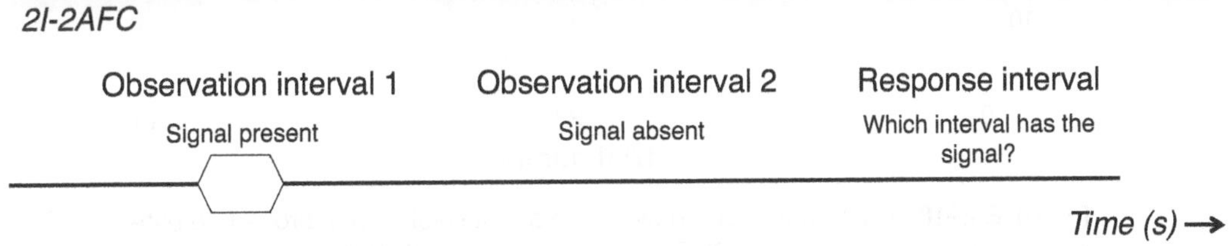

2I-2AFC

Observation interval 1 — Signal present

Observation interval 2 — Signal absent

Response interval — Which interval has the signal?

Time (s) →

FIGURE 2–17. Illustration of a single trial of a 2-Interval/2-Alternative Forced-Choice (2I-2AFC) paradigm for a detection experiment. The signal is present in the first interval.

predetermined for the clinical method: the starting signal level, the step size, and the criterion for stopping the staircase. In many cases, researchers estimate auditory abilities for a variety of tasks, such as the discrimination tasks that are discussed in subsequent chapters in this book, and so they must choose these parameters to make these measurements. No matter the task, some of the same procedural principles that apply for the clinical method are the same, including familiarization and sufficient sampling of the psychometric function. The researcher, however, is not always interested in using a highly efficient method and may sacrifice efficiency for better test-retest reliability.

Experiments commonly use either a *2-down, 1-up* or a *3-down, 1-up* staircase procedure to estimate threshold. In the 2-down, 1-up procedure, a listener must make a correct decision on two consecutive trials before the task difficulty increases. A single error causes the task to become easier. In contrast, three consecutive correct decisions are required for the task difficulty to increase in the 3-down, 1-up procedure. In these procedures, threshold is determined by averaging the signal levels at the reversals, or the stimulus levels at which listeners' responses switched direction. When other parameters of the staircase procedure are selected appropriately, in theory, the 2-down, 1-up procedure estimates 71% correct and 3-down, 1-up estimates 79% correct. As with the clinical procedure, the *starting signal level* should be higher than the final threshold estimate in order to familiarize the listener. Figure 2–18 shows the adaptive staircase procedure applied to auditory detection. Here, the starting signal level is 65 dB SPL, well above the final threshold of 43 dB SPL. The *step size*, which is 5 dB in Figure 2–18, also must yield presentation levels that sample

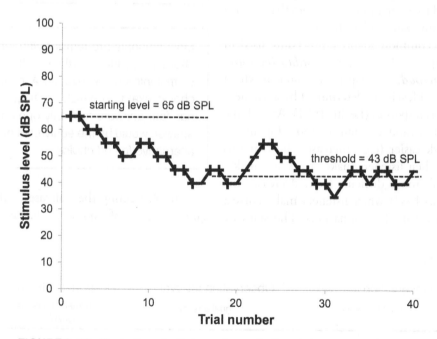

FIGURE 2–18. Illustration of a 2-down, 1-up adaptive staircase procedure estimating a threshold of 43 dB SPL. The stimulus level in dB SPL is plotted versus the trial number. A "+" sign indicates a correct response and a "–" sign indicates an incorrect response.

the psychometric function. Finally, the experimenter needs to determine when to end the threshold estimation procedure, or the *stopping rule*. Usually, research experiments end the procedure after a certain number of trials or after a certain number of reversals. Stopping after a fixed number of trials ensures that every threshold estimate will take roughly the same amount of time, but ending after a fixed number of reversals ensures that the psychometric function has been sampled a specific number of times. The threshold is often estimated by averaging the signal level at the positive and negative reversals, or from the reversals at the end of the ascending trials. Figure 2–18 shows a staircase that ended after 40 trials.

Note also that whereas efficiency is a requirement for the clinician, it is not always the highest priority of the researcher. In some cases, the researcher can sacrifice efficiency to achieve better test-retest reliability than may be possible, or even warranted, in the clinic. Thus, a staircase procedure, when implemented in the research lab, may include many more trials or reversals than would be used in a clinical application. One additional feature of the implementation of psychoacoustic procedures in the laboratory is that thresholds are always measured more than once, generally, at least three times. The repeated measurements allow experimenters to assess the reliability of the threshold estimate.

Signal Detection Theory and Its Applications to Clinical Audiology

The Framework

When measuring threshold and other auditory perceptual abilities, we are often interested in the *auditory sensitivity* of the listener, essentially what the ear *can do*. However, we must also consider the *response proclivity* of the listener, or *how* the listener responds to the

stimuli. We also refer to response proclivity as *response bias*, more explicitly defined as the listener's tendency to say, "Yes, I heard something." Listeners may come to the laboratory or the clinic with different motivations, conscious and unconscious, and these factors must be considered in any psychoacoustic or audiological assessment.

To illustrate the impact of response bias, let us consider more closely a *yes/no* detection experiment. A listener is presented with two types of trials: signal-absent trials and signal-present trials. After any given observation interval, the listener must determine whether their internal response (the neural representation of the stimulus) resulted from a signal being present or not. Because there are many variables involved in coding a sound, including environmental and physiological factors, no signal is associated with a deterministic internal response.

Green and Swets (1966) developed a robust framework within which to characterize this problem and termed it *signal detection theory (SDT)*. In this framework, we can consider the internal response generated by a signal (or the absence of one) to be represented by two probability distributions. Figure 2–19 illustrates this concept and shows one probability distribution associated with the absence of the signal (plotted to the left on the axis) and the one associated with the presence of the signal (plotted to the right). Because signal detection theory applies to measurements near threshold, performance is not at 100%, and these distributions overlap to some degree. The greater the overlap (or the smaller the signal level), the more difficult the task will be for the listener and the poorer the auditory sensitivity.

Although the listener does not have control over their sensitivity to a specific stimulus, the listener is tasked with determining whether a signal was presented, based on the internal response alone. Here, we can assume that familiarization and learning over multiple

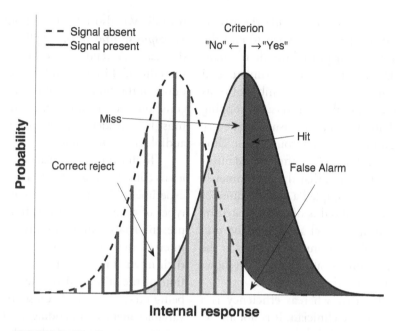

FIGURE 2–19. Illustration of the probability distributions underlying signal detection theory. The distribution on the left (*dashed line*) shows the signal-absent distribution, whereas the distribution on the right (*solid line*) shows the signal-present distribution. The different shaded areas represent four potential signal/response categories. Dark gray = hits (signal present, "yes" response); light gray = misses (signal present, "no" response); white = false alarms (signal absent, "yes" response); and striped = correct rejections (signal absent, "no" response).

trials allow the listener to learn the patterns of activity associated with the signal-absent and signal-present distributions. The theory assumes that the listener establishes a ***criterion***, or an amount of *internal response* above which they will answer, "Yes, I heard a signal" and below which they will answer, "No, I did not hear a signal." The criterion reflects the *response bias* of the listener, the tendency to say, "Yes, I heard a signal." Once the criterion is established, we illustrate it on Figure 2–18 as a vertical line. Although the criterion can be placed anywhere along the *x*-axis, the location of the criterion falls into three distinct categories:

- *Neutral.* This criterion is centered exactly between the two distributions. In this case,

the listener has no bias, or proclivity, to say "yes" more frequently than "no."

- *Conservative (or Strict).* This criterion is anywhere to the right of the neutral criterion and is illustrated in Figure 2–18. In this case, a listener has a stronger tendency to say "no" than to say "yes."

- *Liberal (or Lax).* This criterion is placed to the left of the neutral criterion. Here, a listener is more likely to say "yes" than to say "no."

The criterion separates the two original distributions into four different regions. These regions are determined by whether the signal is absent or present (left vs. right distribution) and whether the listener answers "no" or "yes" (internal response is greater or less than the

2. *Estimating Threshold in Quiet* **41**

criterion). These regions are all labeled on Figure 2–19, and are defined as:

- *Hit (or True Positive).* Listener says "yes" when a signal is present (the dark region).
- *False Alarm (or False Positive).* Listener says "yes" when a signal is not there (the white region).
- *Miss (or False Negative).* Listener says "no" when a signal is present (the light gray region).
- *Correct Rejection (or True Negative).* Listener says "no" when a signal is not there (the striped region).

Under the neutral criterion, a listener will have the highest percent correct (defined as the combined # of hits + # correct rejections divided by the total number of trials). Yet, this listener will have some false alarms due to the overlapping distributions. A listener with a liberal criterion will have a large number of hits, but also a high false alarm rate. In contrast, a listener adopting a conservative criterion will have fewer false alarms (and possibly none) but also fewer hits. Both types of criteria can cause an experimenter to misestimate the threshold.

One additional aspect of SDT is the ***receiver operating characteristic (ROC)***, curve, which is a plot of hits (y-axis) versus false alarms (x-axis). The advantage of the ROC is that it captures all aspects of SDT in a single graph. To illustrate how the ROC can do this, two example ROCs, one from a condition with a high sensitivity (perhaps an easily detected tone) and one with a low sensitivity (perhaps a tone with a lower level), are plotted in Figure 2–20. The sensitivity is reflected by the *bow* of the curve—the more the curve bends toward the upper left corner, the higher the sensitivity. Moving along the ROC curve

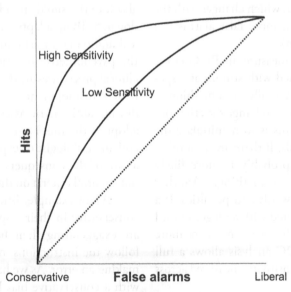

FIGURE 2–20. Two ROC curves, hits plotted versus false alarms, are shown. Greater sensitivity (an easier task) results in an ROC curve with a larger "bow" from the diagonal. When the criterion is conservative (the left side of the plot), false alarms and hits are relatively low. When the criterion is liberal, false alarms and hits are both relatively high.

Signal detection theory has numerous applications in the medical field and is frequently adopted during the development of medical tests. In clinical audiology, newborn hearing screening provides a great example of signal detection theory at work. Newborn hearing screenings are based on a physiological test of cochlear function: the otoacoustic emission, a sound that is generated by the ear in response to a stimulus. Babies who have an otoacoustic emission above a certain level "pass" the newborn hearing screening, and babies whose emission falls below that level or cannot be recorded are "referred" for follow-up testing. The otoacoustic emission varies in size along a continuum, and so the field must decide how big the emission must be to be associated with a pass. Any baby with an emission bigger than that criterion level will pass the test, and any baby with a smaller emission will be referred. The field has determined that identifying hearing loss as early as possible is the primary goal and that missing a baby with hearing loss is far more detrimental than referring babies with good hearing. Thus, newborn hearing screenings adopt a *liberal criterion*. As a result, there are many false positives, and many babies are referred who do not have hearing loss. The hope is that by sending many babies for follow-up testing, the babies who really have hearing loss (the true positives) will not be overlooked (a false negative).

captures the criterion, which changes with the false alarm rate (e.g., more false alarms is a more liberal criterion).

If we want to measure an ROC curve for a listener presented with stimuli at a specific level, we must typically do something to encourage that listener to change the criterion. One way of doing this is to manipulate the percentage of *yes* trials: If there are a lot of *yes* trials, that listener probably is more likely to say, "yes I heard something." Another method is to give rewards and penalties: If a *yes* response is associated with a bigger reward than a *no* response, a listener may also be more likely to say *yes*. ROC analysis allows a full characterization of sensitivity, measured across various criteria.

Application of Signal Detection Theory to Audiometry

The clinical audiologist is very interested in obtaining a rapid, but *accurate,* estimate of absolute threshold. In addition to the 10-dB down, 5-dB up adaptive rule adopted for clinical audiology measurements, which samples the psychometric function, other aspects of clinical procedures are designed to encourage a patient to adopt a neutral criterion. However, during audiometric assessment, listeners can adopt both conservative and liberal criteria, and an audiologist or experimenter should be aware of the consequences of adopting these non-neutral criteria on the threshold estimate.

As an example, listeners may be overly conservative in their responses; perhaps they are exaggerating their hearing loss, do not follow the instructions, or are worried about making an error. As we have seen, the listener with a conservative bias has a decreased tendency to say, "Yes I heard something," and only responds to signals presented at relatively high sensory levels. To illustrate this, a schematic from signal detection theory with an overly conservative criterion is shown in the top panel of Figure 2–21. As before, there

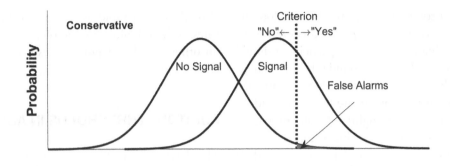

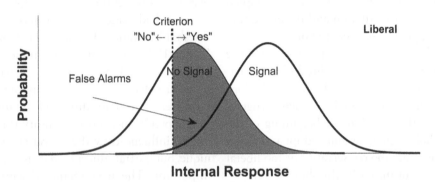

FIGURE 2–21. Two examples of the probability distributions underlying signal detection theory, one with a conservative criterion (*top panel*) and another with a liberal criterion (*bottom panel*). The shaded areas illustrate the region associated with false alarms, and more false alarms are evident for the liberal criterion.

are two distributions that reflect the internal response to *no signal* (shown as the distribution on the left) and the internal response to the *signal* (shown as the distribution on the right). A listener with a conservative criterion requires a higher sensory response to respond to the sound, and therefore we expect their threshold to be higher than true. The region related to false positives is indicated in dark gray and is very small. Shifting the criterion to the right (becoming even more conservative) would effectively eliminate all false positives. In this way a lack of false positives is a potential indicator that a listener has adopted an overly conservative criterion. On the other hand, an extremely liberal responder produces the opposite result: many false positives, as illustrated in the bottom panel of Figure 2–21.

A high false positive rate can make it difficult for an audiologist or experimenter to determine whether a patient response was a hit or a false positive.

Patients adopting either criterion type can lead to difficulty estimating a valid threshold. Those with conservative criteria can produce audiograms with hearing thresholds that are higher (worse) than their true hearing abilities, and the reverse can be true for those adopting liberal criteria. Yet there are facets of the clinical procedure that encourage patients to adopt neutral, or even moderately liberal, criteria such as:

- *Instructions.* Although there is no standard set of instructions for measuring absolute threshold, audiologists commonly give instructions that indicate they are looking for the *softest sound a person can hear*. ASHA guidelines indicate that a participant should respond whenever a sound is heard, no matter how faint (ASHA, 2005). Indirectly, these instructions invite listeners to adopt neutral, or even slightly liberal, criteria.

- *Retesting 1000 Hz.* This is a check to determine the criterion has not changed. If thresholds are lower (better) upon retest, it is possible that the patient initially adopted a conservative criterion and during testing has adopted a more neutral one.
- *Familiarization.* By starting at a level above the patient's estimated threshold, the patient has time to learn the task and adopt a reasonable criterion. If a patient struggles to hear the sound at the beginning of the threshold search, he could adopt a criterion that is either too conservative or too liberal throughout the entire threshold search.
- *Using only ascending runs for threshold estimation.* By using the ascending trials, an audiologist reduces the possibility that responses occur because of anticipation, or a response that occurs because a patient thinks a sound is going to be presented.
- *Randomizing the temporal interval between sounds.* An audiologist can control the time between stimulus presentations, and this manipulation can be very helpful to estimate threshold for patients adopting a liberal criterion. This practice might encourage listeners to adopt a neutral criterion, but if they continue to adopt a liberal criterion, a long temporal separation between stimulus presentations may allow the tester to associate the signal presentation with the response and disambiguate hits from false positives.

In the vast majority of cases, these strategies allow an audiologist to obtain the lowest and most reliable threshold possible. They also allow for a rapid assessment of hearing thresholds and allow an audiologist to focus on other valuable diagnostic tests and aural rehabilitation.

AUDITORY THRESHOLDS IN ADULTS

The development of advanced procedures to measure auditory perception has been refined over the 20th century. By the 1930s, several scientists had made measurements of auditory thresholds at various frequencies (see Sivian & White, 1933 for a summary), but more recent advances in calibration and psychoacoustical procedures have required revisions of the early estimates of absolute threshold. As discussed in Chapter 1 and above, auditory thresholds can be influenced by the measurement technique, but the transducer used is also extremely important. The next section discusses free field versus earphone testing and the effects of hearing loss on absolute threshold.

MAP and MAF

Today, we can measure absolute threshold using a variety of transducers (e.g., loudspeakers, earphones, and bone oscillator). Some of the important measurements of absolute threshold come from comparing thresholds measured in the free field and over headphones. For the *minimum audible field (MAF)* measurements, sounds were presented over a loudspeaker (i.e., in the free field) and calibrated at a location 1 m away from the speaker. Note that for these free-field measures, the listeners were able to use both ears. For the *minimum audible pressure (MAP)* measurements, sounds were presented monaurally (i.e., to a single ear) over headphones, and measurements were based on a calibration reference level at the tympanic membrane.

Figure 2–22 shows recent estimates of the MAP and MAF (ANSI S3.6, 2018; ISO 226, 2003), measured in young adult listeners.

Testing hearing using a bone oscillator is common and necessary for audiometric testing to diagnose whether a hearing loss is conductive or sensorineural.

The MAP/MAF curves in Figure 2–22 illustrate two primary findings:

- *Frequency effects.* The minimum detectable sound pressure level varied as a function of frequency. Notably, the frequency of a pure tone had a large impact on the ability to hear that sound. A higher sound pressure level was needed for detection at both the very low frequencies and the very high frequencies. Both the MAP and the MAF show that thresholds are the lowest for frequencies around 3000 Hz. From this result, we see that adults with normal hearing can detect mid-frequency sounds at lower sound pressure levels than high- or low-frequency sounds. The minimum detectable sound level in dB SPL can vary by more than 30 dB, depending on the frequency tested.

- *Measurement differences.* The free-field measurement (MAF) yielded much lower thresholds than the MAP, with maximum differences in the range of 10 to 15 dB. Three primary factors contribute to this result (Sivian & White, 1933):
  - Listening with two ears versus one. Generally, listening with two ears yields a lower threshold than listening with one,

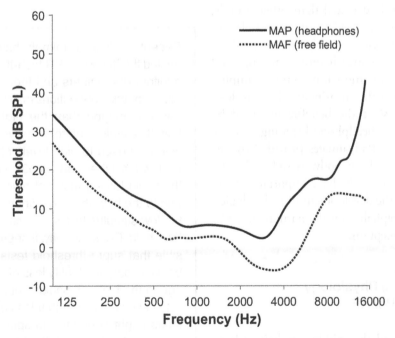

FIGURE 2–22. Absolute threshold curves for minimum audible field (MAF; *solid line*) and minimum audible pressure (MAP; *dotted line*) plotted in dB SPL. Adapted from ANSI S3.6 (2018) and ISO 226 (2003).

but the effect is only about 2 dB (Robinson & Dadson, 1957).

○ Reflections of sound from the body. The body interacts with the sound field, and reflections from the head and torso increase sound level at the tympanic membrane.

○ Gain provided by the pinna and meatus. Headphones eliminate certain resonant properties of the external ear that contribute to sound amplification.

> Visit the companion website for an auditory demonstration of the MAP curve.

These measurements have strong implications for our auditory perception. First, consider the implications for superior audibility between about 2000 and 4000 Hz versus lower and higher frequencies, particularly in the free field. Sounds in this frequency range are more easily detected than other sounds, and therefore are used in sirens and alarms. These frequencies, notably, also contribute substantially to speech understanding, and therefore are the most important to amplify for listeners with sensorineural hearing loss. Second, consider the benefits provided by free field over headphone listening. We are afforded several advantages provided by our external ear and our body, as well as having two ears. Such results have important consequences for the development of technologies, which can capitalize on the natural effects of auditory perception.

Connecting Physiology to the MAP/MAF

The outer and the middle ear have a large influence on the shape of the MAP and MAF. The valley in the MAP/MAF reflects the sound transfer characteristics of the outer and middle ears. Recall that the combined outer and middle ear transfer function has a peak right around 3000 Hz, corresponding to the range of best absolute thresholds. Both structures yield frequency transmission characteristics that vary as a function of frequency, as illustrated in Figure 2–8. On the other hand, the cochlea is thought to transmit sound roughly equally at all frequencies (Rosowski, 1991). Of course, the cochlea is critically involved in the ability to detect sounds, but it has little effect on the shape of the MAP /MAF due to its flat frequency-transmission characteristics. Not surprisingly, then, there is a strong correlation between the MAP /MAF and the transfer characteristics of the outer and middle ears. That peak in the combined outer and middle-ear transfer function has a direct correspondence to the valley in the MAP /MAF curves in Figure 2–22, which is where humans have the best auditory sensitivity.

> Recent studies in animals have suggested that the low-SPR/high-threshold auditory nerve fibers and their associated synaptic connections may be more easily damaged than the high SPR/low threshold auditory nerve fibers when exposed to high levels of sound (Kujawa & Liberman, 2009). Auditory threshold testing may not reveal damage to the high-threshold fibers, due to the low stimulus levels associated with threshold. Consequently, it seems possible that supra-threshold tests would be necessary to identify loss of or damage to the high-threshold fibers. Scientists have speculated that loss of these fibers might contribute to speech perception difficulties in noise, even in the absence of elevated auditory thresholds.

The auditory nerve also has a role in the detection of sounds, as it codes the information on the basilar membrane. For threshold-level stimuli, the only fibers available to code the vibration are the high-SPR/low-threshold fibers. These are the only fibers that respond to sound levels below 20 dB SPL, and therefore, are the only fibers active during threshold testing. These fibers increase their firing rate in response to very low-level sounds, ultimately leading to auditory detection of the tone.

Hearing Loss and Elevated Threshold

The MAP and MAF functions were measured using earphones or loudspeakers as transducers. Both of these transducers activate the air conduction pathway of the ear and involve the entire auditory system. Consequently, conductive (damage in the outer or middle ear) and sensorineural (damage at the level of the cochlea or auditory nerve) hearing loss can have a drastic effect on the MAP and MAF curves. As mentioned earlier, we consider the MAP and MAF curves to be a consequence of the frequency transfer characteristics of the outer, middle, and inner ear. Therefore, it is rather straightforward to make predictions about the effects of hearing losses that alter the transmission characteristics of the components of the ear on the MAP/MAF.

Disordered changes to the function or structure of each component of the ear can yield frequency-specific effects. Changes to the resonant properties of the external ear (such as via growths or malformations) or occlusion (such as via wax or objects) will directly affect hearing in a frequency-specific manner. Changes to the mass or stiffness of the middle ear will also alter the frequency-transmission characteristics of the system and yield frequency-specific effects. Damage to

outer or inner hair cells often produces frequency-specific hearing loss, as certain locations along the length of the cochlea are often impacted more by disease and noise exposure. Each of these disorders will then influence specific portions of the MAP /MAF curves. In many cases, the degree of damage and the location of the damage can be associated with a predictable change in hearing.

Clinical Example: Otosclerosis

All disorders that affect hearing thresholds will influence the MAP and MAF, and here we discuss otosclerosis as an example. Otosclerosis is a condition in which the ossicular bones are resorbed and replaced by a spongy, vascularized bone. In the later stages of the disease, the bony growths lead to fixation of the stapes footplate to the oval window. In the early stages, the disease is considered *stiffness based*, from an acoustics standpoint. That is, the disease increases the stiffness of the middle ear system, which leads to a decreased ability to transmit low-frequency sound. Because the low-frequency gain of the middle-ear frequency-transfer function is diminished, a low-frequency hearing loss will result. Any change in frequency transmission of the ear will raise or the threshold, accordingly. For example, a decrease in sound transmission of 10 dB from 250 to 1000 Hz due to otosclerosis will elevate MAP / MAF thresholds between 250 and 1000 Hz by a corresponding 10 dB. A change like this is illustrated by the unfilled symbols in Figure 2–23, which demonstrates elevated low-frequency MAP thresholds in the presence of early-stage otosclerosis.

As the disease progresses, however, the bony growths add mass to the ossicular chain. Because the increase in mass diminishes sound transmission at high frequencies, high-frequency hearing loss adds to the low-frequency hearing loss. The presence of

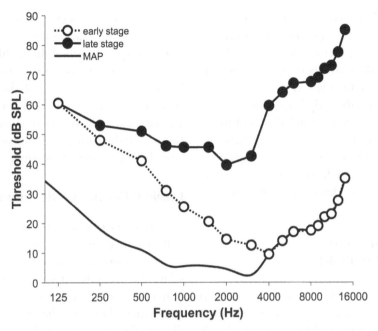

FIGURE 2–23. MAP curves for a patient with early-stage and late-stage otosclerosis. The MAP curve from Figure 2–22 is shown as the solid line for reference. Early- and late-stage otosclerosis curves are shown using unfilled and filled symbols, respectively.

advanced disease will then elevate thresholds in the MAP /MAF functions on the high-frequency side. The effects of later-stage otosclerosis are shown as the filled symbols on the MAP function of Figure 2–23, which demonstrates that the MAP thresholds at all frequencies are elevated.

It is clear from Figure 2–23 that auditory pathology can change the shape of the MAP. However, because the MAP function is not constant across frequencies, we would need to subtract the shifted MAP values from the normative MAP values to determine the threshold change imposed by the auditory pathology. This calculation is fairly straightforward and is visible in Figure 2–23 when the normative MAP values are plotted along with the measured threshold values, but measurements are not conducted in dB SPL in clinical applications, as we discuss in the next section.

Using dB Hearing Level (dB HL)

In clinical situations, we are often interested in knowing how an individual's hearing differs with respect to normative data, or typical auditory behavior. Although the MAP /MAF curves illustrate typical auditory thresholds, they are measured with reference to a fixed acoustic quantity that does not vary with frequency (i.e., the 20 µPa reference for dB SPL). Because the MAP /MAF curves are frequency dependent, using dB SPL as the normative reference can lead to difficulty in observing changes in the curve that might be caused by hearing loss. In audiology, then, the more commonly used dB reference is *dB HL*, referred to as *dB hearing level* or sometimes *dB hearing loss*. Decibels HL is based on a measure of auditory sensitivity based on young adults with typical hearing and uses the MAP or MAF curve as the reference. Thus, any value on the MAP (or MAF) curve becomes 0 dB on the dB HL scale. The following equation applies:

$$\text{dB HL} = \text{dB SPL} - \text{reference threshold in dB SPL (RETSPL)}.$$

Conversions of dB SPL to dB HL depend on the transducer used. Table 2–1 shows values for supra-aural Telephonics (TDH-39) and insert Etymotic ER-3A earphones (ANSI S3.6, 2018 and ISO 389, 2004). In cases when we want to reference the level of a sound to a listener's hearing loss, we can use dB sensation level (dB SL), defined as:

$$\text{dB SL} = \text{dB SPL of the sound} - \text{RETSPL} - \text{dB HL of the individual}.$$

For example, a 1000-Hz tone presented at 80 dB SPL using TDH-39 earphones, to a listener with a hearing loss of 40 dB HL would be at a 73 dB HL presentation level and 33 dB SL (sensation level). Effectively, this sound is 33 dB above the listener's detection threshold.

Using the dB HL reference allows much easier observation of deviations in hearing with respect to what is considered typical.

Plotting data in this way is referred to as the *audiogram*. By normalizing the data, it is more straightforward to visualize the amount of hearing loss. Another major difference between the audiogram and the MAP /MAF curves is that better thresholds are illustrated at the top of the audiogram, and poorer thresholds are indicated at the bottom. To illustrate these two factors, the data from Figure 2–23 are plotted in dB HL in Figure 2–24, at the standard audiometric frequencies of 250 to 8000 Hz. When thresholds are plotted in this way, we observe that this early stage otosclerosis is associated with hearing loss only in the low frequencies and no loss above 3 kHz. On

> The interested reader is referred to the section in Chapter 1 on Auditory Assessment that discusses the historical reasons for plotting the audiogram *upside down* and for using dB HL. Jerger (2009) notes that plotting the audiogram in this way is rather unfortunate because it breaks with scientific convention, where values on *y*-axes are plotted in an ascending manner.

TABLE 2–1. Reference Threshold Values in dB SPL (RETSPL) for TDH-39 and ER-3A Earphones from ANSI S3.6 (2018)

Frequency (Hz)	Reference Threshold in dB SPL		dB HL
	TDH-39	**ER-3A**	
125	45.5	26.0	0
250	25.5	14.0	0
500	11.5	9.5	0
1000	7	5.5	0
2000	9	11.5	0
4000	9.5	15	0
8000	13	15.5	0

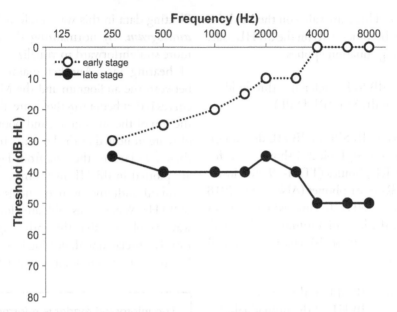

FIGURE 2–24. The auditory thresholds from Figure 2–23 (early-stage and late-stage otosclerosis) are replotted in audiogram format in dB HL.

the other hand, late-state otosclerosis is associated with a hearing loss across the frequency range. Particularly for the late stage otosclerosis case, the audiogram allows easier visualization of how much hearing levels change across the audiometric frequencies.

A common way to quantify the *degree* (or severity) of hearing loss is to categorize absolute thresholds based on ranges of dB HL—the current categories provided by Clark (1981) are shown in Table 2–2. These terms are appropriate for use in describing thresholds among clinicians, but they have been demonstrated to provide little value, and can even be detrimental, in conveying the severity of communication difficulties to both patients and their families. In many cases, particularly in reference to children, these terms lead patients to underestimate the severity of their hearing loss (Haggard & Primus, 1999). Using these categories, however, can provide a general guide for the expected speech understanding difficulties experienced by listeners with sensorineural hearing loss.

TABLE 2–2. Terms Used to Describe Hearing Loss Based on Hearing Levels

Hearing Threshold Level in dB HL	Hearing Loss Label
−10 to 15	Within Normal Limits
16 to 25	Slight Hearing Loss
25 to 40	Mild Hearing Loss
41 to 55	Moderate Hearing Loss
56 to 70	Moderately Severe Hearing Loss
71 to 90	Severe Hearing Loss
91+	Profound Hearing Loss

Source: Clark (1981).

The Impact of Elevated Threshold on Everyday Listening

Considering Erber's (1982) hierarchy of perception, deficits at lower levels in the hierarchy (i.e., detection and discrimination) will be propagated to higher levels. Any listener with an elevated threshold is expected to experience difficulties in recognition and comprehension. As such, the degree of hearing loss will influence the amount of speech that is audible and will also affect the ability to understand speech. A mild hearing loss is expected to impact speech understanding, but to a lesser degree than a more severe hearing loss.

In addition to speech understanding, robust audibility across a wide range of frequencies has been implicated in maintaining an ability to determine which elements of sounds belong together and which elements do not. This **auditory scene analysis** (Bregman, 1990), is a process by which the auditory system organizes sounds into perceptually meaningful elements. The ear can use similarity and differences to determine whether acoustic elements belong together in one sound or are from different sounds. For example, acoustic elements coming from different locations are likely different sounds; acoustic elements that start and stop together may be from the same sound, and two fundamental frequencies may be indicative of two sounds.

Elevated auditory thresholds (poor audibility) cause low-level sounds in the environment to be difficult to hear or inaudible. Because hearing loss is commonly frequency-dependent, one must consider the frequency regions and degree of hearing loss in combination with the frequency and level of the sounds in the environment. In some cases, entire sounds may be inaudible (such as a whisper or a refrigerator hum). Conversational speech is generally considered to have an overall level

of 60 to 70 dB SPL, and so even moderate hearing loss (>40 dB HL; see Table 2–2) can render portions of the speech stimulus inaudible. Further, speech does not contain equal energy across frequency, as illustrated in Figure 2–25, which shows the **long-term average spectrum of speech (LTASS)** measured from 12 languages as the solid line (Byrne et al., 1994). From this figure, we observe that speech energy generally peaks at 500 Hz and is greatest in the frequency range of about 125 to 2000 Hz. The LTASS represents an average across people, and an individual's speech spectrum may deviate from this average, depending on gender, age, and other factors such as speech and voice pathologies.

To illustrate the impact of elevated thresholds on speech, we can compare an individual's audiogram with the LTASS. As an example, consider an individual with a high-frequency sloping sensorineural hearing loss, shown in the inset in dB HL units. To demonstrate the relationship between the audiogram and the LTASS, the audiogram, converted to dB SPL units, is plotted along with the LTASS in the main figure. In the main panel, high thresholds are illustrated at the top of the figure (in contrast to the audiogram). Spectral elements that are higher in level than audiometric thresholds on this plot are audible (those *above* the audiometric threshold), and elements that have levels below the thresholds are not. For this specific audiogram, frequencies above 2000 Hz are not audible to this listener, even though at 2000 Hz, the hearing loss would be described as moderate (45 dB HL).

A listener with an elevated threshold is not likely to hear all components of speech, but the type of speech *information* contained in those elements is also important. Listeners with high-frequency hearing losses, as illustrated here, often will have difficulty perceiving speech sounds with high-frequency content, like the unvoiced fricatives (e.g., /s/ ("seep") or /ʃ/ ("sheep"). Figure 2–25 illustrates a listener

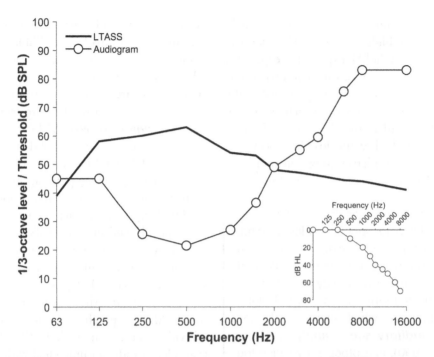

FIGURE 2–25. The long-term average spectrum of speech (LTASS) is plotted along audiometric thresholds in dB SPL for a listener with the audiogram shown in the inset. Adapted from Byrne et al. (1994).

who must rely on speech information below 2000 Hz. In contrast, a listener with a more severe hearing loss or a flat loss will experience different difficulties: A greater portion of the speech may be inaudible and different speech sounds may be affected. Although the interactions are complex and depend on a variety of factors other than audibility (such as age), listeners with moderate-to-severe hearing losses are expected to have confusions among consonants (Bilger & Wang, 1976). Vowel confusions are less common except for those with severe hearing loss (Nábĕlek, 1988), but the cues that are used by listeners with hearing loss may be different from those with normal hearing (Ferguson & Kewley-Port, 2002).

To characterize the effects of reduced audibility on speech understanding, the ***speech intelligibility index (SII)***—a replacement for the Articulation Index—does more than sim-

ply look at the frequencies that are inaudible, it also reflects the information present across the frequencies in speech. It is accepted as a tool for calculating intelligibility of speech and can be used for listeners with normal hearing as well as those with mild-moderate hearing losses (ANSI, S3.5, 2017). The SII assumes that different frequency bands contribute different amounts to the ultimate ability to understand speech, and these differences are characterized via *frequency importance functions*. When a listener has a hearing loss in one of the more important bands, their perception of speech would be affected more than if the loss was in one of the less important bands. Different speech materials and different languages have different SII functions, and so one needs to know the testing materials, the language of testing, the degree of hearing loss, and the shape of hearing loss (i.e., the *configu-*

ration) to fully predict how the hearing loss might impact speech perception. An easy-to-use tool, the ***count-the-dot audiogram***, was developed so that one can quickly calculate and visualize the amount of audible speech information for a particular hearing loss (e.g., Mueller & Killion, 1990). This way, one can estimate the influence of audibility in relation to the information that is present in the speech stimulus on speech perception.

Figure 2–26 illustrates how the count-the-dot audiogram works. In this tool, 100 dots are superimposed on a blank audiogram, and each dot represents roughly 1 percentage point of speech intelligibility. Frequencies that contain more dots (e.g., 1000 to 3000 Hz) contribute more to speech understanding than frequencies with few dots. This example shows an audiogram with a high-frequency loss plotted on a count-the-dot audiogram for English. Counting the dots gives a rough estimate of the speech understanding abilities of the listener, without amplification or auditory assistance. We see that 29 dots are at levels lower than the audiometric thresholds (that is, they are *above* the thresholds on the audiogram). Thus, this listener might be expected to perceive ~70%

of the information available in conversational speech. Count-the-dot audiograms are being developed for other languages, some of which have more emphasis on low frequencies than English (Jin et al., 2017).

Improving audibility (e.g., a talker raising his voice or an assistive device that amplifies sound) will typically improve speech perception. However, supra-threshold factors, particularly those associated with sensorineural hearing loss, begin to impact the perception of sounds in natural scenes, factors which we discuss in subsequent chapters of this text. Even if full audibility is restored, a listener with sensorineural hearing loss would not be expected to have speech perception abilities that are similar to a listener with normal hearing.

Lastly, we should note that speech is a rich and highly redundant signal, allowing a listener to attend to multiple cues to achieve understanding, even when certain portions of the speech are not audible. It is possible for a listener with mild hearing loss to achieve excellent speech perception in quiet, and a listener can use contextual information to *fill in the blanks* during everyday conversations. Yet, we should consider that their hearing loss diminishes the information available to their central auditory system, and even listeners with good speech perception scores expend additional effort to understand speech compared to those with normal hearing.

SUMMARY AND TAKE-HOME POINTS

The measurement of threshold has formed the foundation of the fields of psychoacoustics and audiology. Measurement techniques have illustrated that threshold varies depending on the frequency being tested, the mode of testing (i.e., free field vs. headphones), and the specific measurement technique used. In all cases, the experimenter must be aware that

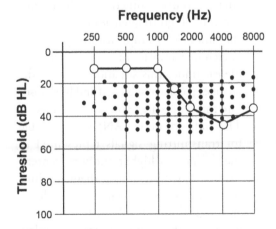

FIGURE 2–26. An audiogram superimposed on a "count the dot" audiogram. Adapted from Killion and Mueller (2010).

perceptual measurements are a consequence of auditory abilities and a listener's response bias. Care and consideration must be taken to reduce or eliminate the effects of a listener bias, or the thresholds being reported may not be valid.

The following are key take-home points of this chapter:

- Pure tones are widely used in audiology and psychoacoustics for measuring absolute thresholds, as they are easily specified with a single amplitude (or decibel value) and a single frequency.
- There are many tests used to measure absolute threshold, with the most common and efficient based on the method of limits. Knowledge of the psychometric function is critical to establish the variables necessary for using the method of limits and related adaptive procedures.
- Signal detection theory provides a theoretical framework within which sensitivity and response proclivity can be measured.
- Absolute thresholds vary depending on the frequency tested, with mid-frequency sounds associated with the lowest absolute thresholds. The shape of these functions is a direct consequence of the transmission characteristics of the outer, middle, and inner ear transfer functions.
- Absolute thresholds collected from free-field measures can be more than 15 dB better than testing over headphones. Acoustic interactions between the sound and the body, amplification by anatomical structures, and binaural effects contribute to these differences.
- Physiological changes to any structure within the peripheral auditory pathway have the potential to lead to hearing loss, which is characterized by elevated thresholds. This hearing loss, in turn, may render portions of environmental stimuli, such as speech, inaudible and make speech more difficult to understand.

EXERCISES

1. Calculate whether a 100-ms pure tone will be sufficiently frequency specific to produce representations independent from one another at the audiometric frequencies of 250, 500, and 1000 Hz. In your answer, consider whether there is overlap of frequencies between the various tones. From an acoustics standpoint alone, would this duration be sufficiently short for testing hearing thresholds?

2. Calculate the dB SPL level for a sound with rms pressure of .0002 Pa. Next calculate the dB SPL level for rms pressure of 0.002 Pa. How many times bigger is the increase in pressure? How many dB bigger is the more intense sound? Do this calculation for 0.02 Pa to establish the relationship between changes in pressure and dB. Discuss this relationship.

3. For the sounds in Exercise 2, what are the dB HL values if the sound was 500 Hz? How about 4000 Hz? Why does frequency impact dB HL but not dB SPL?

4. An increase in middle ear mass (e.g., placement of pressure-equalizing [PE] tubes in the tympanic membrane) will alter the transfer function of the middle ear in the high frequencies by decreasing the amount of amplification provided. Sketch new transfer function of the middle ear under this situation. Discuss the changes you have sketched and how absolute thresholds are expected to change.

5. The auditory nerve (AN) is responsible for transmitting signals represented in the cochlea to higher auditory centers. As mentioned previously, there are three types of AN nerve fibers: low-, middle-, and high-threshold fibers. Consider the impact on the audiogram for a complete loss of low-threshold fibers. Sketch an audiogram (air conduction thresholds only) that would reflect an ear with no

low-threshold fibers. Consider the impact of the loss of high-threshold fibers; sketch an audiogram for an ear with no high-threshold fibers but low-threshold fibers that are intact. Again, air conduction thresholds are ok. Discuss how well the audiogram reflects the function of the entire auditory nerve.

6. List one advantage and one disadvantage of each of the laboratory adaptive staircase procedure and the modified Hughson-Westlake clinical procedure to estimate threshold. Provide a circumstance when each procedure would be preferred with an explanation.

7. Consider the impact of the following decisions as they apply to the staircase procedure for estimating threshold. Discuss whether these decisions may affect the threshold or other test-related factors: (a) Step size too big, (b) Step size too small, (c) Starting level too high, (d) Starting level too low.

8. Discuss the following situations that can occur in audiometry with regards to how the situation might impact the patient's criterion and the subsequent effect on the threshold measured.

   a. Adopting a pattern of stimulus presentations during audiometric testing
   b. Testing a patient with tinnitus
   c. Providing a visual cue to a patient during testing

9. Presbycusis, also known as age-related hearing loss, begins in high frequencies and slowly progresses to lower and lower frequencies. Write about the impact of early-stage presbycusis on the MAP function and later-stage presbycusis on the MAP by providing sketches.

10. Consider the same case presented in Exercise 2–9, but now consider why plotting audiometric thresholds in dB HL, rather than dB SPL, allows a better illustration of the frequencies affected most by the scenario. Discuss the advantages of using dB HL over dB SPL for this particular clinical application.

11. Maria has unilateral hearing loss in which the left ear is completely deaf, and the right has good hearing. Wayne has two ears with good hearing. Sketch predicted MAF functions for Maria and Wayne, and sketch predicted MAP functions for the left ear for both of them. Specifically consider the impact that wearing headphones might have on audiometric thresholds, compared to the free field.

12. Refer back to the LTASS spectrum of speech shown in Figure 2–25 and the audiogram for the listener with a rising hearing loss configuration illustrated in Figure 2–24 (the open symbols for early stage otosclerosis). Sketch the LTASS and then plot the audiogram on the same axes of the LTASS (be sure the audiogram is in dB SPL). What frequencies of the speech will be inaudible to this listener?

13. Repeat exercise 2–12 for the listener with late-stage otosclerosis in Figure 2–24. How does the increased severity of hearing loss and the greater loss at high frequencies influence this individual's ability to hear speech at a conversational level?

14. Plot the audiograms from Figure 2–24 on the "count the dot" audiogram downloaded from the companion website. Discuss how the count the dot audiogram reflects different information from the audibility loss depicted in Figure 2–25.

15. Plot the audiograms from Figure 2–24 on the "count the dot" audiogram downloaded from the companion website. Discuss how the differing amounts of hearing loss affects the speech information available to these two listeners.

Visit the companion website for lab exercises.

REFERENCES

Aibara, R., Welsh, J. T., Puria, S., & Goode, R. L. (2001). Human middle-ear sound transfer function and cochlear input impedance. *Hearing Research, 152*(1–2), 100–109.

American Speech-Language-Hearing Association. (2005). *Guidelines for manual pure-tone threshold audiometry* [Guidelines]. http://www.asha.org/policy

ASA S3.5 (1997; R2017). American National Standard methods for calculation of the speech intelligibility index. American National Standards Institute.

ANSI/ASA S3.6 (2018). American National Standard specification for audiometers. American National Standards Institute.

Bilger, R. C., & Wang, M. D. (1976). Consonant confusions in patients with sensorineural hearing loss. *Journal of Speech and Hearing Research, 19*(4), 718–748.

Bregman, A. S. (1990). *Auditory scene analysis* (Vol. 10). MIT Press.

Byrne, D., Dillon, H., Tran, K., Arlinger, S., Wilbraham, K., Cox, R., . . . Ludvigsen, C. (1994). An international comparison of long-term average speech spectra. *Journal of the Acoustical Society of America, 96*(4), 2108–2120.

Clark, J. G. (1981). Uses and abuses of hearing loss classification. *ASHA, 23*(7), 493–500.

Erber, N. P. (1982). Glenondald auditory screening procedure. *Auditory Training* (pp. 47–71). Alexander Graham Bell Association.

Ferguson, S. H., & Kewley-Port, D. (2002). Vowel intelligibility in clear and conversational speech for normal-hearing and hearing-impaired listeners. *Journal of the Acoustical Society of America, 112*(1), 259–271.

Green, D. M., & Swets, J. A. (1966). *Signal detection theory and psychophysics.* Wiley.

Haggard, R. S., & Primus, M. A. (1999). Parental perceptions of hearing loss classification in children. *American Journal of Audiology, 8*, 83–92.

ISO 226 (2003). Acoustics—Normal equal-loudness-level contours. International Organization for Standardization.

ISO 389 (2004). Acoustics—Reference zero for the calibration of audiometric equipment. International Organization for Standardization.

Jerger, J. (2009). *Audiology in the USA.* Plural Publishing.

Jin, I. K., Kates, J. M., & Arehart, K. H. (2017). Does language matter when using a graphical method for calculating the Speech Intelligibility Index? *Journal of the American Academy of Audiology, 28*(02), 119–126.

Killion, M. C., & Mueller, H. G. (2010). Twenty years later: A NEW count-the-dots method. *Hearing Journal, 63*(1), 10, 12–14, 16–17.

Kujawa, S. G., & Liberman, M. C. (2009). Adding insult to injury: Cochlear nerve degeneration after "temporary" noise-induced hearing loss. *Journal of Neuroscience, 29*(45), 14077–14085.

Kurokawa, H., & Goode, R. L. (1995). Sound pressure gain produced by the human middle ear. *Otolaryngology–Head and Neck Surgery, 113*(4), 349–355.

Levitt, H. (1971). Transformed up-down methods in psychoacoustics. *Journal of the Acoustical Society of America, 49*(2B), 467–477.

Mahomed, F., Swanepoel, D. W., Eikelboom, R. H., & Soer, M. (2013). Validity of automated threshold audiometry: A systematic review and meta-analysis. *Ear and Hearing, 34*(6), 745–752.

Marshall, L., & Jesteadt, W. (1986). Comparison of pure-tone audibility thresholds obtained with audiological and two-interval forced-choice procedures. *Journal of Speech and Hearing Research, 29*(1), 82–91.

Mehrgardt, S., & Mellert, V. (1977). Transformation characteristics of the external human ear. *Journal of the Acoustical Society of America, 61*(6), 1567–1576.

Mueller, H. G., & Killion, M. C. (1990). An easy method for calculating the articulation index. *Hearing Journal, 43*(9), 14–17.

Nábělek, A. K. (1988). Identification of vowels in quiet, noise, and reverberation: Relationships with age and hearing loss. *Journal of the Acoustical Society of America, 84*(2), 476–484.

Palmer, A. R., & Evans, E. F. (1979). On the peripheral coding of the level of individual frequency components of complex sounds at high sound levels. In O. Creutzfelt, H. Scheich, & C. Schreiner (Eds.), *Hearing mechanisms and speech,* (pp. 19–26). Springer-Verlag.

Rhode, W. S. (1971). Observations of the vibration of the basilar membrane in squirrel monkeys using the Mössbauer technique. *Journal of the Acoustical Society of America, 49*(4B), 1218–1231.

Robinson, D. W., & Dadson, R. S. (1957). Threshold of hearing and equal-loudness relations for pure tones, and the loudness function. *Journal of the Acoustical Society of America, 29*(12), 1284–1288.

Robles, L., Ruggero, M. A., & Rich, N. C. (1986). Basilar membrane mechanics at the base of the chinchilla cochlea. I. Input-output functions, tuning curves, and response phases. *Journal of the Acoustical Society of America, 80*(5), 1364–1374.

Rosowski, J. J. (1991). The effects of external and middle-ear filtering on auditory threshold and noise induced hearing loss. *Journal of the Acoustical Society of America, 90*(1), 124–135.

Sachs, M. B., & Abbas, P. J. (1974). Rate versus level functions for auditory nerve fibers in cats: Tone burst stimuli. *Journal of the Acoustical Society of America*, *56*(6), 1835–1847.

Sellick, P. M., Patuzzi R., & Johnstone B. M. (1982). Measurement of basilar membrane motion in the guinea pig using the Mössbauer technique. *Journal of the Acoustical Society of America*, *72*(1), 131–141.

Shaw, E. A. G. (1974). Transformation of sound pressure level from the free field to the eardrum in the horizontal plane. *Journal of the Acoustical Society of America*, *56*(6), 1848–1861.

Sivian, L. J., & White, S. D. (1933). On minimum audible sound fields. *Journal of the Acoustical Society of America*, *4*(4), 288–321.

Speaks, C. E. (2018) *Introduction to sound: Acoustics for the hearing and speech sciences* (4th ed.). Plural Publishing.

von Békésy, G. (1960). *Experiments in hearing*. E. G. Wever (Ed.). McGraw-Hill.

Winter, I. M., Robertson, D., & Yates, G. K. (1990) Diversity of characteristic frequency rate-intensity functions in guinea pig auditory nerve fibres. *Hearing Research*, *45*(3), 191–202.

3

Estimating Thresholds in Noise (Masking)

LEARNING OBJECTIVES

At the end of this chapter, students will be able to:

- Describe the acoustic characteristics of noise and filters
- Discuss the impact of noise on detection of pure tones
- Compare the psychoacoustical techniques used to measure masking
- Explain how masking is used to measure frequency selectivity
- Integrate knowledge of auditory physiology with psychoacoustical masking results in listeners with sensorineural hearing loss.
- Relate changes in frequency selectivity to changes in everyday listening
- Connect the concept of the critical band to clinical masking

INTRODUCTION

The previous chapter covered the psychoacoustic principles underlying the detection of sounds in quiet. However, we rarely spend time in quiet environments and are surrounded by noise of all types, from white noise to speech babble. In almost all cases, the presence of noise leads to difficulties in perceiving the sounds of interest. We call this effect *masking*, broadly defined as the process by which the presence of one sound (the masker) interferes with the perception of another (the signal). In this chapter, we are concerned with the effect masking has on detection ability. However, masking can also be applied to discrimination, recognition, and comprehension.

Two major types of masking are relevant to the perception of sound: *energetic masking*, which occurs when the energy in a masker competes directly with the energy in a signal, and *informational masking*, which occurs when the masker perceptually competes with the signal. Informational masking can be caused from many sources: temporal variations in a stimulus, uncertainty about a stimulus, or even linguistic content. The mechanisms responsible for both types of masking are very different, with energetic masking being traced to a primarily peripheral representation and informational masking typically mediated by central processes. This chapter focuses on the mechanisms responsible for energetic masking.

Several factors dictate whether one sound will mask another, including the power of the masker compared with the signal, the frequency characteristics of the masker compared with the signal, and the temporal structure of the masker relative to the signal. These characteristics will be discussed with a focus on the following aspects of masking:

- *Masking by noise and pure tones.* This section reviews how sound level and frequency content influence the effectiveness of a masker.
- *Frequency selectivity and the auditory filter.* Masking experiments have been central to our understanding of the frequency selectivity of the ear, or the ability of the auditory system to represent one frequency as independent of another. These studies have led to a concept called the auditory filter.
- *The excitation pattern.* The excitation pattern provides a psychological, internal representation of the stimulus spectrum. Its conceptualization has been integral to our understanding of what spectral information is accessible to the auditory system.
- *Masking by fluctuating sounds.* The healthy ear receives benefit from a fluctuating masker, a masker with varied and audible amplitude changes, compared with a steady one.

Many of the early masking studies were critical in the development of the technologies associated with the telephone. The earliest masking studies provide information regarding how various stimuli influence auditory threshold and have provided a great deal of information regarding the representation of frequency in the auditory system, particularly in relation to the frequency-selective nature of the ear. Importantly, masking studies have also been integral in the development of diagnostic audiological techniques. In this chapter, we discuss the role of masking studies in our understanding of auditory processing as well as how sensorineural hearing loss affects the ability to hear masked sounds.

We will discuss the following concepts as they apply to masking in the auditory system:

- Acoustics of noise and filters
- Physiological representation of sounds
- Psychophysical masking in listeners with normal hearing
  - Simultaneous masking by tones and noise
  - Frequency selectivity in simultaneous and forward masking
  - Using masking to infer psychophysical representations of the spectrum (e.g., the excitation pattern)
  - Masking by fluctuating sounds
- Effects of sensorineural hearing loss on masking
  - Reduced frequency selectivity
  - Decreased fluctuating masker benefit
  - Perceptual consequences of reduced frequency selectivity
- Clinical application of masking

ACOUSTICS: NOISE AND FILTERS

Noise

Noise is often referred to as any unwanted sound. However, this definition is not terribly useful in the field of psychoacoustics because it is not associated with an acoustic characterization. This chapter will demonstrate that the acoustic representation of sound is an essential determinant in the ability of that sound to produce masking. Realistically, any sound can be a *noise* and can produce masking, but the amount of masking produced by that sound depends on the relationship between the masking sound (the *masker*) and the sound being detected (the *signal*). The relationship between the sound levels, frequencies, and even the fluctuations within sounds are important. Common masking studies have employed noise maskers that are characterized by a random amplitude structure: white noise and narrowband noise, and so we review the acoustics of these sounds here.

White noise is a very specific type of noise, which is random in nature and has a constant power spectral density. Essentially, this means that when the power spectrum of white noise is plotted, it looks flat across frequency. Within the human hearing sciences, we generally assume that the frequencies contained within the white noise correspond to the range of human hearing, or 20 to 20,000 Hz. Figure 3–1 illustrates the waveform and spectrum of a white noise. We can see large random amplitude fluctuations over time in the waveform represented in Figure 3–1. The spectrum also contains a representation of those fluctuations, but the fluctuations are relatively small, and we generally treat the spectrum of white noise as being flat across frequency, particularly for long-duration white noise.

Unlike a pure tone, which is characterized by amplitude and frequency, we can characterize white noise with a single parameter describing its amplitude. We more commonly describe the amplitude of white noise by one of two primary metrics: the *total power* and the *spectrum level*. The total power calculation weighs all frequencies equally and reflects the overall power of the noise. The total power of a noise stimulus can be calculated directly from the root mean square (rms) pressure using $20\log(P_{rms\text{-}noise}/P_{ref})$. The spectrum level reflects the level within a 1-Hz band and is also sometimes referred to as the *level per*

cycle (LPC) in the field of audiology. Both total power and spectrum level are commonly reported in dB SPL.

Another important noise type is narrowband noise, essentially a band-restricted version of white noise. Because this noise does not contain all frequencies, narrowband noise must always be characterized by at least two parameters in addition to one that represents the power: the *bandwidth* and the *center frequency*. A narrowband noise is fully described by specifying the bandwidth (the range of frequencies in the noise), the center frequency (the frequency at the center of the noise), and the LPC of the noise. A schematic of the spectrum of a narrowband noise is illustrated in Figure 3–2, which also shows the various parameters used to define the noise. A narrowband noise can also be described by the high and low *cutoff frequencies*, which define the highest and lowest frequencies before the noise amplitude is attenuated. These parameters are also labelled in Figure 3–2. It is fairly straightforward to switch between total power and LPC if the noise bandwidth is known, following the equation:

$$\text{Total Power} = 10 \log (BW) + LPC,$$
$$\text{Eq. 3–1}$$

where BW= the bandwidth and LPC = the level per cycle.

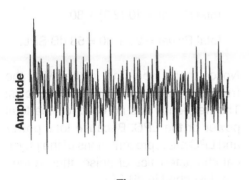

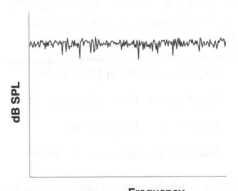

FIGURE 3–1. Plots of the waveform (*left panel*) and spectrum (*right panel*) of white noise.

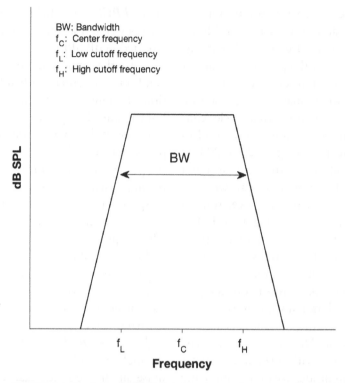

BW: Bandwidth
f_c: Center frequency
f_L: Low cutoff frequency
f_H: High cutoff frequency

BW

dB SPL

f_L f_C f_H

Frequency

FIGURE 3–2. Schematic of the spectrum of a narrow band of noise. The center frequency (f_c), cutoff frequencies (f_L and f_H), and bandwidth (BW) are specified.

In evaluating Eq. 3–1, we can see that the total power will be different for two noises with the same LPC but different bandwidths. For example, we can assume that a white noise has a bandwidth of 20,000 Hz. If the LPC of that noise is 30 dB SPL, the total power can be calculated as follows:

Total Power = 10 log (BW) + LPC

Total Power = 10 log (20000) + 30

Total Power = 10 (4.3) + 30

Total Power = 43 + 30 = 73 dB SPL.

On the other hand, if the bandwidth of the noise is 200 Hz, the total power would be calculated as:

Total Power = 10 log (BW) + LPC

Total Power = 10 log (200) + 30

Total Power = 10 (2.3) + 30

Total Power = 23 + 30 = 53 dB SPL.

Notice that it would not matter what the frequency of the narrowband noise is: The frequency has no effect on the total power or the LPC. Because total power and LPC are representations of the physical characteristics of noise, their values are described in dB SPL.

Filters

Filters have an important role to play in both acoustics and perception, and they are used to modify sound. In many cases, models of auditory perception are based on the concept of filters. For example, we can think of one aspect of hearing loss as a filter because some frequencies are *attenuated* by that hearing loss.

Principles of Filtering

A filter is a device or process that removes or reduces the amplitude of specific components of a stimulus. Filters modify sound by attenuating certain frequency components of a stimulus. Applied to acoustics, a filter will *pass* certain sound frequencies and *attenuate* others. Frequencies that are passed by the filter are unaffected by that filter.

There are four major classes of filters:

- *Low-pass filter.* Passes the low frequencies and attenuates high frequencies.
- *High-pass filter.* Passes the high frequencies and attenuates low frequencies.
- *Band-pass filter.* Passes frequencies within a specified frequency region and attenuates all others.
- *Band-reject filter.* Attenuates frequencies within a specified frequency region and passes all others.

Because we describe filters in terms of their frequency characteristics, they are most easily represented in terms of their *transfer function*, a representation of the gain provided by the filter as a function of frequency. Figure 3–3 illustrates the transfer functions of these four different filter types. The y-axis is gain in dB, which is an indication of how much a filter changes a sound. A 0-dB gain means no alteration in stimulus level, whereas

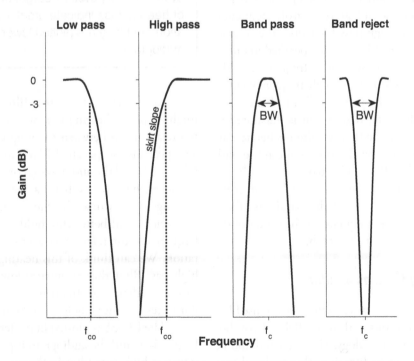

FIGURE 3–3. Schematic transfer functions of different filter types. Variables indicated are f_c = center frequency, f_{co} = cutoff-frequency, and BW = bandwidth. The cutoff frequencies are specified as 3-dB down points.

negative gain implies attenuation. The power of an input (pre-filtered) sound has dB SPL units, and an output (post-filtered) sound has dB SPL units. However, the filter itself is not a representation of sound, and its gain is instead described using dB.

Figure 3–3 shows the transfer functions of the various filter types along with their acoustic descriptors. The cutoff frequencies and the slope of the filter skirt specify low-pass and high-pass filters. Applied to a filter, the cutoff frequency is a boundary in the filter's transfer function at which attenuation begins to occur. In many cases, the cutoff frequency is defined as the point that is 3 dB below the maximum gain, the 3-dB down point. The slope of the skirt indicates how rapidly the filter transitions from passing the signal to attenuating it.

We can observe in Figure 3–3 that the low-pass filter has 0 dB gain in the frequencies below the cutoff frequency (f_{co}) and begins attenuating sound at the cutoff frequency, whereas the high-pass filter does the reverse. The band-pass filter can be specified in one of two ways: using two cutoff-frequencies—the low-frequency and the high-frequency cutoff or the center frequency (f_c) and bandwidth (BW). The latter description is illustrated in Figure 3–3. Note that we often generate narrowband noise by filtering white noise with a band-pass filter. The band reject filter is described in the same manner but, in some sense, is the reverse of the band-pass filter. Here, the center frequency is the center of the rejection band, or the notch.

Hearing Loss as a Filter

There are many ways in which we can use filter characterizations within the field of psychoacoustics and audiology. The outer and middle ears have transfer functions that are band-pass in nature, as the mid-frequencies are boosted more than higher or lower frequencies. On the other hand, the healthy inner ear has a relatively flat frequency-transmission characteristic, and so a filter analysis does not easily apply. However, pathologies in any portion of the ear alter the frequency transmission characteristic of that auditory component, and in many cases these pathologies yield hearing losses in which a filter analogy would apply. For example, a low-frequency hearing loss can be modeled as a high-pass filter, as it attenuates low frequencies and passes high frequencies. Alternatively, a high-frequency hearing loss could be considered a low-pass filter.

We plot an audiogram in a way very similar to filter transfer functions. Audiometric thresholds in dB HL reflect the *change* in hearing from a normative reference, and a threshold of 0 dB HL indicates that sound is not attenuated by the auditory system. Larger amounts of hearing loss indicate greater attenuation, and they are plotted lower on the audiogram.

To illustrate how the filter analogy might apply to hearing loss, we can consider the relationship between the long-term average spectrum of speech (LTASS; discussed in Chapter 2) and the audiogram. For illustrative purposes, here we evaluate a low-frequency hearing loss—worse thresholds in the low frequencies and better thresholds in the high frequencies, also referred to as a *rising* configuration. We can think of this hearing loss as a high-pass filter that attenuates low frequencies more than high frequencies. Figure 3–4 illustrates how hearing loss can be treated as a filter: The LTASS is plotted in the left panel of Figure 3–4, and the audiogram is plotted as if it were a high-pass filter in the middle panel. Note that here, the y-axis is gain, and not the actual hearing thresholds, but we notice that

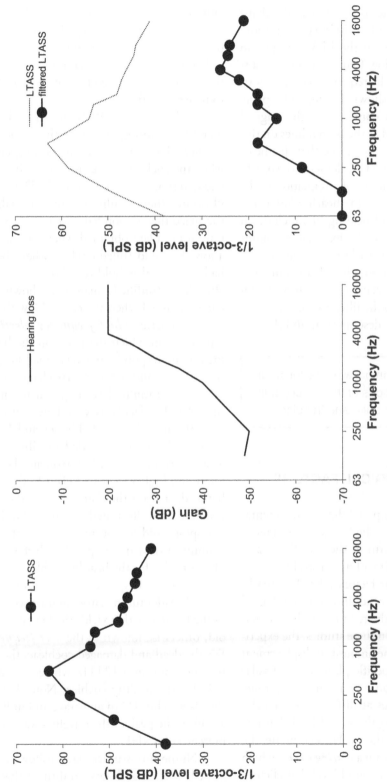

FIGURE 3–4. Illustration of hearing loss as a filter. The left panel illustrates the long-term average spectrum of speech (LTASS). The middle panel illustrates a rising low-frequency audiogram represented as a filter (Gain versus frequency) instead of audiometric thresholds. The right panel plots the filtered speech spectrum (*filled symbols*) along with the original speech spectrum of the left panel (*dotted lines*). Attenuation of the speech stimulus is evident, and greater attenuation is observed in the low frequencies.

the shape of the filter is the same as the shape of an audiogram with a rising configuration. Applying this filter to the LTASS results in attenuation of the low-frequency components more than the high-frequency components, and the result is shown in the right panel of Figure 3–4. For comparison, the original LTASS is illustrated as the dotted lines on this panel. In this way, we can see that this hearing loss has attenuated all elements of speech, with the greater amount of attenuation in the low frequencies where the hearing loss is the greatest. All types of hearing loss include an aspect of filtering, as the loss causes sounds to be more difficult to hear. It is important to recognize, however, that distortions and perceptual deficits accompany sensorineural hearing loss, and so the filter analogy does not provide a complete descriptor of SNHL.

> Visit the companion website for auditory demonstrations of the effects of filtering speech in quiet and in noise.

PHYSIOLOGICAL FACTORS

We observed in Chapter 2 that the representation of vibration on the basilar membrane is primarily in the form of the traveling wave. The shape and size of the traveling wave are both important factors related to masking. Here, we review additional physiological measurements conducted in vivo that are relevant to masking. In these studies, the experimenter measures the amount of displacement (or velocity) at a specific place on the basilar membrane in response to a stimulating tone. By presenting tones at different frequencies and then measuring the sound level that just noticeably vibrates the basilar membrane, the physiologist can obtain a *tuning curve*, which illustrates the lowest sound level that elicits a

vibration plotted as a function of the stimulating frequency. These experiments have also been conducted in the auditory nerve, but rather than measuring vibration, they measure the signal level required to cause a single fiber to increase its firing rate.

Sellick et al. (1982) measured basilar membrane tuning curves in the guinea pig cochlea. They measured the tuning curves when the cochlea was healthy, after threshold had deteriorated, and after death. Figure 3–5 illustrates their results, recorded initially at the place that responded best to an 18-kHz pure tone. Data obtained when the ear had a low threshold (filled circles), when the ear had a higher threshold (unfilled circles), and after death (unfilled squares) are shown. The curve obtained when the ear had low thresholds demonstrates *high frequency selectivity*, a property in which the place on the basilar membrane responds to a very small range of frequencies, and a *band-pass* characteristic. Here, the stimulus level required to vibrate the 18-kHz place was very low, consistent with the low threshold. Higher and higher stimulus levels were needed to vibrate that location as the stimulating frequency became lower and higher than 18 kHz. On the other hand, data from the damaged and the dead cochleae both illustrated a shift in threshold: A response did not occur until a 50-dB SPL stimulus was used, compared with the 10-dB SPL stimulus for the healthy cochlea. We also observe poorer frequency selectivity, indicated by the broader tuning curve, and we see a shift in the frequency that yields the lowest threshold, otherwise known as the *best frequency*. For the dead and damaged cochleae, the best frequency was near 12 kHz, whereas it was 18 kHz for the healthy cochlea. Note that this shift is roughly 1/2 of an octave and indicates a shift in the peak of the traveling wave in the presence of SNHL.

Numerous studies have followed that of Sellick et al. and have confirmed that fre-

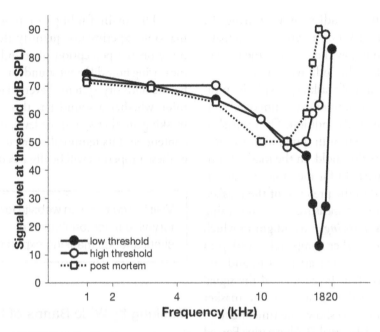

FIGURE 3–5. Basilar membrane tuning curves measured in a healthy cochlea (*filled circles*), after threshold had elevated (*unfilled circles*), and after death (*unfilled squares*). Measurements are from the same basilar membrane location in a single animal. Adapted from Sellick et al. (1982).

quency selectivity is much better than initially reported by von Békésy, due to the damage to the cochlea caused by death in his experiments. Other physiological experiments have also reported tuning curves across a wide range of best frequencies for healthy mammalian species. Universally, those studies showed that the bandwidth (in hertz) of the tuning curves increases with increasing center frequency (Palmer, 1987).

These physiological measures have strong implications for masking, as we observe that a single cochlear location responds to multiple frequencies. Thus, if two frequencies are presented to the ear and they are similar to each other, these two frequencies will vibrate some of the same cochlear locations. We can think of this phenomenon as two tones competing for the same location on the cochlea, and the tone with the greater response would be the dominant one.

INTRODUCTION TO MASKING

Important Concepts

We define *masking* in two ways:

• The process by which sounds are made more difficult to hear by other sounds, or
• The amount by which the threshold of one sound is elevated by another sound.

Unlike physiological experiments, where we can measure the response elicited by a single stimulus, a masking study always involves at least two sounds: a *signal* and a *masker*. The signal is the sound being detected, whereas the masker is the interfering sound. Often the signal is a pure tone, but in principle, it can be any type of sound, such as speech and complex sounds. The same is true for the masker; it can be any type of sound such as noise, speech, or tones. In these studies, by measuring the influence of a masker on a signal, we can make inferences about how the signal or the masker is represented by the auditory system.

The amount of masking is typically measured using two conditions: an unmasked condition and a masked condition. The unmasked condition is detection in quiet, akin to measuring absolute threshold. In the masked condition, the threshold for the same stimulus is then measured in the presence of the masker. Many experiments measured masking using *simultaneous masking*, a paradigm in which the signal and masker completely overlap in time. The masker may start prior to and end after the signal, but the entirety of the signal must fall within the duration of the masker stimulus. Figure 3–6 shows the timeline for a single trial in a 2-Interval, 2-Alternative Forced Choice (2I–2AFC) masking experiment. In this figure, the signal is presented in the first of the two intervals. Recall in a 2I–2AFC experiment, there are two observation intervals: one interval contains the signal and the other does not. The interval containing the signal is selected at random. In a masking experiment, one interval contains the masker and signal, whereas the other interval contains the masker alone. The listener then selects which of these two intervals contains the signal. We can see from Figure 3–6 that the signal occurs within the extent of the masker and only occurs in one of the two intervals. We often consider this experiment as a *detection* one, because a listener is tasked with detecting whether a signal is present.

The main findings of psychophysical masking experiments quantify the effects of noise on the perception of sounds as well as measuring how different sounds are represented by the auditory system. Several factors determine whether a sound has the capability of masking another sound: its level, its frequency content, and its temporal characteristics. Each of these properties will be discussed in turn.

> Visit the companion website for an auditory-visual demonstration of a 2I-2AFC simultaneous masking experiment.

Masking by Wide Bands of Noise

It is intuitive that the sound level of a masker should have a strong effect on its ability to mask sounds. That is, a more powerful masker should produce more masking. This intuition, however, is not quantitative and requires further investigation. For example, intuition cannot address how much masking a given stimulus produces or how changes in the dB SPL of the masker alter the amount of masking. Hawkins and Stevens (1950) reported a very simple but elegant study that addressed portions of these two questions. Their experiment measured the masking produced by a broadband noise (100–9000 Hz) on the detection of pure-tone stimuli with various frequencies. They tested eight different masker levels, ranging from –10 to 60 dB SPL. Data adapted from

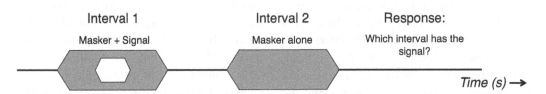

FIGURE 3–6. Schematic of an experimental trial used in a 2I-2AFC task for simultaneous masking.

their experiment are illustrated in Figure 3–7, which shows the threshold of the pure tones measured in the presence of each of the eight maskers as a function of the frequency of the signal. The threshold in quiet is also shown.

The results of Hawkins and Stevens' experiment show the following patterns:

- *Frequency effects.* Masking effects across frequency, although small, were present. At the lowest levels, broadband maskers were able to mask the frequencies between about 1000 and 6000 Hz but not the lower and higher frequencies. For example, the –10 dB SPL masker raised the threshold of the 2000-Hz tone from about 7 dB SPL in quiet to about 11 dB SPL, but that same masker did not shift the threshold of the 250 Hz tone at all. At these low masker lev-

els, these frequency effects could be attributed to audibility, as the level of the noise did not exceed the absolute threshold of the low-frequency tones. Once masking began, however, the same noise masked high frequencies slightly more than low frequencies: the 30 dB SPL masker raised the 500-Hz threshold to 48 dB SPL and the 4000-Hz threshold to 52 dB SPL. This trend was present across all masker levels and amounted to about a 5-dB increase in masking across the audible frequency range.

- *Level effects.* Increasing the masker dB SPL level increased the signal level necessary for detection. Figure 3–7 shows that once masking occurred (that is, once the masker was sufficiently powerful to mask the signal), a 10-dB increase in masker led to a 10-dB increase in masking. For example, at

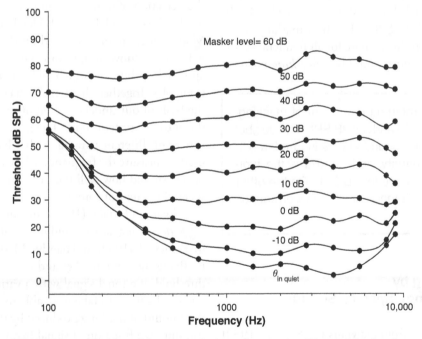

FIGURE 3–7. Masking of pure tones by broadband noise. Thresholds of various frequency tones presented in broadband maskers of different stimulus levels are shown. Solid lines represent curve fits to the data, and the masker levels are reported above the associated masking curve. Adapted from Hawkins and Stevens (1950).

1000 Hz, the 20 dB SPL masker was associated with a 40 dB SPL threshold, and the 30 dB SPL masker caused threshold to be 50 dB SPL.

We can calculate the amount of masking produced by each of these sounds by subtracting the threshold in quiet from the masked threshold. As an example, we can determine how much masking the 20-dB SPL noise masker will have at 2000 Hz:

The threshold in quiet at 2000 Hz is 7 dB SPL.

The 20-dB SPL masker elevates the 2000-Hz threshold to 42 dB SPL.

Amount of masking: 42 dB SPL – 7 dB SPL = 35 dB of masking

The same 20-dB masker, however, produces much less masking at 250 Hz: 39 dB SPL – 25 dB SPL = 14 dB of masking. If we completed this exercise for all frequencies, the resulting figure would be a ***masking pattern***.

> When referring to amount of masking, we use dB and not dB SPL. The decibel level of a sound always is in reference to a quantity, and 20 µPa is the typical reference for dB SPL. On the other hand, differences in dB between sounds use dB.

Masking by Frequency-Specific Sounds

The results from Hawkins and Stevens (1950) illustrate a small, but robust, effect of signal frequency. However, we can better observe the relationship between the frequency of maskers and the frequencies of the signals when experiments are conducted under variable frequency conditions. These experiments measure a property of the auditory system called ***frequency selectivity***, or the ability of the auditory system to represent one frequency as independent of another. From the standpoint of perception, frequency selectivity is defined as the ability to hear one frequency as being separate from another, and is very similar, but not identical, in definition to the same term when applied to physiology.

Wegel and Lane (1924) conducted the earliest experimental work that established the frequency selective nature of the auditory system. They measured the effects of the presence of one tone on the ability to detect a tone of a different frequency. They demonstrated that a masker produced the most masking when it had a frequency similar to that of the signal. Subsequent studies evaluated masking produced by narrow and wide bands of noise on the detection of pure tones and found similar results (Egan & Hake, 1950; Fletcher, 1940). Modern measurements, based on these seminal studies, now adopt somewhat different approaches, but are still based on the same principles. Together, these studies have formed the basis of our understanding of masking in the auditory system today. Here, we discuss a variety of different paradigms that have been used to measure the frequency selective nature of the ear and how well the ear represents the spectral content of sounds.

Egan and Hake (1950) measured *masking patterns* for a narrowband noise with center frequency of 410 Hz and bandwidth of 90 Hz. By fixing the noise masker and measuring the threshold of a tonal signal with a variable frequency, Egan and Hake were able to measure the amount of masking produced by that fixed stimulus as a function of signal frequency. We can consider the masking pattern as a psychological representation of an acoustic stimulus. In some ways, the masking pattern provides a picture of the internal psychological representation of the masker. Egan and Hake measured these masking patterns for this narrowband noise presented at three different levels, 40, 60, and 80 dB SPL, in order to determine if the internal representation of sound was altered by the presentation level. Figure 3–8 illustrates their data and shows the amount of masking plotted as a function of the signal frequency.

Figure 3–8 shows several important findings from Egan and Hake's seminal experiment:

- *Frequency selectivity.* Masking was greatest at signal frequencies nearest the frequencies encompassed by the masker. Signal frequencies that were very distant from those in the masker often experienced no masking.
- *Upward spread of masking.* More masking occurred at signal frequencies higher than the masker than at signal frequencies lower than the masker. We observe this in Figure 3–8 by the asymmetrical shape of the masking patterns. When the signal was lower in frequency than the masker (i.e., signal frequencies <410 Hz), the amount of masking was less than when the signal was higher in frequency than the masker (i.e., signal frequencies >410 Hz). Across all levels tested, more masking was produced when the masker was lower in frequency than the signal than the reverse.
- *Masker level affected frequency selectivity.* Increasing the level of the masker led to more masking and produced greater upward spread of masking. The frequency selectivity of the ear was worse at high levels compared with low.

> Visit the companion website for an auditory demonstration of upward spread of masking.

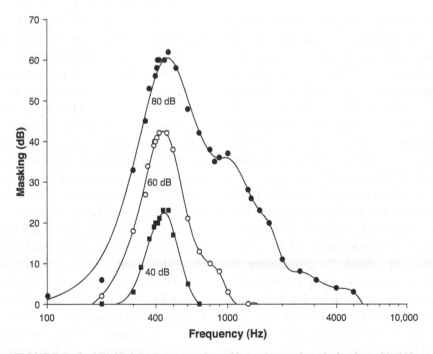

FIGURE 3–8. Masking patterns produced by a narrow band of noise with 410-Hz center frequency and 90-Hz bandwidth. Data obtained at different noise levels (40, 60, and 80 dB SPL) are shown as the different symbols. Adapted from Egan and Hake (1950).

The work of Egan and Hake (1950) allows an estimate of how well the ear is able to resolve different frequencies in the stimulus. Their data illustrate the *frequency selective* nature of the ear in that only frequencies near a signal were able to mask it and **upward spread of masking**, in which low-frequency sounds masked high-frequency sounds greater than the reverse. We can also see substantial nonlinearity: More intense sounds produced greater upward spread of masking. It is impressive how far masking extends for a fairly narrow band of noise, particularly at the high stimulus levels where masking extended multiple octaves!

THE CRITICAL BAND AND THE AUDITORY FILTER

The Critical Band

Fletcher (1940) used a different technique from that of Egan and Hake and used his data to provide the foundation for our modern theory of masking. Rather than measure the masking effects of a fixed masker and vary the frequency of the signal being detected, Fletcher fixed the frequency of the signal and measured the signal's threshold in the presence of different maskers. In this work, Fletcher measured the threshold of a pure tone in the presence of a masker with increasing bandwidth. Importantly, he kept the spectrum level of the noise constant, which led to increases in total noise power as the bandwidth increased. Recall from the section on acoustics in this chapter that the total power of a stimulus is determined by two factors: the spectrum level and the bandwidth. A 10-fold increase in bandwidth leads to a 10-dB increase in the total power. Thus, a 5000-Hz wide noise band is 10 dB more intense than a 500-Hz wide noise band and is 20 dB more intense than a 50-Hz wide noise band. If masking were determined only on the basis of total power, the threshold of a signal added to a band of noise should increase by 10 dB for each 10-fold increase in bandwidth.

Figure 3–9 illustrates an example taken from Fletcher's band-widening experiment, which plots the level of a 2000-Hz signal at threshold as a function of masker bandwidth. The masker was a band of noise centered at 2000 Hz presented at a variety of different bandwidths. Fletcher, however, did not find that the threshold of the signal increased by 10 dB per 10-fold increase in bandwidth! Rather, his experiment showed a very striking finding: For relatively narrow noise bandwidths, signal thresholds did increase as predicted by the power calculation. However, for all of the frequencies he tested, there was always a bandwidth beyond which increases in the masker bandwidth did not lead to further increases in masking. Fletcher dubbed this bandwidth the **critical band**.

Fletcher's data point to frequency selectivity of the ear, just as do the data from Egan and Hake. Fletcher intuited that power at masker frequencies distant from the signal do not produce masking because those masker components do not interact with the signal in the auditory system. Therefore, a band-pass filter analogy might be a great way to describe this aspect of auditory processing. A filter, centered at the signal frequency, only passes certain frequencies that are defined by the critical band. Any frequency outside of the critical band surrounding the signal cannot mask that signal. This is why thresholds did not change as the masker bandwidth was widened beyond the critical band.

Fletcher also noted that the size of the critical band tended to increase with increasing frequency. Data that illustrate the bandwidth of the critical band are plotted as a function of frequency in Figure 3–10. For frequencies up to about 500 Hz, the size of the critical band is fairly constant, but then it increases with increasing frequency. As a result, we see that

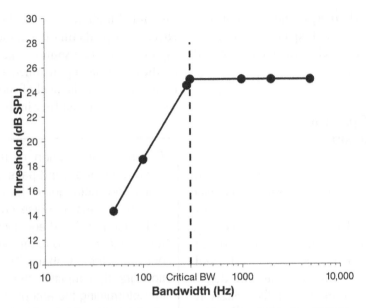

FIGURE 3–9. Band-widening data. The threshold of a 2000-Hz signal is plotted as a function of the bandwidth of a masking noise. The dashed line indicates the estimated critical bandwidth. Adapted from Fletcher (1940).

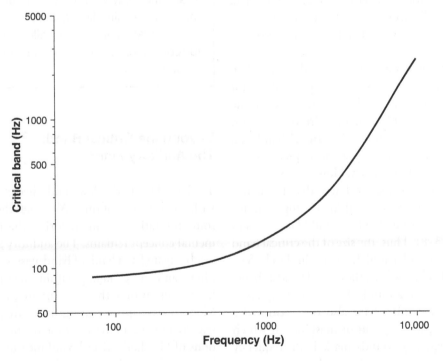

FIGURE 3–10. The size of the critical band plotted as a function of the center frequency. Adapted from Zwicker (1961).

the frequency selectivity of the ear is not constant and gets worse as frequency is increased, as long as frequency selectivity is characterized in terms of hertz.

The Power Spectrum Model of Masking

Using his experiments on the critical band, Fletcher developed the *power spectrum model of masking*, which first posits that the ear functions like a bank of band-pass auditory filters, with many individual filters tuned to specific center frequencies. Secondly and importantly, after filtering, the only determining factor of masking effectiveness is the power of the masker that falls within the critical band (or filter) surrounding the signal being detected. Increases in the power within the critical band will yield increases in the signal level needed for detection. This model accounts for Fletcher's original (1940) data and is still in use today due to its success in predicting masking data for experiments that have used steady-state maskers.

We will note failures of this model in later sections of this chapter, particularly for fluctuating sounds. However, some of the limitations of this model are already apparent. First, Fletcher defined the critical band as a single value used to represent frequency selectivity for each frequency. However, even in the early experiments, we knew that frequency selectivity worsened with increasing stimulus level (as illustrated in Egan and Hake's data in Figure 3–8). Thus, the size of the critical band should be wider at higher stimulus levels. Second, Fletcher defined the critical band as being symmetrical around the signal frequency. However, studies have also demonstrated a robust upward spread of masking, in which low-frequency sounds mask high-frequency sounds to a greater degree than the reverse. Although Fletcher's critical band concept has

substantial limitations, it has been extremely effective in predicting the amount of masking of steady-state sounds, like white noise, on the detection of pure tones. This topic and its application to the field of audiology is discussed in more detail later in this chapter.

> Fletcher's description of the critical band assumed band-pass characteristics and rectangular shape. This filter would pass all noise components within the passband equally as well as fully remove all components that fall outside of the passband. This assumption greatly simplifies the calculation for determining the amount of masking produced by a noise stimulus. Fletcher was acutely aware that his definition of the critical band did not fully describe masking data but remember that Fletcher did not have computers to easily model his data. As a result, he made these simplifying assumptions, but those assumptions still allowed him to robustly predict data on masking by steady sounds.

Beyond the Critical Band: The Auditory Filter

To date, Fletcher's views and theories have withstood the test of time. Although there are some limitations to his theories, the fundamental concept remains: The auditory system can be treated as a bank of band-pass auditory filters, and energy falling within one of those filters determines the amount of masking. Modern descriptions of auditory frequency selectivity have addressed some of the limitations of Fletcher's critical band measurement. First, modern techniques and computers now allow us to characterize auditory filters using many parameters, such as their asymmetry and their dependence on stimulus level. Second, auditory filters are typically measured using a variation of Fletcher's band widening experiment, called the ***notched-noise method***.

Patterson (1976) developed the notched-noise method to measure the shape of the auditory filter. This method uses a masker that is two bands of noise (~300-Hz wide or so) with a spectral notch placed between them. The tone to be detected (the signal) has a frequency that falls within the spectral notch. Rather than vary the bandwidth of the noise as Fletcher did, the bandwidth of the spectral notch is varied. Larger notches will lead to less masking compared to smaller notches, due to

fewer masking components falling within the theoretical auditory filter surrounding the signal frequency. One advantage of this method is that asymmetrical placement of the notch around the center frequency can allow measurement of a filter that is asymmetrical.

Visit the companion website for an auditory-visual demonstration of a notched-noise experiment.

A schematic illustrating this experiment and the type of data resulting from this experiment are shown in Figure 3–11. The left panel

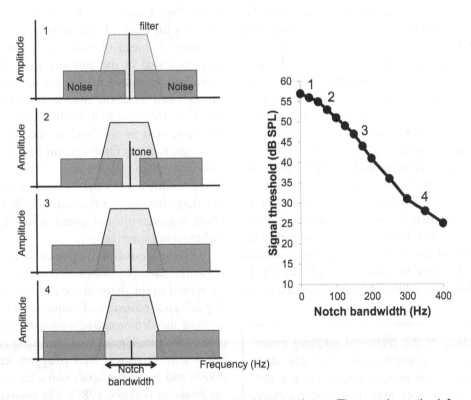

FIGURE 3–11. Illustration of the notched-noise experiment. The panels on the left illustrate various acoustic conditions used in the notched-noise method, from a narrow notch (*panel 1*) to a wide notch (*panel 4*). The right panel illustrates data obtained from the notched-noise method at 1000 Hz with signal thresholds from the various notch bandwidths indicated from #1–4. These thresholds decrease with increasing notch bandwidth. Data are adapted from Patterson (1976).

shows four schematics of the stimuli used. In all cases, a signal tone (illustrated by the line spectrum) is plotted with the notched noise (indicated by the dark gray shaded areas). The different panels illustrate increasing notch bandwidths from panel 1 (top) to panel 4 (bottom). Increasing the size of the notch bandwidth leads to less noise falling in the filter (illustrated by the light gray shading) and a better detection threshold. The signal level at threshold is illustrated by the decreasing signal amplitude. The right panel of Figure 3–11 illustrates the signal threshold as a function of increasing notch bandwidth as we progress from panel 1 to panel 4, as obtained by Patterson (1976). The specific examples shown in the left panel of Figure 3–11 are indicated by the corresponding numbers on the data graph. We see that thresholds decreased with increasing notch bandwidth in Patterson's experiment.

The auditory filter can be calculated by applying the power spectrum model of masking to estimate the shape and characteristics of the auditory filter. To estimate the auditory filter, one must make some initial assumptions about the auditory filter, such as an approximation of the shape and size of the filter. We then pass the stimuli through this hypothetical filter, and, using the power at the output of the filter, estimate the signal level at threshold for various notch bandwidths. By comparing the predicted data with the actual obtained data, we can revise the parameters selected for the auditory filter. When the predicted data yield

a good match to the obtained data, we have an estimate of the auditory filter. Parameters that are commonly estimated are the bandwidth of the filter and the slope of the high-and low-frequency skirts.

Figure 3–12 shows auditory filters obtained by Rosen and Baker (1994), who used the notched-noise method at multiple stimulus levels to estimate the shape of the auditory filter centered at 2000 Hz. Following convention, auditory filters are plotted in terms of gain, and are normalized to 0 dB gain at their center frequency. From this figure, we see that at low levels, the auditory filter is relatively symmetric. However, as level increases, the auditory filter becomes increasingly shallower on the low-frequency side in comparison to the high-frequency side, which does not change with level. This asymmetry accounts for upward spread of masking, as the low-frequency side of the auditory filter allows more low-frequency masker energy to pass through and mask the tone being detected, which in this case is a 2000-Hz tone. We also note that as the level of the stimulus increases, auditory filters become broader and more asymmetric (Rosen et al., 1998). These changes with level occur exclusively on the low-frequency skirt of the auditory filter and result in greater upward spread of masking at higher stimulus levels.

Psychoacoustical frequency selectivity measures have physiological correlates that are related to the shape of the traveling wave. Physiological estimates of frequency selectivity have also demonstrated *asymmetry* (Sellick et al., 1982; see Figure 3–5), *increasing bandwidth with increasing level* (Ruggero et al., 2000), and *increasing bandwidth with increasing frequency* (Palmer, 1987). The correlation between physiological measurements and psychophysical measurements supports the idea that the frequency selectivity measured psychophysically is a consequence of basilar membrane tuning.

Many of the historical auditory filters are not physiologically plausible, and they were used because we did not have a filter that mimicked auditory physiology well. We have much better filters available today, particularly the *gammachirp* auditory filter (Irino and Patterson, 1997).

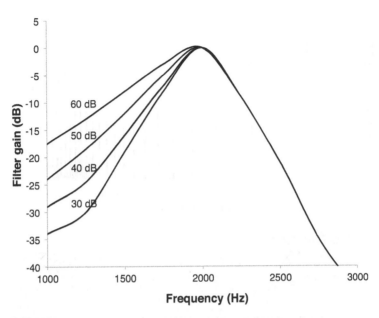

FIGURE 3–12. Plots of auditory filters measured at multiple stimulus levels at 2000 Hz. Adapted from Rosen and Baker (1994).

Auditory filter bandwidths are commonly reported in terms of their equivalent rectangular bandwidth, or ERB. This value quantifies the bandwidth in terms of an equivalent filter that is rectangular in shape. Other measurements of bandwidth can also be used, such as one defined using the 3-dB down points, which correspond to measures from the filter skirts defined by the frequency at which the attenuation is 3 dB. However, the ERB is much more commonly adopted in psychoacoustic literature.

THE EXCITATION PATTERN

Auditory filters provide a unique opportunity for illustrating the representation of sounds from a perceptual standpoint. In particular, by using the power spectrum model of masking, we can approximate the spectral informa-tion as it is represented in the auditory sys-tem. Because auditory filters are not perfectly frequency selective (i.e., they pass more than one frequency), each spectral component of a stimulus is not represented with perfect fidel-ity by the ear. One method of representing sounds to illustrate their *internal* rather than acoustic representation is the ***excitation pat-tern***, a depiction of the excitation evoked by a sound stimulus plotted as a function of the filter center frequency (Zwicker, 1970). The excitation pattern is essentially a multichannel implementation of the power spectrum model of masking. An excitation pattern is generated by passing any stimulus through a bank of auditory filters with varied center frequencies. The excitation is calculated as the power in dB at the output of each auditory filter. This exci-tation value in dB is then plotted as a function of the center frequency of that auditory filter, yielding the excitation pattern.

Figure 3–13 illustrates how an excitation pattern is calculated for the vowel sound /i/ (as in "h<u>ee</u>d") with a fundamental frequency

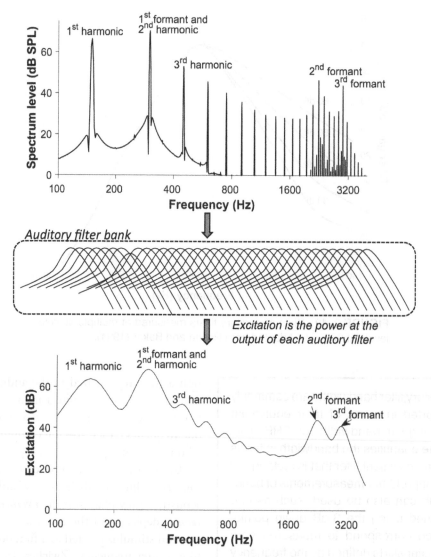

FIGURE 3–13. The power spectrum (*top panel*) and excitation pattern (*bottom panel*) of a harmonic complex modeled after the vowel /i/ ("h<u>ee</u>d") for listeners with normal hearing. The middle panel illustrates the auditory filter bank used to estimate the excitation pattern.

of 150 Hz. The first three harmonics and the first three spectral prominences, the formants, are labelled on the spectrum (top panel) and excitation pattern (bottom panel). Notice the spectrum and excitation patterns are plotted on a logarithmic frequency axis; this is a common practice due to the logarithmic spacing of the basilar membrane. In the spectrum, we

can observe many of the 150-Hz harmonics, which are shown as separate lines at least up to 2000 Hz. We also can see a robust presence of the formants: There are distinct spectral peaks around 300 Hz, 2200 Hz, and 3000 Hz.

The excitation pattern, on the other hand, provides a smoothed representation of the power spectrum. The representation of the individual harmonics and the formants, although easily visible in certain frequency regions, are not nearly as pronounced as in the spectrum. Figure 3–13 illustrates two major differences between the spectral representation and the excitation patterns:

- *Only low-frequency harmonics are visible as peaks in the excitation pattern.* The representation of the low-frequency harmonics is not as robust in the spectrum. Harmonics 1 through 8 or 10 are evident as distinct bumps in the excitation pattern, and these bumps gradually smooth as frequency increases. Harmonics 1 to 8 are considered *resolved*, whereas harmonics 10 and above are considered *unresolved*.
- *The representation of the formants is smoothed in the excitation pattern.* Whereas the formants are well-represented in the excitation pattern, they are slightly smeared and not as pronounced as in the stimulus.

The excitation pattern can also illustrate the impact of masking on the internal representation of the spectrum. Figure 3–14 illustrates the excitation pattern for the /i/ ("heed") of Figure 3–13, but in the presence of a moderate-level noise. In the spectrum (solid line), we observe evidence of harmonics 1 to 5 or so, and the formants at 300, 2200, and 3000 Hz. Regarding the excitation pattern, however, each individual auditory filter passes a portion of vowel as well as a portion of the noise stimulus. The result is a smoother excitation pattern compared with the one obtained without noise and has a representation of only a few harmonics, which are smeared in comparison to the spectrum. The excitation of the first formant is relatively unaffected by the noise, as the level of the formant is well above the level of the noise. However, the 2nd and 3rd formants have less pronounced representations in the excitation pattern, and the effects of noise on their representations are drastic.

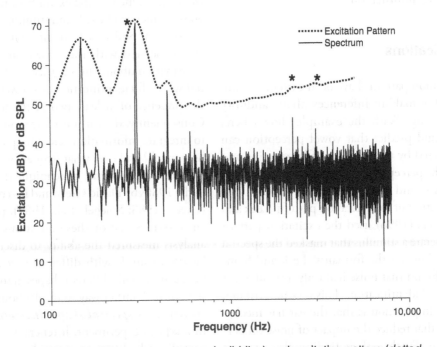

FIGURE 3–14. The power spectrum (*solid line*) and excitation pattern (*dotted line*) for the vowel /i/ ("h<u>ee</u>d") when presented in noise. The asterisks denote the locations of the formants.

Within the excitation pattern, both formants are smeared and reduced in amplitude, and the spectral valley is not as deep.

The excitation pattern provides a great deal of intuition about the representation of sound by the ear, as it reflects the imperfect frequency selectivity of the ear as well as the changing frequency selectivity with increasing frequencies. The imperfect frequency selectivity of the ear is illustrated by the overall smoothing of the spectrum in the excitation pattern. The frequency effects are also illustrated, as the individual harmonics become more smeared together in the high versus the low frequencies. In summary, the excitation pattern provides a psychoacoustical/perceptual representation of the spectrum and simply reflects the information that *may be available* to the ear using known estimates of frequency selectivity. The excitation pattern, however, does not reflect the information that the ear actually uses in perceptual tasks or how the ear uses that information.

Implications

Excitation patterns have been extremely valuable for making inferences about auditory processing. With the example shown here, we could predict that vowel perception can be altered by the presence of large noise, and that the perception of the high-frequency formants would be the most degraded. In one application of the excitation pattern, Leek and Summers (1996) used the excitation pattern to generate a stimulus that masked the spectral valley, but not the formants. Leek and Summers found that noise had only a small effect on vowel identification. This is rather striking, as the implication is that the ear has mechanisms that reduce the impact of noise on perception. Further, their finding also suggests that the spectral valley is not nearly as important for vowel identification as the represen-

tation of the formants. Such results provide fuel for a hot debate in the speech perception literature, as there is also evidence in support of a whole spectrum model for vowel perception (Ito et al., 1999; Molis, 2005). Excitation patterns have also been greatly helpful in our understanding of auditory representations of listeners with SNHL, as discussed in a later section of this chapter.

Profile Analysis

Excitation patterns provide a representation of the spectrum from a psychological perceptive. However, an excitation pattern is only a representation of a *best-case* scenario and does not measure how well the auditory system is able to *use* the information that is represented. As we have observed, many sounds in the environment are broadband in nature, and the acoustic cues are often distributed across frequency. One specific example of this is the vowel, which is a broadband stimulus containing spectral peaks, or formants. The frequencies associated with these formants provide information about the identity of the vowel, but successful identification of a vowel requires the presence of at least two of the formants. Consequently, the ear must have some ability to integrate information across frequency, but how much? and over what frequency range?

Profile analysis, a technique developed in the 1980s by David Green and his colleagues (Green, 1988; Spiegel et al., 1981), provided answers to some of these questions. Profile analysis measured the ability to discriminate between sounds with different spectral profiles, sounds with different shapes in the power spectrum. Another way to think about profile analysis is as *spectral-shape discrimination*. In a typical experiment, listeners would hear stimuli with different spectral profiles and would indicate the one with a target spectral profile. Green's experiments showed that we can discriminate spectral profiles across a very wide frequency range (effectively the entire audible bandwidth) and that our perception benefits from distributed spectral information across frequency. Yet, Berg and Green (1990) expanded on the profile-analysis technique and showed that while human listeners indeed benefited from added information across the audible bandwidth, they did not use all of the spectral information for discrimination. In general terms, they found that listeners performed worse than *best-performance* models, suggesting loss of some spectral information in the perceptual process. Although profile-analysis experiments supported the view that the ear represents the entire stimulus spectrum, they also demonstrated that the ear does not always use this information efficiently, and essentially loses some of the spectral information in the coding process. We can view this interpretation in light of the excitation pattern, which only provides a picture of the information available to the ear.

PSYCHOPHYSICAL TUNING CURVES AND SUPPRESSION

A different way to characterize frequency selectivity is the *psychophysical tuning curve (PTC)*, similar in concept to the physiological tuning curve. The PTC has been used to illustrate additional nonlinear effects of auditory processing. Measuring the PTC uses tone-on-tone masking, in which the signal and the masker are both tones. In a typical PTC measurement task, the tone to be detected is <u>fixed in frequency and level</u>, usually around 10 dB above threshold. Then, for various masker frequencies, the experimenter measures the masker level that just masks the tone. When masking is measured in this way, low masker levels are associated with maskers that produce a lot of masking; they are very effective. We generate a PTC by plotting the masker level

needed to just mask the tone versus the frequency of the masker.

Importantly, PTCs have been measured in two different experimental paradigms: *simultaneous masking* and *forward masking*. Up to this point, our discussion has revolved around simultaneous masking, a paradigm in which masker and signal are presented at the same time. In forward masking, the masker is always presented before the signal and the masker and signal <u>never overlap in time</u>. Using forward masking illustrates an important consequence of nonlinear auditory processing on the masking process. Here, we are specifically concerned with how frequency selectivity is measured under both simultaneous and forward-masked scenarios. Yet, due to the temporal nature of the method, we discuss forward masking again in Chapter 5 on temporal processing.

To illustrate this type of masking, Figure 3–15 shows an experimental trial of a forward masking experiment. Although the masker comes before the signal, the masker can make that signal more difficult to hear.

Visit the companion website for an auditory-visual demonstration of a forward masking experiment and an auditory demonstration of forward masking.

Measuring PTCs under forward and simultaneously masked conditions illustrates why we must consider both situations. Moore et al. (1984) measured PTCs for a tone presented at 10 dB SL and at four different frequencies under both simultaneous and forward masked conditions. They found that simultaneous-and forward-masked PTCs have a very similar shape, as shown in Figure 3–16. However, we see a striking difference between the two types of PTCs. The PTC measured using simultaneous masking was broader than the PTC measured using forward masking.

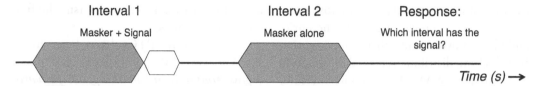

FIGURE 3–15. Schematic of the stimulus presentation sequence used in a 2I-2AFC task for forward masking.

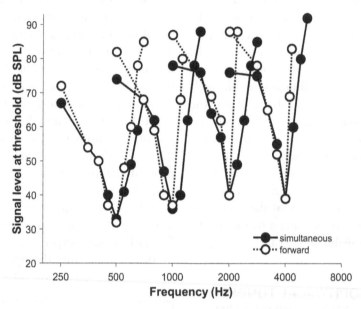

FIGURE 3–16. Example psychophysical tuning curves measured under forward (*dotted lines*) and simultaneous (*solid lines*) masking for four different frequencies. Adapted from Moore et al. (1984).

We also observe evidence of upward spread of masking in the shallower low-frequency tail in both simultaneous-and forward-masked conditions, suggesting that upward spread of masking is a robust property of the auditory system. Although comparisons between psychological and physiological tuning curves can be difficult due to species differences and measurement differences, note how similar the PTCs are in comparison to the physiological tuning curve measured from the basilar membrane in Figure 3–5.

The difference in frequency selectivity obtained using the two methods is a conse-quence of a nonlinear physiological phenom-enon called ***two-tone suppression*** (Sachs & Kiang, 1968; later measured psychophysically by Houtgast, 1974). In brief, the excitation produced by a single tone can be reduced (i.e., suppressed) by the simultaneous presence of a stronger second tone, with the largest effects occurring when the two tones are nearby in fre-quency, but not immediately adjacent (Shan-non, 1976). In masking, then, a strong masker suppresses the signal, effectively lowering the excitation of the signal. Because the masker suppresses the signal, the level of the masker that is needed to mask the signal will be lower than if the signal were not suppressed. As a result, the masker level at threshold is lower in the simultaneous condition than the same masker in the forward-masked condition, where suppression is not active. If we apply this principle to the simultaneously masked PTC, the masker components that fall within the suppressive region around the signal require lower masker levels to mask the signal, causing tuning to appear to be broader than when measured under forward-masking conditions.

Implications

Two-tone suppression may appear to be a negative aspect of auditory processing. In fact, however, it has several benefits related to auditory perception. Under some circumstances, components within a masker can suppress each other, rendering the entire masker less effective. It also leads to improved spectral contrast for broadband stimuli. For example, formants within a vowel suppress components within the valleys, enhancing the spectral representation of the vowel spectrum (because the representation of the valleys is smaller than expected). If we consider two-tone suppression in light of the excitation pattern, the spectral contrast (e.g., the difference between the spectral peak and the valley) could be better compared to that described by the excitation pattern. Auditory filters used for the excitation pattern are measured using simultaneous masking, and therefore might actually underrepresent the spectral information available to the ear!

As a result, we must consider the method used when describing the frequency selectivity of the ear. A fair amount of everyday listening occurs in simultaneous masking situations, and consequently, frequency selectivity measured under these conditions may be most appropriate to include in auditory models. On the other hand, the effects of two-tone

suppression are considerable, and comparison with physiological measurements requires psychophysical measures to be conducted under forward-masked conditions.

MASKING BY FLUCTUATING SOUNDS

Up to this point, our discussion of masking has focused on the masking produced by steady-state sounds. However, as we know, the sounds we encounter in the environment vary in amplitude over time. That is, they fluctuate. An important class of masking experiments focuses on the effects of these fluctuating maskers that have amplitude variations that occur over time. Hall et al. (1984) demonstrated that masking by steady-state noise can be much greater than masking by fluctuating noise, and their data are illustrated in Figure 3–17. In a set of conditions very similar to that conducted by Fletcher (1940), listeners detected a 1000-Hz tone added to steady noise of varied bandwidths. Like Fletcher, Hall et al. found that thresholds increased with increasing bandwidths up to the critical bandwidth and then did not increase more with increasing bandwidth, as shown by the filled circles in Figure 3–17. Hall et al. then imposed fluctuations upon the noise (called *modulation*) and measured thresholds again. In contrast to the results of Fletcher, Hall et al. found that increasing the bandwidth of the modulated noise first increased thresholds but then thresholds decreased as the bandwidth was further increased, as shown by the unfilled circles in Figure 3–17.

Visit the companion website for an auditory demonstration of the difference between detection of a tone in a steady noise versus a fluctuating noise.

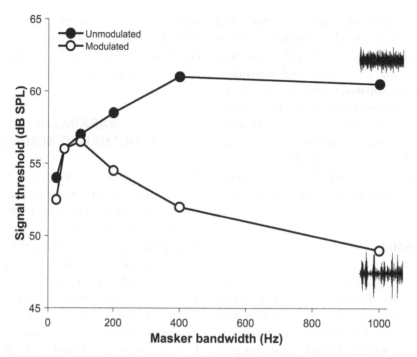

FIGURE 3–17. Thresholds for detecting a pure tone added to a steady band of noise (*filled circles*) and a fluctuating band of noise (*unfilled circles*) as a function of the bandwidth of the noise. Schematics of the noises with a 1000-Hz bandwidth are also illustrated. Adapted from Hall et al. (1984).

We see from Figure 3–17 that the decrease in threshold provided by the fluctuating masker did not begin until the masker bandwidth was greater than the critical band, or around 60 to 100 Hz. The difference in threshold between the steady masker and the fluctuating masker is the *fluctuating masker benefit*. The size of the benefit increased as the bandwidth of the masker increased, with a benefit of over 10 dB for the 1000-Hz wide masker. When the fluctuations across frequency were synchronous, a *release from masking* occurred, meaning thresholds were lower than when stimuli were masked by broadband noise. Data such as these point to problems with Fletcher's power spectrum model of masking, which would have predicted the same thresholds regardless of stimulus fluctuations (Richards, 1992).

To understand Hall et al.'s results, we must first consider how a fluctuating masker may provide benefits to a listener. A fluctuating masker has *dips* or *valleys* in the waveform. These dips provide brief epochs in time that have high signal-to-noise ratios (SNRs), compared with the waveform peaks, and a listener with normal hearing can take advantage of these dips to detect a signal (Buus, 1985). Steady maskers do not have pronounced dips and therefore do not provide opportunities for *dip listening*. To illustrate how this might work, Figure 3–18 shows how the valleys in a masker provide regions of high SNR. Figure 3–18 illustrates a fluctuating masker, plotted along with a signal. The signal is only visible in the masker dips, which therefore have a high SNR. A sophisticated detection system, like the ear, can take advantage of those dips to facilitate detection. Benefits of a broadband modulated masker are not restricted to detecting pure tones, as

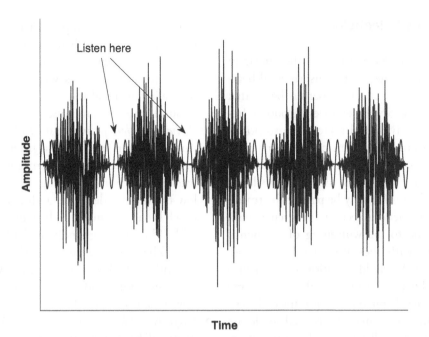

FIGURE 3–18. Illustration of dip listening. A fluctuating masker is shown with a pure tone signal.

they have also been demonstrated for detecting and understanding speech (Miller & Licklider, 1950).

MASKING AND SENSORINEURAL HEARING LOSS

Listeners with sensorineural hearing loss have a common complaint of having great difficulty communicating in noisy environments. This complaint can be partially traced to a greater susceptibility of masking that results from cochlear damage. Deficits in detecting masked sounds have been measured repeatedly in listeners with sensorineural hearing loss, and these are discussed here.

Physiological Factors

Sensorineural hearing loss can be associated with a loss of both outer and inner hair cells within the cochlea. Most listeners with sensorineural hearing loss have either outer hair cell loss or a combination of outer and inner hair cell loss. Loss of the outer hair cells, which are responsible for sharpening the tuning of the traveling wave, leads to a reduction in frequency selectivity in these listeners. This result is evident in the basilar membrane tuning curves provided by Sellick et al. (1982) and illustrated in Figure 3–5, where threshold elevation led to a broadening of frequency selectivity on the basilar membrane. These physiological measurements may be expected to have a direct consequence on the psychoacoustical measurement of frequency selectivity, and we would expect a broadening of the auditory filter in the presence of the loss of outer hair cells. Although loss of the inner hair cells would not affect basilar membrane tuning, their loss may also broaden the psychophysical auditory filter, depending on pattern of fibers that are damaged, and will most definitely raise the threshold for detection.

Frequency Selectivity

Several studies have evaluated the effects of masking in listeners with sensorineural hearing loss, with a general consensus being that listeners with SNHL experience poorer frequency selectivity and a greater susceptibility to masking than their counterparts with normal hearing (Florentine et al., 1980; Leek & Summers, 1993). The high stimulus levels required for testing may be part of the reason for poor frequency selectivity in listeners with SNHL, due to the worsening of frequency selectivity with increasing level. However, even when threshold elevation is taken into account by presenting stimuli at the same sensation levels for the two groups of listeners or when noise masking is used to elevate thresholds of the listeners with normal hearing, listeners with SNHL appear to experience an additional reduction in frequency selectivity due to their auditory pathology.

To illustrate the range and variation of auditory filters measured in listeners with SNHL, five examples of auditory filters obtained from listeners with normal hearing and listeners with SNHL are illustrated in Figure 3–19 (Glasberg & Moore, 1986). Auditory filters obtained from the listeners with normal hearing (top panel) are fairly symmetrical but tend to have a shallower low-frequency skirt compared with the high-frequency skirt, as we have already observed. Note too that there is some variability across listeners in terms of the overall bandwidth and shape. The bottom panel, which plots the auditory filters for the listeners with SNHL shows:

- *Broadening of the auditory filter.* The auditory filters for the listeners with SNHL are broader than for those with normal hearing. One consequence of the broader filter is additional masking in these listeners. Changes to the bandwidth are typically assumed to be approximately two or three times the width of auditory filters measured in listeners with normal hearing. Consequently, listeners with SNHL will need a better signal-to-noise ratio to detect a sound embedded in noise.

- *A shallower low-frequency skirt of the filter.* Auditory filters measured in listeners with SNHL tend to be more asymmetric than in listeners with normal hearing. Typically, the low-frequency side of the auditory filter is much broader than the high-frequency side of the filter, although individual differences exist. The consequence is that these listeners with a shallower low-frequency auditory filter skirt tend to experience greater upward spread of masking.

- *Large variability across listeners.* Measurements of frequency selectivity in listeners with SNHL demonstrate considerable variation in the bandwidth and asymmetry of the filter. Although many listeners present with broader auditory filters, one cannot easily predict from audiometric thresholds how poor frequency selectivity might be (Glasberg & Moore, 1986). The degree of asymmetry exhibited in the auditory filters of listeners with SNHL is extremely variable, and some listeners (like HI2 in Figure 3–19) might exhibit broadening of the high-frequency skirt as well as the low-frequency skirt.

Psychophysical tuning curves obtained in listeners with SNHL demonstrate poor frequency selectivity as well. The poorer frequency selectivity of the listeners with SNHL becomes even more apparent when PTCs are measured under conditions of forward masking, as tuning is not sharper under forward masked conditions for listeners with sensorineural hearing loss (Moore & Glasberg, 1986). Wightman et al. (1977) found that the suppression mechanism is not effective in listeners with sensorineural

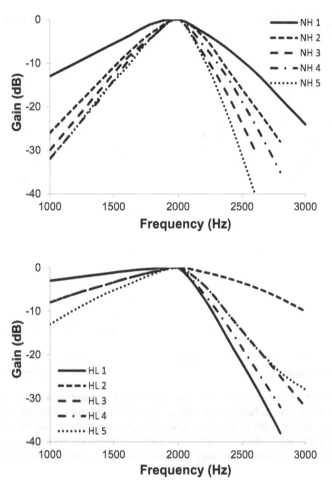

FIGURE 3–19. Auditory filters centered at 2000-Hz are plotted for five listeners with normal hearing (*top panel*) and five listeners with sensorineural hearing loss (*bottom panel*). Adapted from Glasberg and Moore (1986).

hearing loss. Recall that in listeners with normal hearing, suppression caused the simultaneously obtained PTCs to be broader than the forward-masked PTCs (as illustrated in Figure 3–16). Thus, loss of suppression explains why the PTCs are so similar between forward-masked and simultaneously masked conditions. Poor frequency selectivity and loss of suppression would cause listeners with SNHL to experience more masking and a reduction to the important contrasts present in the spectrum.

Excitation Patterns

To illustrate how broadening the auditory filter affects the excitation pattern, the left panel of Figure 3–20 plots the excitation patterns for the vowel /i/ ("h<u>ee</u>d") in an ear with typical frequency selectivity (solid lines) and an ear with filters twice as wide (dotted line). The dashed-dotted lines indicate an excitation pattern with broader filters and an additional sloping high-frequency hearing loss, 20 dB HL

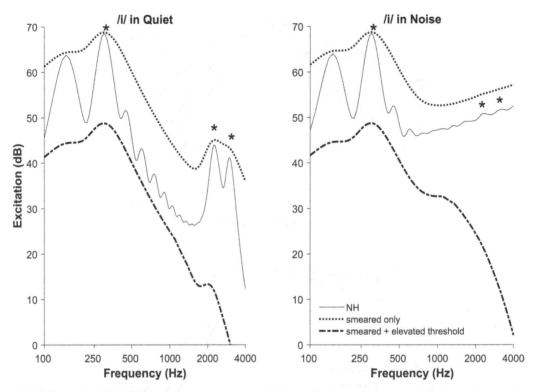

FIGURE 3–20. Excitation patterns for the vowel /i/ ("h<u>ee</u>d") presented in quiet (*left panels*) and in noise (*right panel*). Excitation patterns based on an ear with no hearing loss are shown with the solid lines, and excitation patterns with poorer frequency selectivity are shown as the dotted lines. Excitation patterns with the dashed-dotted lines add attenuation to the smeared excitation patterns, to better simulate the effects of sensorineural hearing loss. Asterisks show the location of the formants.

up to 1500 Hz, sloping to 55 dB HL at 4000 Hz. When comparing the excitation patterns for the vowel stimuli in quiet, we see that the excitation pattern with reduced frequency selectivity (dotted lines) shows that the peaks associated with the individual low-frequency harmonics and the formants are greatly smoothed compared with the typical excitation pattern. Then, when we add on the effects of elevated thresholds (dashed-dotted lines), the overall excitation is reduced. For this hearing loss, even in quiet, the 2nd formant is barely represented, and the 3rd formant is not. On the whole, the broadened auditory filters provide less access to the spectral information present in a stimulus, and elevated thresholds limit the availability even more.

The impact of noise on the excitation pattern for listeners with SNHL is shown in the right panel of Figure 3–20, again along with the excitation pattern for listeners with normal hearing. Because wider auditory filters pass more of the noise, the spectral contrasts are obscured even more than for listeners with normal hearing. Notably, the two high-frequency formants are essentially completely obscured by the noise. When examining the excitation pattern that includes elevated thresholds (dashed-dotted lines), we see very little spectral information available to this listener, other than the first formant.

Many stimuli in the environment contain relatively small spectral contrasts, and this illustration of the excitation pattern suggests that reduced frequency selectivity can have a real impact on the perception of sounds in our environment. Further, even small reductions of spectral contrast may be problematic when stimuli are masked. Reduced frequency selectivity by listeners with sensorineural hearing loss is generally considered to translate into difficulties understanding both speech in quiet and speech in noise.

Masking by Fluctuating Maskers

The difficulties imposed by sensorineural hearing loss are not restricted to steady noise. Listeners with sensorineural hearing loss have been demonstrated to receive much less benefit from fluctuating maskers than those with normal hearing, and in some cases receive no fluctuating masker benefit at all (Bacon et al., 1998; Festen & Plomp, 1990). The reduced benefit can be attributed to several different factors, with a primary factor being that the dips in the fluctuating stimulus are rendered inaudible by sensorineural hearing loss. Thus, the ear with hearing loss does not have the opportunity to take advantage of high-SNR temporal epochs. Other factors related to hearing loss are also likely involved, such as alterations in the representation of the waveform, which is discussed in more detail in Chapter 5. The inability to take advantage of temporal fluctuations in a masker leads to substantial deficits for everyday listening and is a major contributor to difficulties understanding speech in noise.

Perceptual Consequences of Reduced Frequency Selectivity

A reduction in frequency selectivity may lead to deficits in perceiving sounds that require a robust representation of the stimulus spectrum. As such, one might expect a connec-

tion between reduced frequency selectivity and difficulties with speech perception, as spectral information is an important cue to identify certain speech sounds. To address this question, Baer and Moore (1993) simulated reduced frequency selectivity and found that even very poor frequency selectivity (six times worse) had only a very small effect on speech understanding in quiet. On the other hand, however, Baer and Moore observed very large effects of reduced frequency selectivity for that same speech signal presented in noise. Reduced frequency selectivity has also been linked to poor abilities to understand speech in noise for people with SNHL (Festen & Plomp, 1983; Dubno et al., 1984).

One way to think about this is that poor frequency selectivity of the ear with SNHL increases the susceptibility to masking by other sounds. If we consider the auditory filter as the model of frequency selectivity, a doubling of the bandwidth of that filter, which is also a reduction in frequency selectivity, will increase the masked threshold of a tone by approximately 3 dB, and additional increases in the bandwidth further increase the masked threshold. Whereas a change in masked threshold of 3 dB might seem relatively small, it can make a huge difference for speech perception. For reference, a 3 dB decrease in the signal-to-noise ratio can be associated with a decrease in speech understanding of 20 to 60 percentage points, which could drastically influence the ability of an individual to participate in a conversation. In this way, diminished frequency selectivity could increase the difficulty of speech understanding in noise listening situations.

Notably, hearing loss reduces the fluctuating masker (FLM) benefit, which allows listeners with normal hearing to benefit from modulated background noises such as speech. To illustrate the importance of the FLM in speech understanding and how loss of the FLM can be impacted by SNHL, data from

Festen and Plomp (1990) are plotted in Figure 3–21. Festen and Plomp measured sentence understanding in a modulated (fluctuating) and steady noise for listeners with normal hearing and SNHL. Figure 3–21 shows performance plotted as a function of the SNR. For listeners with normal hearing, the psychometric function for the steady masker is to the right at *higher* SNRs than for the modulated masker, meaning that the fluctuating masking provides a benefit (about 5 dB) to the listeners. Another way to think about this is that performance is higher for the FLM than the steady masker. If we look at the SNR of –8 dB, we observe that performance was 80 percentage points higher for the modulated than the steady masker! On the other hand, the listeners with sensorineural hearing loss required overall higher SNRs to achieve the same level of speech understanding as the listeners with

normal hearing, and they did not benefit from the FLM at all. In fact, their performance in the fluctuating masker was slightly worse than performance in the unmodulated masker. We can see this because the psychometric function for the steady masker is to the left at *lower* SNRs than for the modulated masker. Their study provided clear evidence that listeners with SNHL cannot take advantage of the fluctuations in a masker to the same degree as listeners with normal hearing.

Lastly, reduced frequency selectivity is also associated with upward spread of masking, which can be problematic for both speech in quiet and speech in noise. To better understand this, we first must look at the acoustics of speech. First, as we have observed, speech itself has a peak at 500 Hz, and the long-term average spectrum of speech has a roll-off of about –9 dB per octave above 500 Hz

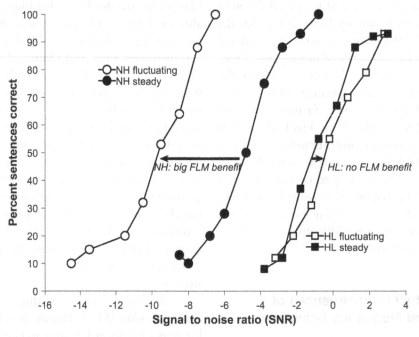

FIGURE 3–21. Illustration of the fluctuating masker benefit for sentence understanding for listeners with hearing loss (*squares*) and listeners with normal hearing (*circles*). Percent sentences correct is plotted versus the SNR for a steady noise (*filled symbols*) and fluctuating noise (*unfilled symbols*). Adapted from Festen and Plomp (1990).

(recall Figures 2–25 and 3–4), meaning that speech progressively decreases in level as frequency increases. Second, the frequencies that are most important to speech tend to be in the range of 1000 to 4000 Hz. This is illustrated in the count-the-dot audiogram of Figure 2–26, in which the most dots are concentrated between 1000 and 4000 Hz. Within speech, the low-frequency components, such as the harmonics produced by a speaker's voice and the first and second formants of vowels, are commonly higher in level than higher-frequency elements such as unvoiced fricatives (e.g., /s/, "seep", and /ʃ/, in "sheep") or stop consonants like /p/ ("peep") and /k/ ("keep"). Thus, the elements that provide the energy to speech (i.e., the vowels) effectively can mask (via upward spread of masking) the elements that are important to understanding speech. Lastly, environmental noise also tends to have a low-frequency emphasis, and upward spread of masking by the low-frequency components of noise on speech can impair the ability to hear and identify the information-carrying elements of speech.

Increased susceptibility to upward spread of masking exacerbates the above scenarios and has been shown to be associated with poorer speech perception in quiet (Hannley & Dorman, 1983) and in noise (Klein et al., 1990). In addition, if a listener has low-frequency hearing loss and requires amplification of low frequencies, upward spread of masking effects are expected to be even greater because those low frequencies are amplified. In this case, the amplified low-frequency sounds can provide additional masking of the high-frequency elements of speech that are necessary for speech understanding. As such, upward spread of masking can complicate fitting hearing aids for listeners with low-frequency hearing loss. One successful rehabilitation strategy for these individuals is to reduce the amount of gain prescribed in the low frequencies, but modern hearing aids also adopt numerous tech-

nologies, such as multi-channel adaptive noise reduction and directionality, which also can be used to reduce upward spread of masking.

Summary of Effects of SNHL on Masking

Taken together, we see that listeners with sensorineural hearing loss experience a reduction in frequency selectivity, a greater susceptibility to masking, and reduced effects of two-tone suppression compared with listeners with normal hearing. Impaired frequency selectivity directly contributes to a reduced representation of the spectrum and leads to greater susceptibility to masking. Loss of two-tone suppression also reduces the representation of spectral contrast, and the inability to take advantage of stimulus fluctuations significantly degrades the ability to detect and understand sounds in a variety of noisy environments. All of these factors contribute to difficulty understanding speech, particularly in noise.

CLINICAL IMPLICATIONS OF MASKING

The principles of masking are also an integral component to an audiological assessment. Whenever a patient presents with an asymmetry between the ears, audiologists apply the principles of masking when obtaining an audiogram. All transducers coupled to the head (e.g., earphones or a bone oscillator) can allow sound to *cross over* via bone conduction from the test earphone to the non-test (contralateral) cochlea. Any time a patient has an asymmetry in hearing, the audiologist evaluates whether cross-hearing (in which the non-test ear responds to the sound rather than the test ear) can occur. If necessary, the audiologist applies the principles of masking to ensure that the threshold measurements reflect the sensitivity of the ear being tested. When masking is used in audiogram measurement, it is used to shift the threshold of the non-test ear to a level that does not allow the non-test ear to detect the tone presented to the test ear. The maskers used for clinical masking are derived explicitly from Fletcher's work on the critical band, and critical band theory governs masking in audiology in the following ways:

- *Masker bandwidth.* When masking pure tones in clinical applications, the maskers used must have bandwidths that exceed the critical band. A masker narrower than the critical band would be insufficient as a masker for diagnostic audiology.
- *Masker effectiveness.* The size of the critical band is a necessary component to determine how effective a masker can be. Because the audiologist is interested in the effectiveness of the masker rather than its total power, maskers are considered in terms of their **effective masking level**, dB EML. The effective masking level is the dB HL value to which threshold is shifted in the presence of a noise at that dB EML.

The bandwidths of the maskers used for clinical masking are all wider than the critical band. If a masker is too narrow, it can sound like a tone or it can have audible fluctuations. These wider maskers also ensure sufficient masking across individuals with and without hearing loss and at high stimulus levels.

For example, if a patient's absolute threshold is measured in quiet at 10 dB HL, and then this patient's threshold is measured in the presence of a 40-dB EML noise, the threshold will become 40 dB HL in that noise. On the other hand, a patient with an absolute threshold of 60 dB HL will not experience any masking by this noise, as absolute threshold is greater than the dB EML of the noise. Although it is likely that this patient cannot hear this noise, sometimes a patient may hear a noise that produces no masking of the test frequency, because the masker could contain audible frequencies outside of the critical band.

Effective masking level is determined by the spectrum level of the noise, the critical band at the test frequency, and a conversion from dB SPL to dB EML, which can be calculated in the following way:

$$dB\ EML = 10\log(CB) + LPC - RETSPL, \qquad Eq.\ 3\text{--}2$$

where CB = critical bandwidth, LPC = level per cycle of the noise, and RETSPL = the reference threshold in SPL. RETSPL values and critical band values are given in Table 3–1.

Using Eq. 3–2 as a guide, we can see that increases in the LPC of the noise will increase its masking effectiveness. However, we also see that increasing the noise bandwidth beyond the critical band will not lead to increases in masker effectiveness. The noise bandwidth is not a component of Eq. 3–2. This equation only applies for maskers that have bandwidths greater than the size of the critical band.

We can calculate the dB EML of the following stimulus: a 1000-Hz wide noise, centered at 500 Hz, presented at a 40-dB LPC over TDH-39 headphones.

Using Eq. 3–2 and the TDH-39 entries in Table 3–1,

$$dB\ EML = 10\log(50) + 40 - 11.5 = 45.5\ dB\ EML.$$

This masker can shift any threshold for a pure tone <45.5 dB HL to 45.5 dB HL. Any threshold that is greater than 45.5 dB HL will not be affected by this masker.

TABLE 3–1. Reference Thresholds in dB SPL for TDH-39 Earphones and Critical Band Values in Hz

Frequency (Hz)	Reference Threshold in dB SPL		Critical Bandwidth (Hz)
	TDH-39	**ER-3A**	
125	45.5	26.0	70
250	25.5	14.0	50
500	11.5	9.5	50
1000	7	5.5	64
2000	9	11.5	100
4000	9.5	15	200
8000	13	15.5	400

Sources: RETSPL values are from ANSI S3.6 (2018) and critical bandwidth values are from Hawkins and Stevens (1950).

SUMMARY AND TAKE-HOME POINTS

A variety of different stimuli can mask other stimuli. The relationship between the frequencies, level, and fluctuations of the masker and the signal being detected are important. Higher-level maskers with frequencies near the signal have the greatest effect in elevating the signal's threshold. Upward spread of masking also increases as stimulus level increases. Listeners with normal hearing receive a release from masking when maskers fluctuate, as they can rely on brief temporal epochs with high signal-to-noise ratios in order to detect signals or identify speech sounds. Sensorineural hearing loss greatly impacts masking, with listeners experiencing greater masking effects, increased upward spread of masking, and a reduction in the fluctuating masker benefit.

Fletcher's findings have had a far-reaching impact on our understanding of masking by the ear and its ability to represent the spectrum of sounds. His critical band theory and the power spectrum model of masking are still used to calculate masking effectiveness for audiological applications, and excitation patterns use his principles to characterize how a sound might be represented by the auditory system. Although Fletcher's theory was not perfect, it has had a profound impact on our understanding of the frequency selective nature of the ear.

The following are key take-home points of this chapter:

- Masking experiments have demonstrated that the level, frequency, and fluctuations of a masker are influential in its ability to mask a signal. Experiments that have manipulated the bandwidth of stimuli and other acoustic characteristics have illustrated that healthy ears are very frequency selective and have a robust ability to represent the spectral content of a stimulus. These findings have influenced the selection of maskers used in clinical audiometry.
- Frequency selectivity in listeners with normal hearing worsens with increasing stimulus level and with increasing center frequency.
- All listeners experience upward spread of masking, in which low-frequency sounds mask high-frequency sounds greater than the reverse.

- The excitation pattern provides a representation of the internal spectral information available to the auditory system.
- Sensorineural hearing loss causes a reduction in frequency selectivity, leading to a greater susceptibility to masking, greater upward spread of masking, and more difficulty understanding speech in noise.
- Listeners with normal hearing receive benefits from fluctuating maskers; these benefits are lost to listeners with sensorineural hearing loss.

EXERCISES

1. Calculate the total power for three different noises all having an LPC = 40 dB SPL. Bandwidth = 100 Hz, 1000 Hz, and 10,000 Hz. Using your calculations, discuss how increasing the bandwidth by a factor of 10 alters the total power in the noise.

2. You are outside doing a hearing screening by measuring the ability of a patient to detect a 1000-Hz pure tone. However, there is an annoying sound in the background, specifically a tonal sound with a frequency of roughly 8000 Hz. You can hear this sound, but it is likely at a moderate sound pressure level. Do you think that the presence of this background sound influence your threshold measurement at 1000 Hz? Discuss.

3. In a general sketch, convert (approximately) the 20- and 60-dB masking functions represented in Figure 3–7 to a masking pattern. This will be a graph showing amount of masking in dB, plotted as a function of the frequency of the signal being detected. Using your result, discuss how increasing the masker level affects masking at the different signal frequencies.

4. Sketch predicted data for a listener with normal hearing for the following notched

noise experiment. The signal to be detected is 1000 Hz in a noise with a notch. Thresholds for this signal are measured at different notch bandwidths (placed symmetrically around the signal frequency): 0, 25, 50, 75, 100, and 200 Hz. The experiment is conducted at two masker levels: one high (e.g., 80 dB SPL) and one low (e.g., 30 dB SPL). Your sketch should illustrate the following:
   a. The condition (high or low level) that produces the most masking for the 0-Hz notch (i.e., no spectral notch)
   b. The condition (high or low level) that yields less frequency-specific data
   In your sketch, you should consider the size of the auditory bandwidth at 1000 Hz and the effects of level on masking and the auditory bandwidth.

5. Sketch excitation patterns for a pure tone for the following types of listeners. Be sure to pay attention to your axis labels and consider both the effects of audibility and frequency selectivity.
   a. A listener with normal hearing
   b. A listener with 40 dB of conductive hearing loss (hint: A conductive hearing loss only attenuates the sound; it does not distort it.)
   c. A listener with 40 dB of sensorineural hearing loss

6. Sketch excitation patterns for a harmonic complex containing frequencies of 300, 600, 900, 1200, 1500, 1800, 2100, 2400, 2700, and 3000 Hz (all harmonics have the same amplitude) for the following types of listeners. Be sure to pay attention to your axis labels and consider both the effects of audibility and frequency selectivity.
   a. A listener with normal hearing
   b. A listener with 40 dB of conductive hearing loss (hint: A conductive hearing loss only attenuates the sound; it does not distort it.)
   c. A listener with 40 dB of sensorineural hearing loss

7. Using your sketches from Exercise 3–6, discuss which listener will experience the most detrimental effects of noise on perceiving this harmonic complex and why.

8. Auditory filters provide straightforward ways to determine how much a single tone will influence the detection of another tone. Using the auditory filter for a listener with normal hearing shown in Figure 3–12 (the 60-dB curve), calculate the level of the following tones that are passed through this filter. Using the numbers, discuss whether the 1500-Hz tone or the 2500-Hz tone will have a greater masking effect on the 2000-Hz tone. Explain whether your calculations are consistent with upward spread of masking.
   a. 1500 Hz presented at 60 dB SPL
   b. 2000 Hz presented at 60 dB SPL
   c. 2500 Hz presented at 60 dB SPL

9. Discuss the concept of upward spread of masking and explain why this concept might lead to problems with low-frequency amplification in hearing aids.

10. Assume a situation in which a listener with sensorineural hearing loss receives linear amplification that ensures audibility but does not exceed uncomfortable levels (essentially, the sound is made to be louder). Will this form of amplification reduce the masking of speech by environmental sounds?

11. Discuss whether simple linear amplification could increase the fluctuating masker benefit for listeners with sensorineural hearing loss.

12. Calculate the total power and the dB EML for a noise band 500 Hz wide centered at 2000 Hz with an LPC = 30 dB SPL. Do the same for a noise band that is 5000 Hz wide and centered at 2000 Hz. Discuss which of these noises is a more effective masker. After that discussion, consider whether one of these maskers is more efficient at masking than the other. Discuss the factors that you considered.

Visit the companion website for lab exercises.

REFERENCES

ANSI/ASA S3.6 (2018). *American National Standard Specification for Audiometers.* American National Standards Institute.

Bacon, S. P., Opie, J. M., & Montoya, D. Y. (1998). The effects of hearing loss and noise masking on the masking release for speech in temporally complex backgrounds. *Journal of Speech, Language, and Hearing Research, 41*(3), 549–563.

Baer, T., & Moore, B. C. (1993). Effects of spectral smearing on the intelligibility of sentences in noise. *Journal of the Acoustical Society of America, 94*(3), 1229–1241.

Berg, B. G., & Green, D. M. (1990). Spectral weights in profile listening. *Journal of the Acoustical Society of America, 88*(2), 758–766.

Buus, S. R. (1985). Release from masking caused by envelope fluctuations. *Journal of the Acoustical Society of America, 78*(6), 1958–1965.

Dubno, J. R., Dirks, D. D., & Morgan, D. E. (1984). Effects of age and mild hearing loss on speech recognition in noise. *Journal of the Acoustical Society of America, 76*(1), 87–96.

Egan, J. P., & Hake, H. W. (1950). On the masking pattern of a simple auditory stimulus. *Journal of the Acoustical Society of America, 22*(5), 622–660.

Festen, J. M., & Plomp, R. (1983). Relations between auditory functions in impaired hearing. *Journal of the Acoustical Society of America, 73*(2), 652–662.

Festen, J. M., & Plomp, R. (1990). Effects of fluctuating noise and interfering speech on the speech reception threshold for impaired and normal hearing. *Journal of the Acoustical Society of America, 88*(4), 1725–1736.

Fletcher, H. (1940). Auditory patterns. *Reviews of Modern Physics, 12*(1), 47–66.

Florentine, M., Buus, S., Scharf, B., & Zwicker, E. (1980). Frequency selectivity in normally hearing and hearing-impaired observers. *Journal of Speech, Language, and Hearing Research, 23*(3), 646–669.

Glasberg, B. R., & Moore, B. C. (1986). Auditory filter shapes in subjects with unilateral and bilateral cochlear impairments. *Journal of the Acoustical Society of America, 79*(4), 1020–1033.

Green, D. M. (1998). *Profile analysis: Auditory intensity discrimination.* Oxford Science.

Hall, J. W., Haggard, M. P., & Fernandes, M. A. (1984). Detection in noise by spectro-temporal pattern analysis. *Journal of the Acoustical Society of America, 76*(1), 50–56.

Hannley, M., & Dorman, M. F. (1983). Susceptibility to intraspeech spread of masking in listeners with sensorineural hearing loss. *Journal of the Acoustical Society of America, 74*(1), 40–51.

Hawkins Jr., J. E., & Stevens, S. S. (1950). The masking of pure tones and of speech by white noise. *Journal of the Acoustical Society of America, 22*(1), 6–13.

Houtgast, T. (1974). *Lateral suppression in hearing* [Doctoral dissertation, Free University, Amsterdam].

Irino, T., & Patterson, R. D. (1997). A time-domain, level-dependent auditory filter: The gammachirp. *Journal of the Acoustical Society of America, 101*(1), 412–419.

Ito M., Tsuchida, J. & Yano, M. (2001). On the effectiveness of whole spectral shape for vowel perception. *Journal of the Acoustical Society of America* 110(2), 1141–1149.

Klein, A. J., Mills, J. H., & Adkins, W. Y. (1990). Upward spread of masking, hearing loss, and speech recognition in young and elderly listeners. *Journal of the Acoustical Society of America, 87*(3), 1266–1271.

Leek, M. R., & Summers, V. (1993). Auditory filter shapes of normal-hearing and hearing-impaired listeners in continuous broadband noise. *Journal of the Acoustical Society of America, 94*(6), 3127–3137.

Leek, M. R., & Summers, V. (1996). Reduced frequency selectivity and the preservation of spectral contrast in noise. *Journal of the Acoustical Society of America, 100*(3), 1796–1806.

Miller, G. A., & Licklider, J. C. (1950). The intelligibility of interrupted speech. *Journal of the Acoustical Society of America, 22*(2), 167–173.

Molis, M. R. (2005). Evaluating models of vowel perception. *Journal of the Acoustical Society of America, 111*(2), 2433–2434.

Moore, B. C., & Glasberg, B. R. (1986). Comparisons of frequency selectivity in simultaneous and forward masking for subjects with unilateral cochlear impairments. *Journal of the Acoustical Society of America, 80*(1), 93–107.

Moore, B. C., Glasberg, B. R., & Roberts, B. (1984). Refining the measurement of psychophysical tuning curves. *Journal of the Acoustical Society of America, 76*(4), 1057–1066.

Palmer, A. R. (1987). Physiology of the cochlear nerve and cochlear nucleus. *British Medical Bulletin, 43*(4), 838–855.

Patterson, R. D. (1976). Auditory filter shapes derived with noise stimuli. *Journal of the Acoustical Society of America, 59*(3), 640–654.

Richards, V. M. (1992). The detectability of a tone added to narrow bands of equal-energy noise. *Journal of the Acoustical Society of America, 91*(6), 3424–3435.

Rosen, S., & Baker, R. J. (1994). Characterising auditory filter nonlinearity. *Hearing Research, 73*(2), 231–243.

Rosen, S., Baker, R. J., & Darling, A. (1998). Auditory filter nonlinearity at 2 kHz in normal hearing listeners. *Journal of the Acoustical Society of America, 103*(5), 2539–2550.

Ruggero, M. A., Narayan, S. S., Temchin, A. N., & Recio, A. (2000). Mechanical bases of frequency tuning and neural excitation at the base of the cochlea: Comparison of basilar-membrane vibrations and auditory-nerve-fiber responses in chinchilla. *Proceedings of the National Academy of Sciences, 97*(22), 11744–11750.

Sachs, M. B., & Kiang, N. Y. (1968). Two-tone inhibition in auditory-nerve fibers. *Journal of the Acoustical Society of America, 43*(5), 1120–1128.

Sellick, P. M., Patuzzi, R., & Johnstone, B. M. (1982). Measurement of basilar membrane motion in the guinea pig using the Mössbauer technique. *Journal of the Acoustical Society of America, 72*(1), 131–141.

Shannon, R. V. (1976). Two-tone unmasking and suppression in a forward-masking situation. *Journal of the Acoustical Society of America, 59*(6), 1460–1470.

Spiegel, M. F., Picardi, M. C., & Green, D. M. (1981). Signal and masker uncertainty in intensity discrimination. *Journal of the Acoustical Society of America, 70*(4), 1015–1019.

Wegel, R., & Lane, C. E. (1924). The auditory masking of one pure tone by another and its probable relation to the dynamics of the inner ear. *Physical Review, 23*(2), 266.

Wightman, F. L., McGee, T., & Kramer, M. (1977). Factors influencing frequency selectivity in normal and hearing-impaired listeners. In E. F. Evans & J. P. Wilson (Eds.), *Psychophysics and physiology of hearing* (pp. 295–306). Academic Press.

Zwicker, E. (1961). Subdivision of the audible frequency range into critical bands (Frequenzgruppen). *Journal of the Acoustical Society of America, 33*(2), 248.

Zwicker, E. (1970). Masking and psychological excitation as consequences of the ear's frequency analysis. In R. R. Plomp & G. F. Smoorenburg (Eds.), *Frequency analysis and periodicity detection in hearing* (pp. 376–394). Sijthoff.

4

Loudness and the Perception of Intensity

LEARNING OBJECTIVES

Upon completing this chapter, students will be able to:

- Apply appropriate methodology to loudness measurement
- Compare the strengths and weaknesses of the different methods used to assess loudness perception
- Describe the effects of intensity, frequency, and bandwidth on loudness
- Discuss the implications of Weber's law for tones and noises
- Relate the effects of SNHL to loudness perception
- Evaluate the role of changes to loudness perception on everyday listening

INTRODUCTION

Sounds in our environment are associated with numerous perceptual dimensions, and to fully understand perception, we must evaluate our perception in terms of more than just the ability to detect sounds. One of these perceptual dimensions is the *loudness* of sounds, defined as the attribute of auditory sensation by which sounds can be ordered on a scale ranging from soft to loud. Loudness is a primary component of auditory sensation, and its concept is intuitive to anyone who can hear. In our everyday lives, we assess how loud a sound is and whether one sound is louder than another. Loudness is a perceptual correlate of sound *intensity*, the power per unit area of a sound, and the mechanisms by which sound intensity is coded by the ear are of fundamental importance to understanding the loudness percept. We have already captured one of these facets in our discussions of absolute threshold, but the relationship between loudness and intensity and frequency is also relevant to our understanding of auditory function. For example, degraded perceptions of intensity can lead to speech identification errors, particularly for speech elements that contain varied intensities across frequency, such as vowels or fricatives.

The healthy ear has an exceptional ability to represent many sound intensities—from approximately 0 dB SPL (threshold) to 120 dB

SPL (the level above which damage generally occurs). This 120-dB range of hearing maps to a range of audible intensities of a **trillion to one**! Yet even though our ear can code intensities across this range, our ear is able to detect changes in intensity that are smaller than 1 dB! Taken together, the studies on the representations of intensity by the ear, via loudness and intensity discrimination experiments, illustrate the truly exceptional abilities of the ear.

The perception of loudness has been measured in multiple ways and is affected by several acoustic variables. The following chapter discusses the following aspects of loudness:

- *Loudness growth.* In this section, we will evaluate the relationship between loudness and sound intensity, including the techniques and the measurement units.
- *Equal loudness contours.* The loudness of a sound also depends on its frequency. Here, we review how we know that sounds around 3000 Hz are louder than higher- and lower-frequency sounds when presented at the same sound pressure level.
- *Spectral loudness summation.* In this section, we evaluate the role that stimulus bandwidth has on the loudness of sounds.
- *Intensity discrimination.* The previously mentioned aspects of loudness all establish the relationship between acoustic variables and the loudness of sounds. Intensity discrimination experiments, on the other hand, measure the just noticeable difference in intensity between two sounds.

It is worth noting that loudness and intensity are two distinct concepts. Loudness is a psychological perception associated with sound and is a perceptual quantity. We cannot measure it directly—we can only measure the loudness of a sound in the context of other sounds. Further, loudness measurements rely on human reports of loudness. Consequently,

the techniques employed to measure loudness are quite different from those used to measure sound level. This chapter reviews several psychoacoustic tools that have been developed to assess the perception of loudness.

On the other hand, intensity is an acoustic quantity, and we can measure it directly using a sound level meter. We do not need a human listener to make measurements of sound level. The difference in how we measure loudness versus sound level has implications for how we interpret loudness data and highlights why the terms loudness and intensity are not interchangeable.

In this chapter, we discuss the following concepts, as they apply to loudness perception:

- Acoustics—Intensity and the decibel
- Physiological representation of stimulus level
- Loudness measures in listeners with normal hearing
- Intensity discrimination and Weber's law
- Loudness and intensity discrimination in listeners with SNHL
  - Recruitment
  - Perceptual consequences to everyday listening

ACOUSTICS: INTENSITY AND THE DECIBEL

The decibel is an essential acoustic parameter for this chapter. In Chapter 2, we discussed the relationship between the decibel and sound pressure, but we did not discuss the relationship between the decibel and intensity. Sound intensity and sound pressure are related to one another. Sound pressure is defined as force per unit area (pascals or N/m²) and can be measured via movement of the diaphragm of a microphone used with a sound level meter. In contrast, sound *intensity* is the power carried by the sound waves per unit area and has units of watts/m². For the purposes of this course, intensity and pressure can be calculated from one another following this equation:

$$I = p^2/Z,$$

where I is the intensity of sound, p is the rms pressure of the sound, and Z is the impedance of air. The impedance of air is a constant, and is about 400 Rayls (1 Rayl = 1 N·s/m³) at 20° C. Because intensity and pressure are related, we can calculate decibels using either the pressure (P_1) or intensity (I_1) of that sound using either dB SPL = 20 log(P_1/P_{ref}) or dB IL =10 log(I_1/I_{ref}), where P_{ref} is the reference pressure 20 μPa and I_{ref} is the reference intensity of 1×10^{-12} W/m², where W = watts. Note that dB SPL is the ***sound pressure level*** in decibels and dB IL is the ***intensity level*** in decibels. However, for the applications in this text, dB SPL = dB IL, and dB SPL will be used exclusively throughout this text.

Visit the companion website to see a calculation demonstrating dB SPL = dB IL.

PHYSIOLOGICAL REPRESENTATION OF STIMULUS LEVEL

Because it is well-established that the perception of loudness and the intensity of sound are intimately related to one another, we should discuss the representation of sound intensity in the auditory system. Although physiological measures will never be able to measure loudness, as loudness is a perception, physiological measurements are crucial for understanding the auditory mechanisms that ultimately lead to loudness. Coupling psychophysical with physiological measurements can facilitate our understanding of loudness perception.

Basilar Membrane Vibration

Stimulus intensity is represented within the cochlea by the size (the displacement) and velocity of the vibrations on the basilar membrane. Johnstone and Boyle (1967) made some of the first in vivo measurements of basilar membrane responses, and Rhode (1971) reported the first in vivo ***input-output (I-O)*** functions.

To illustrate the characteristics of basilar membrane response, in vivo measurements from Ruggero and Rich (1991) are plotted in Figure 4–1. They placed a small bead on a chinchilla's basilar membrane and measured the vibration of that bead when the basilar membrane was stimulated with sound. By stimulating the ear with sound presented at various sound levels (in dB SPL) and measuring the velocity of the bead as a function of the dB levels, Ruggero and Rich obtained basilar membrane (BM) I-O functions in the chinchilla. They measured basilar membrane responses in two important conditions. The first measurement was conducted in a healthy, intact chinchilla cochlea. They then treated the cochlea with furosemide, a reversible ototoxic agent that altered the function of the outer hair cells, and measured the basilar membrane response again. Examining Figure 4–1, we see:

- *A compressive function in the healthy ear.* In the healthy cochlea, basilar membrane velocity increased rapidly at the low stimulus levels. Once a moderate stimulus level was reached, velocity increased more slowly, and then increased quickly again at the highest levels. The region at moderate levels is considered the ***compressive nonlinearity*** of the ear, as basilar membrane vibration grows more slowly than at the lower levels.
- *Damage altered the I-O function.* Damage to the outer hair cells altered the lowest level at which a velocity could be recorded (e.g., it elevated the threshold of response at this

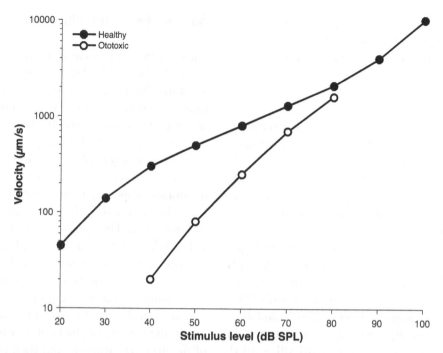

FIGURE 4–1. Basilar membrane velocity is plotted as a function of stimulus level. The solid line indicates the basilar membrane Input-Output (I-O) function in a healthy cochlea. The dashed line indicates the I-O function after treatment with the ototoxic agent. Adapted from Ruggero and Rich (1991).

location). Damage also altered the slope of the I-O function, which became steeper than in the healthy cochlea.

Because the shape of the basilar membrane I-O function changes when outer hair cells are selectively altered, we can infer that healthy outer hair cell function is responsible for the compressive nonlinear shape of the basilar membrane I-O function. When damage to the outer hair cells occurs (such as via treatment by furosemide or another mechanism), we can expect that the shape of the basilar membrane I-O function will change and become steeper. The sound pressure level associated with the smallest amount of detectable vibration (e.g., the threshold of vibration) also increases. The place of maximum excitation also shifts basally as the intensity of a stimulus increases (McFadden, 1986).

Auditory Nerve Responses

The auditory nerve is responsible for coding the vibration of the basilar membrane and provides a neural representation of stimulus level in the auditory system. Rate-level functions for the different fiber types are shown in Figure 4–2, to reiterate how the different fibers in the auditory nerve code for different stimulus levels. Auditory nerve fibers are characterized based on their spontaneous firing rate (SPR), with low (15% of fibers), medium (25% of fibers), and high (60% of fibers) spontaneous firing rates.

Figure 4–2 shows that each of the three different fiber types (low-, medium-, and high-SPR fibers) increase their firing rate as the stimulus level increases. The threshold of each of the fiber types, the stimulus level that causes a detectable increase in firing rate from spontaneous, is also different. As a result, dif-

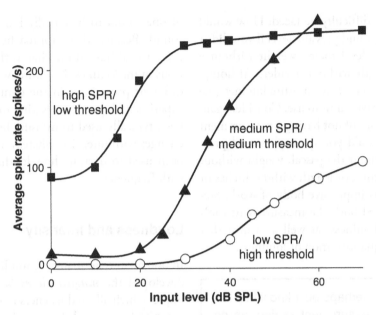

FIGURE 4–2. Auditory nerve rate-level functions for the three different Type I auditory nerve fibers, classified by their spontaneous firing rate (SPR). Based on data from Winter et al. (1990).

ferent fibers will respond by different amounts depending on the level of the stimulus. For example, a sound at 15 dB SPL will only cause the high-SPR fibers to fire. On the other hand, a stimulus presented at 50 dB SPL will cause all three fiber types to fire: the high-SPR fiber will be in *saturation*, firing at its highest possible rate. The low-SPR fiber will not yet be in saturation and will fire at a lower firing rate than the high-SPR fiber. Although all fibers will fire to a 50 dB SPL stimulus, they will not all code an increase in stimulus level. Only the medium and high threshold fibers will have an increase in firing rate if the stimulus level increased from 50 dB SPL. In this way, we see two physiological codes for stimulus level: the firing rate of individual fibers and the pattern of firing rates across the three different fiber types.

LOUDNESS PERCEPTION

A primary question in the loudness literature is how loud one sound is compared with another sound. As we have discussed, we cannot measure the loudness of a sound directly, but we do have techniques that allow the assessment of the relative loudness between sounds. Stanley S. Stevens pioneered the study of measuring the subjective quantity of loudness and had great interest in the relationship between intensity and loudness. It is easy to intuit that increasing stimulus intensity will increase loudness, but Stevens was interested in quantifying how loudness varied with intensity. He asked questions such as:

- If sound pressure level changes by 10 dB, how much does loudness change?
- Is a 10 dB difference in sound pressure level associated with the same loudness difference if a stimulus is presented at a low level versus a high level?

At the time Stevens was conducting his research, there were no psychophysical tools available to measure the loudness of sounds.

Consider the difficulty he faced: How would you measure sound pressure level if you didn't have a sound level meter, weight without a scale, or length without a ruler? Although Stevens had no tools to measure loudness, he also did not have a unit to use. Consider again the implications of not having a measurement unit: How would you quantify sound pressure level without the pascal, weight without pounds or grams, or length without inches or meters? In his impressive body of work, Stevens developed both the measurement tools to quantify loudness, as well as a unit that allowed the quantification of loudness.

Stevens is perhaps best known for his work on measurement scales, as he is the one who identified four different scales: nominal, ordinal, interval, and ratio. A nominal scale requires placing data into categories without an order (e.g., hair color, gender, days of the week, etc.). An ordinal scale is a ranking, but the distance between the ranks is not specified (e.g., a Likert scale, degree of happiness). An interval scale is also ranked, but the distance between points is meaningful (e.g., temperature, GRE score), and does not have a true zero. A ratio scale has order, meaningful distance between points, and a true zero (e.g., length, age). Examples of these scales are prevalent throughout this book. For example, a yes/no decision uses a nominal scale. Categorical loudness scaling (discussed in this chapter) is an ordinal scale. The pitch of a sound in mels (Ch. 6) is likely an interval scale, and percent correct is a ratio scale.

Measuring loudness has been approached from two different directions: rating the relative loudness of sounds and matching the level of one sound to be equally loud as another sound. Because these approaches have been used to address somewhat different questions in the loudness literature, we discuss the different procedures in the context of their experimental questions. Rating methods have been typically used to measure how loudness changes with intensity, whereas matching has been used to measure how loudness changes with frequency.

Loudness and Intensity

In one of Stevens' many accomplishments, he developed the ***magnitude estimation*** technique, which allowed listeners to estimate the magnitude of sounds by providing numerical values corresponding to the size of their perception as the intensity of the stimulus was varied. When the magnitude estimation technique is applied to measuring loudness, listeners hear a sound and assign a number (or rating) to that sound according to its perceived loudness. Consequently, we sometimes also call these procedures ***rating*** or ***scaling***. When loudness is measured in this way, the resulting function that relates the ratings to stimulus intensity is a ***loudness growth function***.

Visit the companion website for an auditory-visual demonstration of magnitude estimation.

Stevens' Power Law

Using magnitude estimation, Stevens (1956) and later investigators measured the growth of loudness in human listeners with normal hearing for 1000-Hz pure tones. In this type of experiment, listeners hear two tones: a reference tone (a 40-dB SPL tone) followed by a test tone. In different experimental conditions, test tones are presented at a range of levels. Listeners are told that the reference tone (a 1000-Hz tone presented at 40 dB SPL) should be assigned a rating of 1. Stevens defined this reference sound as one **sone**, the unit of loudness. Listeners then rate the relative loudness of other tones compared with that reference. For example, a sound twice as loud would be assigned a value of 2 and a sound half as loud would be assigned a value of .5. Using this approach, the numbers resulting from magnitude estimation only have meaning in the context of each other and in the context of the number assigned to the reference. If a listener assigned a value of 2 in a magnitude estimation experiment, we could determine that 2 is double that of 1, but the 2 by itself is meaningless. A sound with a loudness of two sones is twice as loud as a sound with a loudness of one sone, but we do not know the absolute loudness of either of those sounds.

Data adapted from experiments such as this are illustrated in Figure 4–3 as the filled symbols, which shows that the loudness in sones increases as the sound level increases.

For levels above about 30 dB SPL, the function also looks like a line, so we might be tempted to conclude that there is a proportional, linear relationship between loudness and sound level in dB SPL. However, notice that the y-axis is plotted on a logarithmic scale, and a 10 dB change is associated with a doubling of loudness. As a result, Stevens (1956) noted that loudness and intensity (in W/m^2) have a **power law relationship** at moderate to high stimulus intensities.

Together, the loudness growth function of Figure 4–3 illustrates several striking findings when we evaluate the data obtained between 30 and 90 dB SPL:

- *Increasing sound level increases loudness.* Increasing sound by 10 dB doubles the loudness. For any dB SPL value above 40, increasing by 10 dB doubles the sones. For

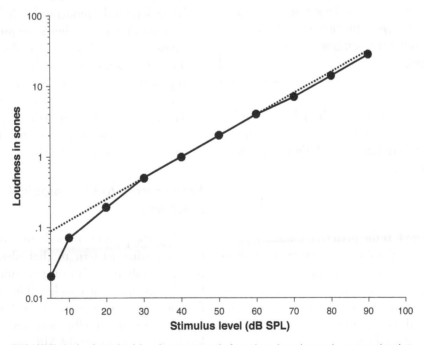

FIGURE 4–3. A typical loudness growth function. Loudness in sones is plotted as a function of stimulus level in dB SPL. The dotted line represents growth predicted by Stevens' power law. Data are similar to those reported by Hellman and Zwislocki (1961), but who used dB SL.

example, if we increase the decibel level of a sound from 40 to 50 dB SPL, the loudness goes from one sone to two sones, a doubling of loudness. Changing the sound level 50 to 60 dB, the loudness changes from 2 to 4 sones, and so on. Decreasing the sound level by 10 dB also halves the loudness.

- *A power relationship between sound intensity and loudness.* When loudness ratings are plotted on a logarithmic scale against sound pressure level in dB SPL, the data fall on a line. This indicates that there is a power relationship between the perceived loudness of a stimulus and the intensity.

> Whether data are plotted on logarithmic or linear scales is important for making inferences about the relationships between dependent (the measured) and independent (the experimentally manipulated) variables. In the case of loudness growth functions, we could plot either axis on linear scales. The different ways of plotting the data would yield different shapes of the same function.

Today, we refer to the relationship between loudness and stimulus intensity as **Stevens' power law**, which follows the following equation:

$$L \alpha I^{0.3}, \qquad \text{Eq. 4–1}$$

where L is the perceived loudness, and I is the physical intensity. This equation illustrates a power law because the *intensity is raised to some power.* Note that α is a symbol indicating proportionality. Equation 4–1 indicates that a 10 dB change in sound level produces a doubling of loudness.

Referring to Figure 4–3, we must also consider the change in the loudness growth

> The power relationship between loudness and intensity predicts a line on log-log axes (note that dB SPL is calculated by taking the log of an intensity, so in a sense, the x-axis is logarithmically spaced), we can take the logarithm of both sides of the equation:
>
> $$\log (L) \alpha \log (I^{0.3})$$
>
> using the law of logarithms: $\log(x^n) = n \log(x)$, then
>
> $$\log(L) \alpha 0.3\log(I).$$
>
> This equation has a similar format to a line: $y = mx$, where m is the slope (0.3). Thus, if we plot this relationship on log-log axes, we will see a line.

function that occurs at low levels. We observe here that the loudness growth function has a steeper slope at low sound levels compared with the slope at the moderate levels. The dotted line on Figure 4–3 shows the predictions for Stevens' power law, and we observe that for low levels, loudness growth is more rapid than growth at the higher stimulus levels and does not follow Stevens' power law. It is now well established that the growth of loudness is more rapid at low levels than at moderate ones (Hellman & Zwislocki, 1961).

Relationship to Physiological Measures

Notably, the pattern of loudness growth follows a similar pattern to that observed in basilar membrane input-output functions of healthy mammalian cochlea. The BM I-O functions presented in Figure 4–1 illustrate a rapid growth of vibration amplitude at levels below 30 to 40 dB SPL and a slower growth of vibration at moderate to high levels. Such similarity between these two measurements suggests that the magnitude of basilar membrane vibration contributes strongly to the perception of loudness and that there is a strong correlation between the amount of basilar membrane vibration and loudness for pure tones. Thus, sounds that yield more vibration on the basilar membrane should be louder than sounds that yield less vibration.

However, we must also consider that loudness is a perception that is not only a consequence of basilar membrane vibration. The central auditory system has a clear role in the representation of loudness and includes mechanisms that transform basilar membrane vibration into perception. The next step in the pathway, of course, is that of the auditory nerve. Unlike the pattern observed for vibration measured at a single place on the basilar membrane, however, a single auditory nerve fiber is not enough to explain loudness growth.

One of the issues here is the very large **dynamic range of hearing**, which encompasses sound levels ranging from those near threshold (e.g., 0 to 10 dB SPL) to the level at which damage or uncomfortably loud sounds are experienced (e.g., 100 to 120 dB SPL). A single locus on the basilar membrane is able to code this large range, as we observed in Figure 4–1. The auditory nerve also codes for stimulus intensity: Figure 4–2 illustrates that increasing stimulus level increases the firing rate of auditory neurons. However, each individual fiber cannot, by itself, provide sufficient information to code the entire dynamic range of the auditory system. If we look more closely at the rate-level functions shown in Figure 4–2, the following observations indicate why a single fiber cannot provide the code for all stimulus levels represented by the auditory system:

- *Dynamic ranges of fibers are less than 60 dB.* None of the auditory nerve fibers that are depicted have a dynamic range close to 100 dB. In fact, Palmer and Evans (1979)

showed that only about 10% of fibers have a dynamic range greater than 60 dB.

- *Most auditory nerve fibers are saturated at high stimulus levels.* That is, when the stimulus level is high, increases in stimulus level do not increase the firing rate. A fiber that is in saturation will not be able to indicate when the stimulus level has changed. Because most auditory nerve fibers (60%) are low-threshold fibers and another 25% are mid-threshold fibers, most are in saturation at moderate and high levels.

- *Different fibers are needed to code for low and high stimulus levels.* The high-SPR fibers code for low levels and the mid-and low-SPR fibers represent the higher stimulus levels. All fiber types are necessary to represent the level of sound from 0 to 100 dB SPL.

Thus, the code for loudness must be more sophisticated than a simple increase in firing rate within a single fiber, and the responses to multiple fibers must be involved in the coding of the dynamic range of the auditory system. Low stimulus levels can only be coded by low-threshold fibers, and except for the very lowest stimulus levels, multiple fibers will fire in response to even a low-level stimulus. Higher stimulus levels will lead to the involvement of multiple fibers, including the high-threshold fibers. Psychophysical modeling also implicates the involvement of many fibers to code the full dynamic range of hearing (Viemester, 1988).

An implication of this work, then, is that damage to any of the various types of auditory nerve fibers should alter the perception of loudness. Although we currently have no mechanism to assess the health of various fiber types in humans, damage to the low-threshold fibers will impact threshold measurements and loudness near threshold. Abnormal loudness perception of high-level sounds might implicate loss or damage to high-and mid-threshold fibers.

Other Measurement Techniques

Magnitude estimation is known to have several problems, particularly related to the poor reliability of the measurements and large variability in results across listeners (Algom & Marks, 1984). Many experimenters have attempted to circumvent such issues by using a variety of different procedures. Loudness growth functions can also be measured using a *magnitude production* technique. In contrast to magnitude estimation, where the listener rates the loudness of a sound, the listener adjusts the level of a sound to a certain loudness. For example, one might adjust the level of a test sound so that it is twice as loud as a reference sound. Typically, the *method of adjustment* is used for this approach, as the listener has control over the test stimulus. Results tend to be similar to those collected using magnitude estimation.

Today, magnitude estimation is more likely to be conducted using *cross-modality scaling*, in which a listener rates the loudness of a stimulus by adjusting the length of string or a slider on a computer monitor. The advantage of this procedure is that length is represented using a true ratio scale (for example, 2 inches is double the length of 1 inch), whereas rating (assigning a number) does not necessarily result in a ratio scale even if listeners are instructed to use one (e.g., a loudness rating of 2 is twice as loud as a rating of 1). However, these methods remain fairly time consuming, and these procedures do not eliminate all of the criticisms of magnitude estimation techniques.

In cases where we need more rapid estimates (such as clinical applications), another alternative is *categorical loudness scaling*, in which there is no explicit reference (Garner, 1953). Clinicians and scientists may use these procedures to measure the level at which sound is uncomfortably loud (the *uncomfortable loudness level; ULL*) or the level at

which sound is most comfortable. In this procedure listeners are given a set of terms ranging from "very soft" to "painfully loud," and they use those terms to categorize the loudness of the sounds they hear. This procedure has been adapted for clinical use due to its ease and speed of administration, and an example of the categories commonly used in clinical applications is shown in Figure 4–4 (Hawkins et al., 1987). Here, the different categories are also illustrated with different sized boxes to reinforce the differences between the categories for patients. In these procedures, a clinical

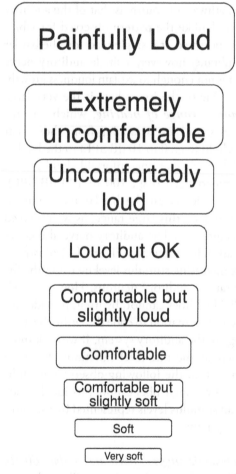

FIGURE 4–4. Categories used in categorical loudness scaling procedures. From Hawkins et al. (1987).

version of this procedure would begin testing at a low stimulus level and the stimulus level would be increased until the listener rates the sound as comfortable or uncomfortably loud, depending on the application.

> Visit the companion website for an auditory-visual demonstration of a measurement of loudness using categorical loudness scaling.

Loudness and Frequency

Equal-Loudness Contours

Other methods are also commonly used to assess loudness, with a ***matching***, or ***loudness balancing***, procedure being one of the easiest to implement and interpret. In this procedure, rather than measuring the relative loudness of a sound using a rating procedure, the *method of adjustment* is used in which the listener adjusts the level of a sound so that its loudness matches that of a reference sound.

In a common implementation of the *loudness balancing* procedure, we measure the level of a sound of interest (the test stimulus) that matches the level of a 1000-Hz stimulus (the reference stimulus). For these studies, a 1000-Hz tone is always the reference sound, and it is presented at some fixed stimulus level (e.g., 40 dB SPL). The two sounds (the 1000-Hz reference and the test stimulus) are always presented in succession (never simultaneously) and sometimes to opposite ears if the listener has normal hearing. In a typical experiment, the *method of adjustment* is used where the listener adjusts the level of the test sound so that its loudness is equal to that of the reference sound. The level of the 1000-Hz tone in dB SPL is the ***loudness level*** of the test sound, measured in ***phons***. If the refer-

ence sound is a 40-dB SPL, 1000-Hz tone, the test sound would have a loudness level of 40 phons. However, if the reference were presented at 70 dB SPL, the test sound would have a loudness level of 70 phons.

If tones are used as the test stimuli, this procedure allows measurement of ***equal-loudness contours***, functions that illustrate the sound level as a function of frequency associated with equal loudness, and first measured by Fletcher and Munson (1933). In their experiment, Fletcher and Munson fixed the level of a 1000-Hz reference tone and, using loudness balancing, asked listeners to adjust the level of a test tone until it was perceived as being equally loud to the reference tone. They repeated this measurement for multiple frequencies and reference levels. For a given reference level, then, they achieved a single equal-loudness contour. Data adapted from Fletcher and Munson are illustrated in Figure 4–5.

Each function in Figure 4–5 represents a set of sounds that have the same loudness level. For example, sounds on the 40-phon curve were equally loud and had a loudness level of 40 phons. Note in particular that the equal-loudness contours were not flat and depended on frequency. For example, a 3000-Hz tone presented at 35 dB SPL had the same loudness level as a 10,000-Hz tone presented at 48 dB SPL. From Fletcher and Munson's data, we can conclude that the frequency of a sound impacts its loudness, with sounds between 3000 and 5000 Hz perceived as louder than other frequencies when presented at the same dB SPL level. This simple illustration demonstrates that sound pressure level (or intensity) and loudness are not the same. Taking any curve for reference, we can make the following inferences:

- *Strong frequency effects are present.* Sounds between about 3000 to 6000 Hz can be presented at lower sound pressure levels than

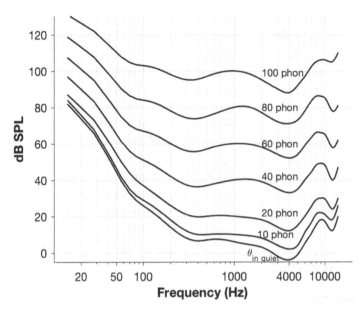

FIGURE 4–5. Equal-loudness contours. Each contour represents a series of stimuli having the same loudness in phons, with the bottom-most curve labeled absolute threshold (θ) in quiet. Adapted from Fletcher and Munson (1933).

sounds at other frequencies to be equally loud. Generally speaking, then, we consider tones at these frequencies to be louder than tones at many other frequencies.

• *Patterns follow middle and outer ear amplification.* Equal-loudness contours follow similar patterns to the amplification provided by the outer and middle ears. There are some subtle differences in the shape of the equal-loudness contours as the stimulus level is increased, particularly at low frequencies. However, generally speaking, the patterns are similar across the different levels.

Over the years, the equal-loudness contours have been revised, with contemporary data included in the International Standard (International Organization for Standardization, 226, 2003). These equal-loudness contours are very similar to Fletcher and Munson's data illustrated in Figure 4–5. Even today, these contours are commonly called *Fletcher-Munson* curves.

There are many practical implications for equal-loudness contours. First, the data above suggest that the loudness of sounds across frequency is predominantly determined by the characteristics of the outer and middle ear. Disorders in these structures will alter the relationship between the loudness of sounds across frequency. Second, equal-loudness contours have many practical implications and are used in the design of alarms and sirens and in numerous audio production applications. Further, the A-weighted decibel (dB A) uses the 40-phon loudness contour to calculate a decibel metric that approximates the sound level as represented by the human ear. Interestingly, dB A provides a better assessment of a specific sound's potential for causing hearing loss than dB SPL and is, therefore, often used to describe the sound level in industrial environments and for noise dosing.

Bandwidth Effects: Spectral Loudness Summation

The intensity and frequency of sound are not the only factors that determine the loudness —the bandwidth is also a factor. The influence of bandwidth on loudness is referred to as *spectral loudness summation*. It is important to also understand the effects of changing stimulus bandwidth on the loudness of sounds, particularly because we listen to a variety of different sounds with different bandwidths on a regular basis and we use both narrowband and broadband sounds in audiometric testing. Zwicker et al. (1957) first demonstrated that loudness depends on bandwidth, using the loudness balancing technique. Their listeners adjusted the level of a comparison noise (centered at 1420 Hz with a 2300-Hz band-

width) so that it matched the level of a test noise centered at 1420 Hz but had a variable bandwidth. A subset of their data is presented in Figure 4–6, which shows data collected at four levels. Note that Zwicker et al. had listeners adjust the level of the comparison stimulus, rather than the test stimulus. As a result, within a single curve, louder sounds are plotted higher on the y-axis in Figure 4–6. Figure 4–6 illustrates the following effects:

- *Loudness increased with increasing bandwidth.* For the narrowest bandwidths, the loudness level of the test stimuli was relatively constant with increasing bandwidth. However, at a certain bandwidth (corresponding to a value very similar to but somewhat greater than the critical band), the loudness level of the test stimuli began

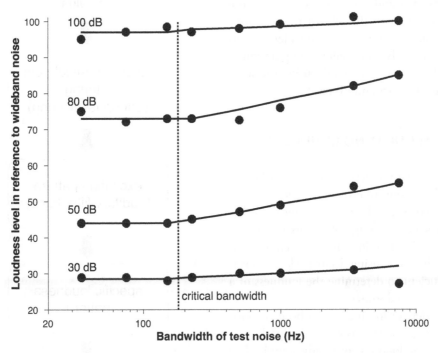

FIGURE 4–6. Spectral loudness summation. The matching sound pressure level in dB SPL of a comparison noise (2300-Hz wide centered at 1420 Hz) is plotted a function of the bandwidth of a test noise centered at 1420 Hz. Data from four different test stimulus levels (30, 50, 80, and 100 dB SPL) are indicated. Adapted from Zwicker et al. (1957).

to increase as the bandwidth increased. It is worth pointing out that the dB SPL of the test stimuli remained constant, so the increase in loudness was not associated with an increase in the power present in the stimuli. The increase in loudness must be created by the auditory system.

- *Loudness changes with bandwidth were greatest at moderate stimulus levels.* The rate of change of loudness with bandwidth was not constant across levels. It was most rapid at 50 and 80 dB and less rapid at the high and low levels.

The take-home message, then, is that wide bandwidth stimuli are louder than narrow bandwidth stimuli when presented at the same dB SPL level. These results again highlight that loudness and sound pressure level are not the same. Further, when assessing the loudness of sounds, we must consider more than the power or dB SPL of the stimulus. These issues are taken into consideration in loudness models, which allow computation of a sound's loudness of sounds, using the spectral characteristics and dB levels.

CALCULATING LOUDNESS

There are many practical situations where it would be helpful to estimate the loudness of sounds. For example, using loudness models has impacted the design of alarms and acoustic spaces. Because loudness and sound level are not the same, using decibel calculations is not sufficient to determine the loudness of a particular sound source.

Models of loudness have been demonstrated to provide reasonable ballpark estimates of the loudness of steady sounds. The work of Brian Moore and colleagues (e.g., Moore et al., 1997) now forms the basis of a standard for calculating the loudness of steady sounds, published by the Acoustical Society

of America (ANSI 3.4, 2007). These models are based on the premise that the loudness of a sound is based on the total neural activity evoked by the sound; greater neural activity leads to a louder sound. Because we have no direct way to measure or quantify total neural activity in the human auditory system, a model of neural activity forms the basis of the loudness estimate. These models are psychophysical in nature and are based on psychophysical, not physiological, data. Figure 4–7 illustrates the steps involved in calculating the loudness of sounds.

The steps of the loudness model are as follows:

1. *Stimulus filtering by outer and middle ear transfer functions.* The consequence of this

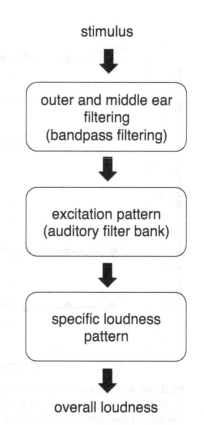

FIGURE 4–7. Flow chart illustrating the steps involved in models used to calculate loudness.

step is adding gain to frequencies between about 600 and 4000 Hz.

2. *Filtered stimulus transformed into an excitation pattern.* Recall that an excitation pattern is calculated by passing a stimulus through a bank of auditory filters consisting of different center frequencies. The power at the output of each auditory filter is calculated.

3. *Excitation pattern transformed into a specific loudness pattern.* This process essentially converts the excitation pattern into a loudness density pattern. The decibel level in each filter band is converted into a specific loudness, which has the units of sones per equivalent rectangular bandwidth (ERB, a measure of auditory filter bandwidth). Essentially, the compressive nonlinearity of the ear and the width of the auditory filter are taken into consideration to establish the specific loudness for each auditory filter.

4. *Loudness calculated from the area under the specific loudness pattern.* This calculation gives the total loudness of a sound.

To illustrate the process of the loudness model, two example stimuli are shown as they are passed through the different steps of the model in Figure 4–8. Each of these example stimuli has a similar loudness, in order to show how the loudness model might predict the loudness of two sounds that are very different in overall level and bandwidth. The first sound is a 57 dB SPL, 1000-Hz tone (shown with the solid line), and the second is a band-limited noise (shown with the dotted line) with a total power of about 43 dB SPL. These two sounds are similar in their loudness (3.4 sones) and loudness levels (56.8 phons), as determined by the loudness model.

The top panel of Figure 4–8 illustrates the spectrum of these sounds. The middle panel shows the excitation patterns of these two sounds, which is a model of the internal representation of these two stimuli. Finally, the bottom panel illustrates the specific loudness pattern. The pure tone has a higher dB SPL level, excitation, and maximum specific loudness than the noise. However, the noise has a wider bandwidth and is therefore subject to spectral loudness summation. The area under the two specific loudness pattern curves is the same for the tone and the noise, which is why the two stimuli have the same loudness.

The loudness model is based on many decades of psychophysical data, and it predicts the loudness of steady-state sounds rather well. It is also clear from the loudness model that sounds can be loud because of multiple reasons; sounds may be loud because of high presentation levels or because of a wide bandwidth. As the field progresses, we may be able to use loudness models to estimate how loud sounds might be for a listener with sensorineural hearing loss or for sounds that fluctuate. The applications are numerous. We could use such models to select the best ring tone that would allow you to hear an emergency phone call or to program a hearing aid for attending a symphony versus a lecture.

REACTION TIME AS A MEASURE OF LOUDNESS

Reaction time is a correlate of loudness that has garnered favor in the past few years, and reaction time has the potential to provide a less subjective correlate of loudness than magnitude estimation. If reaction time, the time it takes to respond to a stimulus, varies in a predictable way with loudness, then reaction time could be used as a fast and possibly more reliable estimate of the loudness of sounds. This metric has strong potential application for animal studies, as animals cannot provide loudness estimates, but animal studies are critical to understanding the physiological mechanisms that underlie loudness perception.

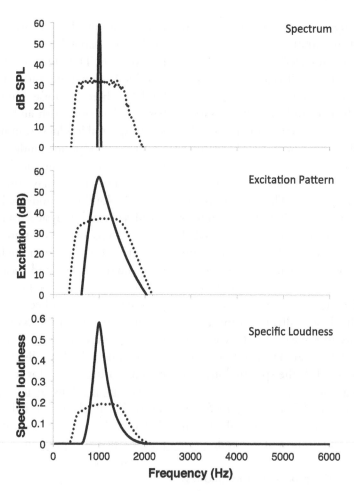

FIGURE 4–8. Illustration of loudness model calculations. Two stimuli (a pure tone and band of noise) that have the same loudness are passed through the model. The pure tone is represented by the solid line, and the noise is represented by the dotted line. Each panel represents the output at a different stage of the loudness model.

In a detection experiment, the reaction time is defined as the amount of time required for a listener to detect a stimulus (e.g., by pressing a button), and it is generally measured from stimulus onset. Although reaction time is not commonly considered a psychoacoustic measure, reaction time measurements have become increasingly valuable for assessing components of auditory processing. Notably, reaction time experiments allow

measurements for detection of sounds across a broad range of stimulus levels. Psychoacoustic detection experiments do not allow this, as the relevant measures for detection are either absolute threshold or percent detected. A typical psychometric function only covers a range of about 10 to 15 dB. Reaction times, on the other hand, can be measured to sounds presented at levels across the full dynamic range of hearing.

In the simplest reaction time experiment, a listener responds to a stimulus as accurately and as quickly as possible. Chocholle (1940) was one of the first to demonstrate that the reaction time to a stimulus decreases (gets faster) as the sound pressure level increases, as shown in Figure 4–9. Chocholle also demonstrated that equal-loudness contours obtained using reaction times closely resemble those measured using the loudness balancing technique adopted by Fletcher and Munson (1933). Many years later, Humes and Ahlstrom (1984) showed that loudness growth measured using magnitude estimation was correlated with loudness growth measured using reaction time. Recent measurements show that the correlation between reaction time and loudness only holds for moderate to high stimulus levels, but not so for low stimulus levels (Schlittenlacher et al., 2017). Wagner et al. (2004) further demonstrated that spectral loudness summation measured using reaction times also follows patterns similar to those observed using loudness balancing. Taken together, there is converging evidence that reaction time provides an indirect measure of loudness, at least for moderate to high stimulus levels.

Because loudness can be difficult to measure, using alternative methods such as reaction time to characterize loudness has value for research and clinical purposes. Certain populations, like animals or people with significant language disabilities, cannot always provide loudness judgments like those described in this chapter. Consequently, using reaction time as a correlate of loudness has been gaining traction in animal models and has proven valuable in establishing animal models for auditory disorders (Lauer & Dooling, 2007). Reaction time measures are beginning to become more widespread in human testing as well. For example, recent studies have applied reaction time techniques in the development of models of *hyperacusis*, an increased sensitivity to sounds. Reaction times would be expected to be faster in the presence of hyperacusis, and therefore reaction time may provide a fast and reliable way to measure loudness in large groups of people.

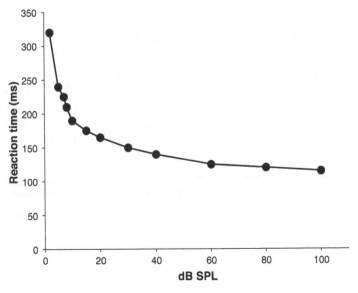

FIGURE 4–9. Reaction time data are plotted as a function of stimulus level in dB SPL. Adapted from Chocholle (1940).

INTENSITY DISCRIMINATION

Due to the problems with both rating and matching studies, other investigators have approached the study of the auditory representation of intensity by using discrimination experiments. In these cases, the researchers measure the *just noticeable difference (JND)* in intensity. Recall that the JND is the smallest difference that is discriminable by the ear and is also known as the *difference limen*. These experiments fall in a long series of psychoacoustic studies that evaluate the capabilities of the ear. In these experiments, the primary question is, "What is the smallest intensity change that the ear can detect?" These experiments also ask whether the JND is a constant across intensities or whether it varies.

Weber's Law

A common method to measure the JND for intensity is to conduct an *intensity discrimination* experiment in which a listener hears two sounds, and one of the stimuli (the reference) has a specific intensity (I) and the other (the test stimulus) has a higher intensity (I+ ΔI), where ΔI is the change in intensity between the reference and the test stimulus. An example of an experimental trial for an intensity discrimination experiment is illustrated in Figure 4–10. Although the intensity of the stimulus is varied, the listener's task is perceptual, and so selects the stimulus that is perceived as being louder. The experimenter uses standard psychophysical techniques (such as 2I–2AFC and an adaptive staircase procedure) to measure the JND in terms of ΔI. When only the intensity of stimulus is varied, we can also call this experiment *increment detection*.

It can be difficult to generate an intuition for this type of experiment, so rather than considering intensity discrimination of sound for the time being, let us consider a weight-lifting experiment. A weightlifter is given a weight and is asked to determine the next size weight needed to determine that one of the weights is bigger than the other. The weightlifter experiments with numerous weights and determines that she can tell the difference between a 10-lb. and an 11-lb. weight. Next, that same weightlifter is given a 50-lb. weight and determines the size of the weight that is just noticeably heavier. Again, she experiments and determines that she can tell the difference between a 50-lb. and a 55-lb. weight. Finally, she does this at 100 lbs. and discovers that she can differentiate between 100 and 110 lbs.

Note that there is a trend here: as the size of the weight increases, the amount needed to differentiate between weights increases. However, the increase occurs in a systematic way —for each weight lifted, the just noticeable weight difference is a change of 10% (a proportion of 0.1) in the weight. In this case, the pattern is 10 versus 11, 50 versus 55, and 100 versus 110 lbs., or a 10% difference in weight across the various baseline weights. If the JND

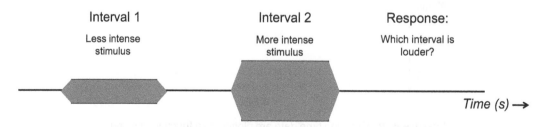

FIGURE 4–10. Illustration of an experimental trial in an intensity-discrimination experiment.

is defined as the just noticeable difference in weight, the JND equals 1, 5, and 10 lbs. for the various weights. However, if we describe the JND as a percentage, the JND equals 10%, 10%, and 10% for the various weights. This pattern is now commonly known as *Weber's law*, which states that the just noticeable change in a stimulus is a constant ratio (or percentage) of the original stimulus. Weber's law is characterized by the following equation:

$$\Delta S/S = k,$$

where ΔS is the just detectable change, S is the size of the original stimulus, and k is a constant. This quantity, $\Delta S/S$, is commonly called the *Weber fraction*.

Visit the companion website for an auditory demonstration of an intensity discrimination experiment.

Ernst Heinrich Weber (pronounced Vay-burr) conducted the experiments needed to formulate the law. However, his student Gustav Fechner formulated the law mathematically and named it after his mentor.

Weber's Law Applied to Intensity Discrimination

Now that the weightlifting analogy provides an intuition of Weber's law, we can apply the same concept to an intensity discrimination experiment. Note that in these experiments, the size of the stimulus is characterized by the intensity (I) of the sound in W/m^2, not the decibel value of the sound, as this is important for understanding and interpreting Weber's law. Here, the JND is defined as ΔI, or the

difference in intensity between two sounds. Applied to intensity discrimination, then, the Weber fraction is $\Delta I/I$.

Intensity discrimination has been measured as a function of stimulus intensity for both tonal and noise stimuli, with surprising results. However, in order to fully understand and appreciate the results, we must consider the different ways of representing performance. Several metrics are commonly used in the research literature, and a brief overview of them is provided here. Understandably, the use of multiple acoustic descriptors can be frustrating to a student, but it is often unclear to a researcher which metric is the best to describe auditory perception, as there is not always a standard unit to use. Predictions of Weber's law are illustrated in Figure 4–11:

- *JND as ΔI.* We can report the JND as ΔI and plot that JND as a function of intensity, I. If we plot data in this way, the JND would increase as the stimulus level increases and the line relating ΔI to I would be an <u>increasing line</u>. The left panel of Figure 4–11 illustrates this prediction.
- *JND reported as the Weber fraction.* We can also report the JND in terms of the Weber fraction, $\Delta I/I$, and plot the Weber fraction as a function of intensity or dB SPL. Because Weber's law predicts that the Weber fraction is a constant, the resulting plot would be a <u>horizontal line</u> regardless of whether the x-axis was plotted using intensity units or dB SPL, as shown in the right panel of Figure 4–11.
- *JND reported as a decibel difference.* It can also be convenient to plot the JND as a dB transformation of the Weber fraction, such as $10\log(\Delta I/I)$ or $10\log[(\Delta I/I)+1]$. Conveniently, the latter transformation is the decibel difference between two sounds, often called ΔL in dB. For these transformations, Weber's law again predicts the plot would still be a <u>horizontal line</u> regardless of

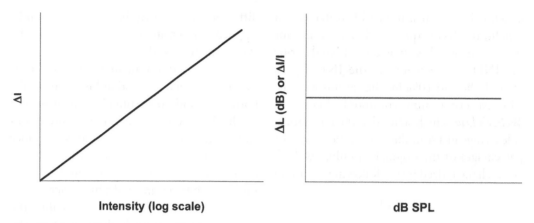

FIGURE 4–11. Predictions of Weber's law using different acoustic quantities. The left panel illustrates ΔI plotted as a function of I. The right panel illustrates ΔL or ΔI/I plotted as a function of dB SPL.

the units for the x-axis (e.g., they could be intensity units, I, or dB SPL). This prediction is shown in the right panel of Figure 4–11 and occurs because the Weber fraction is a constant.

To test whether Weber's law holds for auditory intensity discrimination, Miller (1947) measured intensity discrimination for a noise stimulus across a large range of stimulus levels. Data adapted from his report are shown in Figure 4–12 as the filled, black symbols. Figure 4–12 plots the JND in terms of the decibel difference (ΔL in dB) as a function of the intensity of the noise stimulus in dB sensation level (SL). Note that the other data plotted on this figure are discussed next.

Miller's data illustrate the following:

- *Weber's law held for noise at moderate-to-high levels.* That is, the function relating ΔL to dB SL was a horizontal line, as long as sound levels were above about 20 dB SL. We observe no change in the Weber fraction as the stimulus level increases. We can interpret these data to indicate that the JND in intensity is a <u>proportion of the intensity</u> of the stimulus.

- *Weber's law did not hold at low stimulus levels.* Here, the Weber fraction decreased with increasing level, suggesting that intensity discrimination became proportionally easier with increasing level. Miller's listeners were particularly poor at intensity discrimination for the very low-level sounds.

Humans are exceptional at their ability to tell whether two sounds are louder than one another—note that these thresholds are less than ½ of a decibel—particularly in light of the dynamic range of the auditory system being over 100 dB!

Twenty years before Miller made his measurements for noise, Riesz (1928) measured whether Weber's law holds for tones. However, his experiment did not use the intensity discrimination paradigm described here and instead relied on modulation detection. Yet, Reisz's experiment suggested that Weber's law may not hold for tonal stimuli and that intensity discrimination continues to improve proportionally as stimulus level increases, even for moderate and high levels. Jesteadt et al. (1977) conducted a comprehensive follow-up study that adopted an intensity discrimination procedure. They measured the Weber fraction

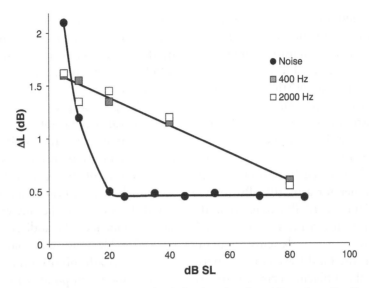

FIGURE 4–12. Intensity discrimination data for white noise stimuli and pure tones. ΔL in dB is plotted as a function of the dB SL of the stimuli. Noise data are adapted from Miller (1947). Tone data are adapted from Jesteadt et al. (1977).

for tones at multiple stimulus frequencies and stimulus levels. Data obtained at 400 and 2000 Hz are plotted along with Miller's in Figure 4–12 as the square symbols. Jesteadt et al.'s data look rather different from those of Miller, as the functions for pure tones are not horizontal lines, but rather they have negative slopes. Jesteadt et al. actually measured seven different tone frequencies, with the same results for all frequencies. From their data, along with those of Reisz, we conclude that:

- *Weber's law did not hold for tones.* In fact, the JND, when expressed as a proportion of the intensity of the stimulus, decreased with increasing intensity across the audible range. This phenomenon is called the ***near miss to Weber's law***. Note that we observe this result only for tones and not noise at levels greater than 20 dB SL.
- *The Weber fraction was not dependent on frequency.* The overall sensitivity for intensity discrimination did not vary with frequency,

and the slope of the near miss to Weber's law was constant across the frequencies up to about 10 kHz.

Explanations for the Near Miss

The near miss to Weber's law is a consequence of the ability of the central auditory system to take advantage of multiple pieces of information across frequency, and it highlights that basilar membrane vibration and auditory nerve firing rate together do not provide enough information to understand the perception of loudness. The central auditory system has a clear role.

To better understand why the near miss happens, consider the following example. For a pure tone at 2000 Hz presented at 60 dB SL, the JND for intensity discrimination (ΔL) is approximately 0.9 dB (see Figure 4–12). The JND for this pure tone is larger than the JND for noise, suggesting that when noise is presented, the auditory system can use multiple frequency regions to discriminate between sounds with different intensities. To illustrate how the ear might be able to improve its detection with increasing stimulus level, we look to the excitation pattern, which provides a psychoacoustical representation of the spectral information available to the ear.

Figure 4–13 illustrates two excitation patterns, one calculated from a 60-dB SPL tone and another for a 64-dB SPL tone at 1000 Hz. Figure 4–13 illustrates that the 64-dB excitation pattern has a higher maximum excitation and extends across more frequencies than the 60-dB excitation pattern. At 1000 Hz, the difference between the two excitation patterns is about 4 dB. However, as the auditory filter center frequency increases, the difference between the two excitation patterns also increases. The excitation pattern associated with the higher-level stimulus has a greater spread of excitation, and due to upward spread of excitation, the spread of excitation is most pronounced on the high frequency side. As an illustration, the high frequency edge of the excitation pattern corresponding to 2250 Hz represents an excitation difference of about 8 dB.

Using these patterns, we can envision how the ear may be able to use information across frequency in order to determine which of the two tones is more intense than the other. The auditory filters higher in frequency contain much more information about the intensity difference than the one centered at the signal frequency. The auditory filters greater than 2250 Hz, however, do not have any representation of the 60-dB stimulus, but there is a small amount of power passed through the auditory filters in the 64-dB stimulus. These auditory filters are considered *off-frequency* and provide a very robust representation of the dB difference between two sounds. As more and more auditory filters become involved in representing the stimulus, the ear effectively has more and more information with which to

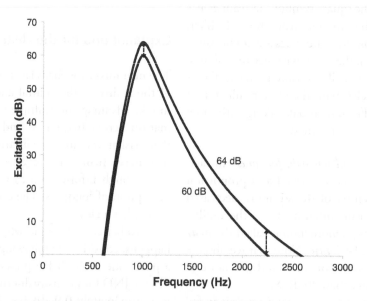

FIGURE 4–13. Excitation patterns for two tones at 60 and 64 dB SPL. The difference between the excitation patterns is larger on the high-frequency side of the excitation pattern when compared to the peak, illustrated by the two arrows on the figure.

determine whether one sound is more intense than another.

Note that because the excitation pattern of a pure tone is asymmetric and spreads to higher-frequency regions more than low-frequency regions, the high-frequency edge has been hypothesized to be the most important. This idea has been tested in several different experiments, all of which used experimental manipulations designed to block the high-frequency spread of excitation. The logic is that if the high-frequency edge provides additional information cueing an intensity change, blocking this information should restore Weber's law.

Schroder et al. (1994) measured intensity discrimination in which they blocked the high-frequency spread of excitation using noise bands. They also tested Weber's law using listeners with steeply sloping SNHLs (listeners with very good hearing in the low frequencies but significant hearing loss in the high frequencies). Both experimental manipulations restored Weber's law; that is, the Weber fraction did not improve with increasing stimulus level in either experiment. Florentine et al. (1987) measured intensity discrimination for the extended high frequencies, where spread of excitation could not occur due to basilar membrane mechanics. Their results at very high frequencies also demonstrated support for Weber's law. Taken together, there is strong support for the notion that the near miss results from the ear's ability to use multiple frequency regions across the excitation pattern to code for intensity.

EFFECTS OF SENSORINEURAL HEARING LOSS ON LOUDNESS

Loudness Recruitment

Sensorineural hearing loss (SNHL) has a robust and profound effect on loudness, with a primary effect being abnormally rapid growth of loudness. Fowler (1928) was the first to report that listeners with SNHL experienced loudness perceptions that ranged from very soft to uncomfortably loud, similar to listeners with normal hearing, but over a smaller range of decibel levels due to reduced audibility. He referred to this phenomenon as **loudness recruitment**. Numerous studies have followed Fowler's initial observations, and an illustration of loudness growth in listeners with SNHL is illustrated in Figure 4–14, which shows a sample loudness growth function for a listener with 40 dB of sensorineural hearing loss plotted along with a loudness growth for a listener with normal hearing. Loudness growth functions like this one are typically measured using pure tones as stimuli.

Figure 4–14 shows some clear differences between the loudness growth functions in these two listeners, summarized as follows:

- *Rapid growth of loudness in SNHL compared with normal hearing.* The slopes of the two functions are strikingly different. Loudness for listeners with sensorineural hearing loss grows much more quickly than loudness for listeners with normal hearing.
- *Similar loudness at very high stimulus levels.* Regardless of the presence of hearing loss, the loudness at high levels is similar for the two groups of listeners. The functions tend to converge at levels around 80 to 90 dB HL. The consequence of this is that the level at which sound becomes uncomfortable (the **loudness discomfort level, LDL,** or the **uncomfortable loudness level, UCL**) is similar for listeners with normal hearing and those with sensorineural hearing loss.

The slope of the loudness growth functions (loudness in sones vs. dB SPL), then, is steeper for the listeners with SNHL than for listeners with normal hearing. Hellman and Meiselman (1993) found that the slopes of

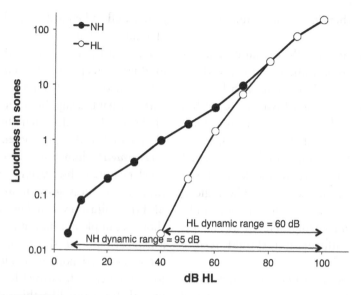

FIGURE 4–14. Loudness growth functions a normal-hearing listener (*filled circles*) and for a listener with a 40-dB HL sensorineural hearing loss (*unfilled circles*). The dynamic ranges of hearing of the two listeners are labeled.

loudness functions increased with the degree of sensorineural hearing loss. For losses of 60 dB of greater, slopes were at least twice that in normal hearing listeners, but more typically were four or five times greater. They also noted considerable variability in loudness growth across listeners, suggesting that we cannot exactly predict loudness growth from degree of hearing loss. However, all listeners with sensorineural hearing loss experienced some degree of loudness recruitment. Taken together, there is clear experimental evidence for loudness recruitment in listeners SNHL, although wide variability exists across listeners.

A complementary way to think about loudness recruitment is to consider the ***dynamic range*** of the ear with SNHL and the ear with normal hearing. The dynamic range, defined

Although we commonly accept that listeners with SNHL experience loudness recruitment, recent experiments have questioned this finding. A somewhat controversial idea is related to the loudness of sounds at and near threshold for listeners with SNHL. These measurements can be difficult to make, but work by Buus and Florentine (2002) suggests that the loudness of sounds at and near threshold may be higher for listeners with SNHL than for those with normal hearing. Essentially, listeners with SNHL appear to perceive sounds near their threshold as being louder than listeners with normal hearing. Buus and Florentine have named this particular phenomenon ***softness imperception***. This phenomenon occurs in conjunction with the abnormally rapid growth of loudness observed for levels between 10 dB SL and about 80 dB SPL.

as the difference between LDL and threshold, is also illustrated on Figure 4–14 for each hypothetical listener. Note that magnitude estimation techniques do not allow measurement of the LDL (see the upcoming section on measuring the LDL). However, for now, we can assume that the LDL corresponds to a loudness of about 100 to 200 sones, or roughly 100 dB HL. With this assumption, the dynamic range of the listener with normal hearing is 95 dB (or 5 dB HL to 100 dB HL). On the other hand, the listener with SNHL has a threshold of 40 dB HL and an LDL of 100 dB HL, and therefore, has a dynamic range of 60 dB. Thus, we see that the dynamic range, also illustrated in Figure 4–14, is smaller for the listener with SNHL. Because the LDL does not change with SNHL, the greater the hearing loss, the smaller the dynamic range. Yet, most listeners with SNHL will experience a similar range of loudness across their dynamic range, from about 0.02 sones to about 100 sones.

It is important to recognize that the dB level associated with loudness discomfort does not decrease with SNHL. Listeners with mild to moderately severe sensorineural hearing losses generally have LDLs very similar to listeners with normal hearing. Although LDLs can be highly variable across listeners, even

with normal hearing, we do not consider listeners with sensorineural hearing loss to be more sensitive to high-level sounds. Thus, the full range of loudness—from very soft to very loud—is squeezed into a dynamic range much smaller than that of listeners with normal hearing. The consequence, then, is a steeper slope for the function relating loudness to stimulus level in dB.

Loudness growth functions have shapes very similar to BM I-O functions measured in animals with healthy cochleae, but we also observe a correlation in the shape of damaged input-output functions and the loudness growth measured in listeners with SNHL. Note the strong similarity between the loudness growth data of Figure 4–14 and the data on BM vibration in an animal with auditory damage (e.g., Figure 4–1) due to loss of outer hair cells. Loss of outer hair cells impacts the shape and slope of the basilar membrane I-O function in a way very similar to loudness growth functions measured in listeners with SNHL. This correlation and the presence of loudness recruitment in listeners with mild and moderate SNHL, who presumably have predominantly outer hair cell loss, suggest that loss of outer hair cells contributes to loudness recruitment.

On the other hand, loss of inner hair cells, as they do not interact with basilar membrane vibration, has no effect on the shape of the BM I-O function. Psychophysically, however, loss of inner hair cells will elevate the threshold and would be expected to impact the perception of loudness because of a reduced input to the auditory nerve. Although there is no current way to assess the relative contribution of inner and outer hair cells to a specific listener's hearing loss, hearing losses greater than 60 or 70 dB HL likely involve inner hair cell loss in addition to outer hair cell loss. For many of these listeners, the loudness of sounds, even at high levels, does not approach the loudness measured in listeners with normal hearing (see

> Diagnostic audiology has capitalized on the different growth of loudness measured in listeners with normal hearing and those with SNHL to assess retro-cochlear disorders. It is expected that listeners with SNHL have recruitment if their loss is cochlear in origin. However, if a listener with SNHL does not present with recruitment, the loss may be caused by retro-cochlear pathology, like an auditory nerve tumor. Such tests are now replaced by physiological tools.

Smeds and Leijon, 2010 for a discussion). This phenomenon is sometimes called *under recruitment*, *partial recruitment*, or *incomplete recruitment*. These listeners will overall experience softer sounds compared with listeners with less hearing loss. As a result, it can be extremely difficult, and sometimes impossible, to restore full loudness perception for some of these listeners using amplification.

To summarize, listeners with mild-moderate sensorineural hearing losses typically experience loudness recruitment, in which the loudness of sounds tends to grow more rapidly than for listeners with normal hearing. Yet, mild-moderate sensorineural hearing loss is not typically associated with abnormal loudness discomfort levels. On the other hand, listeners with severe-to-profound losses can experience under recruitment and may perceive all sounds as being relatively soft compared with the loudness perception of listeners with normal hearing and mild-moderate losses.

We can use loudness growth data to emphasize why caution must be taken to not interchange the terms loudness and intensity. Consider Figure 4–14 and a stimulus presented at 20 dB HL. This stimulus is soft to the listener with normal hearing but inaudible to a listener with sensorineural hearing loss. Thus, it would be a mistake to refer to this stimulus as soft—it is only soft to the person who is able to hear it!

Perceptual Consequences of Loudness Recruitment

As discussed, most listeners with sensorineural hearing loss generally perceive sounds to be softer than listeners with normal hearing when those sounds are presented at the same sound pressure level. This observation primarily applies to sound levels below 80 dB SPL, such as conversational speech, which is typically 60 to 70 dB SPL. Figure 4–14 illustrates how this might come about. For example, a sound presented at 60 dB SPL would be perceived as approximately 6 sones by a listener with normal hearing, whereas a listener with SNHL will perceive the sound to be about 2 sones. Sounds at 80 dB SPL and above will be perceived to have similar loudness for both listeners. Thus, for sounds below about 80 dB SPL, listeners with SNHL will perceive the same dB SPL sounds as being softer than listeners with normal hearing.

That said, as we have discussed, listeners with SNHL also experience loudness recruitment in which loudness grows quickly with input sound level, and the recruitment will cause the range of loudness perceptions encompassed by many sounds to be larger than experienced by a listener with normal hearing. Whereas many sounds may overall be perceived as softer for listeners with sensorineural hearing loss, recruitment can be associated with difficulties in everyday listening, particularly as many sounds in the environment fluctuate over time, such as speech and music.

It has been hypothesized that loudness recruitment may lead to deficits in speech perception, due to the distortion of the speech envelope imposed by the SNHL. In this way, recruitment distorts natural loudness relationships *within a sound*, and when paired with other perceptual changes associated with SNHL, such as elevated thresholds and reduced frequency selectivity, the representation of a speech stimulus is far from that represented by a healthy ear. Yet, it has been difficult to establish the specific impact of loudness recruitment on speech perception by listeners with sensorineural hearing loss. Recruitment, elevated auditory thresholds, and reduced frequency selectivity co-occur in the presence of sensorineural hearing loss, as all are caused by a loss of or damage to outer hair cells.

One approach taken to determine if loudness recruitment impacts speech perception has been to process speech using a simulation of loudness recruitment, and then to present the processed speech signal to listeners with normal hearing. In one example of this approach, Moore and Glasberg (1993) processed speech using a loudness recruitment model, presented the altered speech to listeners with normal hearing, and then measured speech perception abilities under different degrees of simulated recruitment. Moore and Glasberg demonstrated a detrimental impact of loudness recruitment on speech intelligibility, particularly when the recruitment simulation was coupled with a simulation of elevated absolute threshold. However, most research has not been able to directly link loudness recruitment with disruption to speech understanding in individuals with SNHL. As such, a connection between loudness recruitment and a reduction in speech perception ability has not been clearly established. Other studies have even argued that loudness recruitment has little-to-no effect on speech understanding (Byrne, 1996; Souza, 2002). In support of this are Souza's (2002) findings in which compensating for recruitment using hearing aids had no effect on speech understanding in quiet or in noise. As such, it is plausible that the central auditory system and associated neural areas have mechanisms in place to compensate for such distortions in the representation of speech.

Loudness recruitment does have the potential to impact the ability to understand speech in fluctuating noise. The loss of outer hair cells that causes recruitment also alters the representation of fluctuating sounds when compared to an ear with intact outer hair cells. In this case, an ear with outer hair cell damage will experience greater envelope fluctuations than the healthy ear. These enhanced fluctua-

tions are thought to increase the amount of simultaneous and forward masking for fluctuating maskers. As a result, loss of outer hair cells can negatively influence the *fluctuating masker benefit*, as discussed in Chapter 3, but the connection between the reduced benefit and loudness recruitment, per se, has not been established.

Measuring Loudness Discomfort and Hyperacusis

As has been mentioned, hypersensitivity to sounds, or ***hyperacusis***, is not a common consequence of SNHL. That is, most people with SNHL do not experience hyperacusis. Hyperacusis is typically considered a separate pathology from SNHL, and it can also be present in listeners with normal hearing. Hyperacusis can, and often does, occur in the presence of sensorineural hearing loss, and it is also commonly, but not always, associated with tinnitus. Many patients are aware that they have a heightened sensitivity to sounds, but patients may also believe that they have hyperacusis, even if their experiences fall within normal ranges. Thus, it is important to fully document a patient's response to intense and moderate-level sounds to verify whether hyperacusis is indeed present.

To assess whether a patient is experiencing hyperacusis, a measurement of loudness discomfort levels (LDLs) is sometimes made, as discussed in the recommendations of ASHA (n.d.) and the British Audiology Society (2022). LDLs are also often measured as a component of hearing aid fitting to establish maximum hearing aid output levels. A common clinical approach to measure LDLs is to apply a straightforward ascending method of limits, with clear instructions and loudness anchors that are easy for patients to understand (Cox et al. 1997). Aspects of this procedure are similar to categorical loudness scaling, discussed previously. In this case, the tester is specifically looking for the level at which a sound is deemed "uncomfortably loud." A common procedure initially developed by Hawkins et al. (1987) provides a listener with seven-to-nine loudness categories with words ranging from "very soft" to "painfully loud," as illustrated in Figure 4–4. Presentation begins at a level that targets the *soft* category (a level approximately 20 dB SL but may be lower depending on the degree of hearing loss). Upon hearing the sound, the patient categorizes the loudness using the scale provided. Stimulus level is increased in 5-dB steps, or possibly 2-dB steps for a patient with a very small dynamic range, until the patient indicates that the sound is uncomfortably loud. Patients with hyperacusis may have LDLs that are below 85 to 90 dB SPL, although LDLs alone are perhaps not sufficient to diagnose hyperacusis (Sheldrake et al., 2015).

> Note that there are other terms in operation with the same meaning as LDLs: uncomfortable loudness levels (UCLs or ULLs) or threshold of discomfort (TD). Which term to use is a large discussion among scientists and professionals. If one follows the convention to use the term that corresponds with the measurement, UCL or ULL is probably more appropriate than LDL or TD, because patients are typically asked to find a level that is uncomfortable. Whereas LDL is commonly used in United States, ULL is the recommended terminology by the British Society of Audiology.

SUMMARY AND TAKE-HOME POINTS

Loudness is a perceptual quantity that, although correlated with stimulus intensity, is also influenced by other acoustic factors, such as frequency and stimulus bandwidth. Loudness is measured using techniques based on rating and matching, and these different techniques can be used to make inferences about the growth of loudness with increasing intensity (rating experiments) and the influence of frequency on loudness (matching experience). In comparison to listeners with normal hearing, listeners with sensorineural hearing loss experience a more rapid growth of loudness with increasing intensity but do not generally experience different loudness discomfort levels. As rating and matching experiments adopt methods that yield variable and sometimes biased results, intensity-discrimination experiments are also commonly used to assess the representation of intensity in the auditory system.

The following points are key take-home messages of this chapter:

- Loudness is measured using magnitude estimation and quantified in sones. It increases with intensity and follows patterns very similar to basilar membrane input-output functions. Loudness and intensity have a power law relationship, and a 10-dB change in sound level corresponds to a doubling of loudness.
- The loudness level measured using loudness balancing is quantified in phons. The loudness level depends on frequency and follows patterns very similar to the frequency/gain characteristics of the outer and middle ears. The loudest sounds, when presented at equal SPLs, are in the 3 to 5 kHz range.
- Loudness depends on stimulus bandwidth. For bandwidths greater than a critical band, loudness increases with increasing bandwidth, a phenomenon called spectral loudness summation. A sound can be loud because of a high sound level or because it has a broad bandwidth.
- Weber's law predicts that the just detectable amount of intensity is proportional to the intensity of the sound ($\Delta I/I = k$). Weber's

law holds for noise at moderate-to-high levels but not for low levels or for tones. Tones exhibit a near miss, in which $\Delta I/I$ or ΔL decreases with increasing intensity, a finding related to off-frequency listening.

- Listeners with sensorineural hearing loss experience rapid growth of loudness, referred to as recruitment. Their loudness discomfort levels are the same as those of listeners with normal hearing, except among those with severe SNHL who experience under-recruitment.

- Loss of outer hair cells is the primary contributor to recruitment, and although we know that outer hair cell loss contributes to difficulty understanding speech, whether this is related to loudness recruitment itself, is still to be determined.

EXERCISES

1. Using loudness growth functions, determine how much louder a 50 dB SPL sound is than a 30 dB SPL sound. Is this the same relationship for 50 dB versus 70 dB SPL? Or 70 dB versus 90 dB SPL? (All have a 20 dB range.) Discuss. In your answer, be sure to consider the implications of the units for loudness: A sound at 4 sones is twice as loud as a sound at 2 sones, and a sound at 8 sones is twice as loud as a sound at 4 sones.

2. Using equal-loudness contours, determine the dB SPL values of 200, 2000, and 8000 Hz tones when they are equally loud at 60 phons.

3. Using equal-loudness contours, determine the loudness level (in phons) of 200, 2000, and 8000 Hz tones when they are presented at 40 dB SPL. Which of these tones is louder when presented at the same sound pressure level? Discuss.

4. You are going to a concert next week, and you expect that sound levels will exceed 100 dB SPL. To protect your hearing, you purchase a set of musicians' earplugs, which have a constant attenuation of 25 dB at all frequencies.

   a. Using the equal-loudness contours given in Figure 4–5, discuss whether these earplugs will change the natural loudness relationships across frequency that will occur in the concert.

   b. Your friend purchases foam earplugs with the following attenuation characteristics (Table 4–1). Do you expect that he will have the same experience at the concert that you will? Again, use the equal-loudness contours to discuss. Consider, in particular, whether his perception will be dominated more by low or high frequencies.

5. Using equal-loudness contours, sketch a loudness growth function (in phons) for a 250-Hz tone. Compare that loudness growth function to that at 1000 Hz. Using your results, discuss why we would not use phons as a unit to measure loudness growth.

6. Provide three different examples indicating why loudness and intensity are not interchangeable terms.

7. Sketch loudness growth functions for a listener with 50 dB of conductive hearing

TABLE 4–1. Attenuation Characteristics of Earplugs

	Frequency (Hz)					
	250	500	1000	2000	4000	8000
Attenuation (dB)	15	15	20	25	30	40

loss. (Hint: the conductive hearing loss will only attenuate the sound.) When drawing your sketch, pay attention to use correct axis labels. From your sketch, what is the dynamic range? What is the LDL? Explain your answers using your knowledge of auditory physiology.

8. Why do listeners with typical SNHL experience LDLs that are similar to listeners with normal hearing?

9. Discuss how loudness recruitment might impact speech understanding in quiet.

10. Sketch loudness growth functions for a listener who demonstrates partial recruitment. In this case, the patient has 60 dB of sensorineural hearing loss. Label the dynamic range on your sketch.

11. Using only loudness as a guide, discuss the impact on loudness perception of providing amplification for a patient who experiences partial recruitment and another patient who does not, but has the same degree of hearing loss.

12. Sketch a loudness growth function consistent with a listener (with normal hearing) who experiences hyperacusis at all stimulus levels. Label the dynamic range on your graph.

> Visit the companion website for lab exercises.

REFERENCES

Algom, D., & Marks, L. E. (1984). Individual differences in loudness processing and loudness scales. *Journal of Experimental Psychology: General, 113*(4), 571.

American National Standards Institute. (2007). ANSI 3.4. Procedure for the computation of loudness of steady sounds.

American Speech-Language-Hearing Association. (n.d.). *Tinnitus and hyperacusis.* http:// www.asha.org/Practice-Portal/Clinical-Topics/Tinnitus-and-Hyperacusis/

British Society of Audiology (2022). *Recommended procedure determination of uncomfortable loudness levels.* http://www.thebsa.org.uk/resources/determination-uncomfortable-loudness-levels/

Buus, S., & Florentine, M. (2002). Growth of loudness in listeners with cochlear hearing losses: Recruitment reconsidered. *Journal of the Association for Research in Otolaryngology, 3*(2), 120–139.

Byrne, D. (1996). Hearing aid selection for the 1990s: Where to? *Journal of the American Academy of Audiology, 7*(6), 377–395.

Chocholle, R. (1940). Variation des temps de réaction auditifs en fonction de l'intensité à diverses fréquences. *L'année psychologique, 41*(1), 65–124.

Cox, R. M., Alexander, G. C., Taylor, I. M., & Gray, G. A. (1997). The contour test of loudness perception. *Ear and Hearing, 18*(5), 388–400.

Fletcher, H., & Munson, W. A. (1933). Loudness, its definition, measurement and calculation. *Bell Labs Technical Journal, 12*(4), 377–430.

Florentine, M., Buus, S. R., & Mason, C. R. (1987). Level discrimination as a function of level for tones from 0.25 to 16 kHz. *Journal of the Acoustical Society of America, 81*(5), 1528–1541.

Fowler, E. P. (1928). Marked deafened areas in normal ears. *Archives of Otolaryngology, 8*(2), 151–155.

Garner, W. R. (1953). An informational analysis of absolute judgments of loudness. *Journal of Experimental Psychology, 46*(5), 373–380.

Hawkins, D. B., Walden, B. E., Montgomery, A., & Prosek, R. A. (1987). Description and validation of an LDL procedure designed to select SSPLSO. *Ear and Hearing, 8*(3), 162–169.

Hellman, R. P., & Meiselman, C. H. (1993). Rate of loudness growth for pure tones in normal and impaired hearing. *Journal of the Acoustical Society of America, 93*(2), 966–975.

Hellman, R. P., & Zwislocki, J. (1961). Some factors affecting the estimation of loudness. *Journal of the Acoustical Society of America, 33*(5), 687–694.

Humes, L. E., & Ahlstrom, J. B. (1984). Relation between reaction time and loudness. *Journal of Speech, Language, and Hearing Research, 27*(2), 306–310.

International Standards Organization. ISO 226 (2003). *International Standard normal equal-loudness contours.*

Jesteadt, W., Wier, C. C., & Green, D. M. (1977). Intensity discrimination as a function of frequency and sensation level. *Journal of the Acoustical Society of America, 61*(1), 169–177.

Johnstone, B. M., & Boyle, A. J. F. (1967). Basilar membrane vibration examined with the Mössbauer technique. *Science, 158*(3799), 389–390.

Lauer A. M., & Dooling, R. J. (2007). Evidence of hyperacusis in canaries with permanent hereditary high-frequency hearing loss. *Seminars in Hearing, 28*(4), 319–326.

McFadden, D. (1986). The curious half-octave shift: Evidence for a basalward migration of the traveling-wave envelope with increasing intensity. In R. Salvi, D. Henderson, R. Hamernik, & V. Colletti (Eds.), *Basic and applied aspects of noise-induced hearing loss* (pp. 295–312). Springer.

Miller, G. A. (1947). Sensitivity to changes in the intensity of white noise and its relation to masking and loudness. *Journal of the Acoustical Society of America, 19*(4), 609–619.

Moore, B. C., & Glasberg, B. R. (1993). Simulation of the effects of loudness recruitment and threshold elevation on the intelligibility of speech in quiet and in a background of speech. *Journal of the Acoustical Society of America, 94*(4), 2050–2062.

Moore, B. C., Glasberg, B. R., & Baer, T. (1997). A model for the prediction of thresholds, loudness, and partial loudness. *Journal of the Audio Engineering Society, 45*(4), 224–240.

Palmer, A. R., & Evans, E. F. (1979). On the peripheral coding of the level of individual frequency components of complex sounds at high sound levels. In O. Creutzfeldt, H. Scheich, & C. Schreiner, *Hearing mechanisms and speech* (pp. 19–26). Springer-Verlag.

Rhode W. S. (1971). Observations of the vibration of the basilar membrane in squirrel monkeys using the Mössbauer technique. *Journal of the Acoustical Society of America, 49*, 1218–1231.

Riesz, R. R. (1928). Differential intensity sensitivity of the ear for pure tones. *Physical Review, 31*(5), 867.

Ruggero, M. A., & Rich, N. C. (1991). Application of a commercially-manufactured Doppler-shift laser velocimeter to the measurement of basilar-membrane vibration. *Hearing Research, 51*(2), 215–230.

Schlittenlacher, J., Ellermeier, W., & Avci, G. (2017). Simple reaction time for broadband sounds compared to pure tones. *Attention, Perception, and Psychophysics, 79*(2), 628–636.

Schroder, A. C., Viemeister, N. F., & Nelson, D. A. (1994). Intensity discrimination in normal-hearing and hearing-impaired listeners. *Journal of the Acoustical Society of America, 96*(5), 2683–2693.

Sheldrake, J., Diehl, P. U., & Schaette, R. (2015). Audiometric characteristics of hyperacusis patients. *Frontiers in Neurology, 6*, 1–7.

Smeds, K., & Leijon, A. (2010). Loudness and hearing loss. In M. Florentine, A. Popper, & R. Fay (Eds.), *Loudness* (pp. 223–259). Springer.

Souza, P. E. (2002). Effects of compression on speech acoustics, intelligibility, and sound quality. *Trends in Amplification, 6*(4), 131–165.

Stevens, S. S. (1956). The direct estimation of sensory magnitudes: Loudness. *American Journal of Psychology, 69*(1), 1–25.

Viemeister, N. F. (1988). Intensity coding and the dynamic range problem. *Hearing Research, 34*(3), 267–274.

Wagner, E., Florentine, M., Buus, S., & McCormack, J. (2004). Spectral loudness summation & simple reaction time. *Journal of the Acoustical Society of America, 116*(3), 1681–1686.

Winter, I. M., Robertson, D., & Yates, G. K. (1990) Diversity of characteristic frequency rate-intensity functions in guinea pig auditory nerve fibres. *Hearing Research, 45*(3), 191–202.

Zwicker, E., Flottorp, G., & Stevens, S. S. (1957). Critical band width in loudness summation. *Journal of the Acoustical Society of America, 29*(5), 548–557.

5

Temporal Processing

LEARNING OBJECTIVES

Upon completing this chapter, students will be able to:

- Discuss the strengths and weaknesses of various measures of temporal processing
- Differentiate between temporal acuity, temporal masking, and temporal integration
- Evaluate the mechanisms of temporal integration
- Explain the relationship between temporal integration and tone durations used for audiometry
- Describe the influence of sensorineural hearing loss and auditory neuropathy on temporal processing
- Relate deficits in temporal processing to everyday listening

INTRODUCTION

The representation of the temporal features of sounds is a key component to auditory processing. Time is an extremely important aspect of both sound and its perception, as all sounds vary over time to some degree, and information in sounds unfolds over time. Note that because sound is a vibration, all sounds, by definition, are characterized by pressure changes occurring over time. However, if the overall amplitude and frequency of a sound remain constant over time (e.g., a pure tone or white noise), the sound is considered a steady one. Sounds with changes in amplitude over time are considered time-varying, or *fluctuat-*

ing, and the limits on the perceptual ability to represent those variations is the focus of this chapter.

This ability to represent the variations in amplitude over time is referred to as ***temporal processing***. Temporal processing is a key component in coding natural sounds and the information contained in them. Consider speech, for example, which contains temporal elements that are important for the differentiation and identification of speech sounds. An ear that can represent the temporal aspects of speech is able to gather more information about a speech signal than an ear that cannot represent the temporal changes across time. Music also contains important temporal

129

elements, as the pattern of note duration and timing between notes yields rhythm. Figure 5–1, which plots a waveform of a speech sentence spoken by a single talker, illustrates the pattern of high-and low-amplitude variations that occur over time. The waveform is of a fluctuating sound and therefore has large amplitude changes over time. The waveform in Figure 5–1 is plotted along with its envelope, which is a representation of the slow temporal variations in the stimulus. This waveform illustrates two aspects of the stimulus that are time dependent: rapid individual pressure variations, commonly called ***temporal fine structure*** or the ***carrier***, and slower changes in the pressure variations, referred to as the ***envelope*** or the ***modulator***. Both of these aspects are labeled in Figure 5–1 for reference. The rapid variations are very important for auditory perception, but we do not typically perceive them as temporal events,

like we do the envelope. Thus, the perception of temporal fine structure is usually not treated as an aspect of temporal processing. On the other hand, we consider the ability to represent stimulus envelope as a component of temporal processing. We will discuss the following aspects of temporal processing in this chapter:

- ***Temporal resolution*** or ***temporal acuity***. This aspect of temporal processing measures the ability of the ear to represent changes in the envelope of sound.
- ***Temporal masking***. Temporal masking is sometimes considered an aspect of temporal resolution and is measured using forward-masking techniques. However, because temporal masking uses masking techniques, whereas the other measures of temporal acuity do not, it is sometimes considered as separate to temporal resolution.

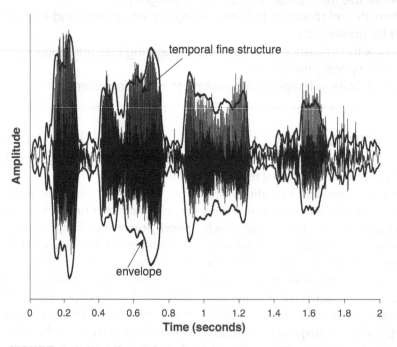

FIGURE 5–1. Waveform of an English sentence. The waveform has numerous amplitude fluctuations over time, demonstrating the nature of fluctuating stimuli in the natural world. The carrier (fine structure) and envelope (modulation) are also shown.

- *Temporal integration*. In this section, we review the ability of the ear to take advantage of increased sound duration.

Perceptual aspects of temporal processing are key elements contributing to our ability to decode both speech and musical signals, and degradations in temporal processing can undermine the ability to understand speech and appreciate music. In addition, the concept of temporal integration plays a role in experimental design for psychoacousticians, but audiologists should be knowledgeable of temporal integration, as the concept is foundational to audiometric testing. Additionally, sensorineural hearing loss can impact some of these abilities, and its influence should be considered when designing experiments or conducting audiometric tests.

We will discuss the following concepts, as they apply to temporal processing:

- Temporal resolution: gap detection and amplitude modulation detection
  - Acoustic considerations
  - Psychoacoustic experiments and methods
- Temporal masking: forward masking
- Temporal integration and its implications for audiology
- Effects of sensorineural hearing loss (SNHL)
  - Temporal resolution and temporal masking
  - Temporal integration
  - Temporal processing deficits and everyday listening
- Auditory neuropathy spectrum disorders (ANSD)

TEMPORAL RESOLUTION: GAP DETECTION

There have been numerous investigations into temporal resolution using a variety of different procedures. Today, we use **gap detection** to provide a rapid and general assessment of the

temporal resolution of the auditory system. In a gap detection task, we measure the *just noticeable duration* of a silent gap embedded into a stimulus.

The Gap Detection Paradigm

Plomp (1964) developed an intuitive paradigm to assess the temporal acuity of the auditory system. Plomp reasoned that perception of a stimulus persists, even after cessation of the acoustic signal. He suggested that the perception of sound decays over time and that persistence of the perception could interfere with the perception of a subsequently occurring sound. Plomp measured this decay using two broadband noise pulses, separated by a silent period, Δt. Plomp measured the minimum detectable silent period, the *gap*—Δt—between the two noise pulses and varied the levels of the two pulses. We now call his paradigm **gap detection.** Figure 5–2 illustrates how gap detection might be implemented in a 2I–2AFC task. One interval contains the stimulus with the gap, whereas the other interval does not. The listener selects which of the two intervals contains the brief gap. Essentially Plomp asked, "What is the smallest gap that can be detected?"

Visit the companion website for an auditory-visual demonstration of a gap detection experiment.

To get a feel regarding why gap detection reflects temporal processing, a schematic adapted from Plomp's paper is illustrated in Figure 5–3, which shows how gap detection provides a measure of the decay of auditory sensation. The upper panel shows a schematic of the stimulus: two noise pulses separated by a silent gap, Δt. The lower panel shows

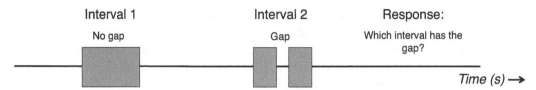

FIGURE 5–2. Illustration of an experimental trial in a gap detection experiment.

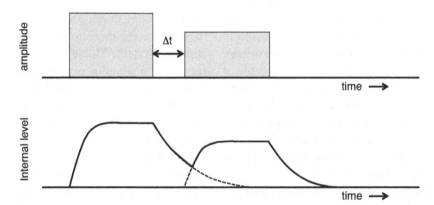

FIGURE 5–3. Illustration of a gap detection experiment, as originally conceptualized by Plomp (1964). The top panel illustrates a schematic of two pulses separated by a silent gap with duration Δt. The bottom panel illustrates the "internal representations" of the two pulses and how they build up and decay over time.

Plomp's visualization of how the amplitude of these stimuli might be represented in the auditory system. This diagram also illustrates how an internal psychological representation of one sound can decay into the representation of the following sound. If the gap between the two sounds is very short, a listener will hear the second sound blend into the first sound and cannot perceive the gap. However, if the gap is sufficiently long, a listener will hear the interruption of the pulse pair. The *just detectable gap* reflects how much temporal separation can be between the two sounds before the first sound has decayed enough to allow for the listener to hear the silent gap in between them.

Although Plomp's original experiment varied the levels of the noise pulses, today we typically set the levels of the noises to be equal, and we measure the minimum detectable gap between two sounds. The longer the gap needed for detection, the greater the decay produced by the first stimulus. Plomp measured *gap detection thresholds* (the just detectable gap) in white noise to be approximately 2 to 3 ms for listeners with normal hearing (Plomp, 1964).

The type of sound used in a gap detection task, be it a pure tone, narrow band of noise, or white noise, has a strong influence on the gap detection threshold. The following sections will discuss the factors that are necessary to interpret the gap detection threshold for only a subset of these sounds, but gap detection has been measured for numerous different stimulus types. For the purposes of this chapter, we place gap detection in two categories: gap detection in *steady* sounds, such as white noise and pure tones, and gap detection in *fluctuating* sounds, such as (relatively narrow) narrowband noise. Experimenters testing both types of stimuli have also attempted to measure gap detection in a frequency-specific way, although with less success. This body of work has demonstrated that the gap detection threshold depends on several stimulus characteristics and is not always 2 to 3 ms. In fact, it is often much higher. The gap detection threshold is affected by stimulus level, stimulus bandwidth, and whether a stimulus is fluctuating or not. These factors are discussed in the sections to follow.

White noise can be considered a steady sound because the random fluctuations are too rapid to be heard as fluctuations. The envelope of white noise is effectively flat, as white noise contains no slow amplitude variations over time. If narrowband noises have relatively wide bandwidths (perhaps greater than about 400 to 500 Hz), they are perceived as steady, but bands of noise with narrower bandwidths may have audible fluctuations and therefore would be fluctuating sounds. Interestingly, very narrow bands of noise can sound remarkably similar to a pure tone.

Visit the companion website for demonstrations of noises with different bandwidths.

Before we can discuss the experimental results, however, we must first consider the acoustic effects of inserting a brief quiet gap in the waveform of a sound stimulus. As we will see below, introducing a temporal gap into a stimulus can alter the spectral characteristics of that sound. Experimenters testing both steady and fluctuating stimuli must consider whether spectral cues are present in their sounds. Should this happen, the gap detection threshold no longer reflects temporal processing but reflects spectral resolution instead. This phenomenon can make it difficult to measure gap detection in a frequency-specific manner.

Gap Detection: Acoustics

Anyone interested in evaluating temporal processing must be mindful of the relationship between the waveform and spectrum—changes to the temporal characteristics of a stimulus can lead to changes in the spectrum, just as the reverse can occur. An example we have already discussed is the time-frequency trade-off: Sounds cannot be brief in time as well as frequency specific. Shortening a sound will lead to additional frequencies present in the sound (i.e., spectral splatter). Applying this same concept to gap detection, abruptly stopping and starting a sound, as happens when a short gap is inserted into a stimulus, can also produce spectral splatter.

If we consider the relationship between the waveform and spectrum, we can observe that placing a silent gap within a stimulus has the potential to introduce spectral changes. Effectively, we can consider a stimulus with a gap as two sequential stimuli. However, because the just noticeable gap between two sounds may be 2 to 3 ms, the first sound must be rapidly turned off and the second sound must be rapidly turned on. Depending on the characteristics of the two sequential sounds, spectral changes can occur. To illustrate how these effects might manifest, Figure 5–4 illustrates the spectra of two noise stimuli (top panels) and 2000-Hz tone stimuli (bottom panels) without gaps (left panels) and with a 2-ms temporal gap (right panels).

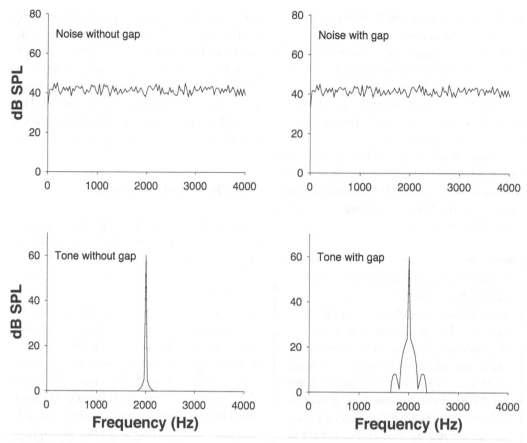

FIGURE 5–4. Illustration of spectra for sounds without 2-ms gaps inserted (*left panels*) and with gaps inserted (*right panels*). The spectra in the top panels are for noise without and with the temporal gap, and the spectra in the bottom panels are for a 2000-Hz tone without and with the temporal gap.

Figure 5–4 shows that when a gap is introduced into a white noise, spectral splatter is negligible, as white noise already has a wide frequency range. The two noise spectra may be slightly different from each other, but using a random sample of white noise each time a stimulus is presented (with or without the gap) prevents the listener from using tiny spectral differences to detect the presence of the gap. We can do this because every sample of white noise is different with unique amplitude fluctuations.

For pure tones, however, the frequencies introduced by the gap change the spectral characteristics of the stimulus. Although tone without the gap is not fully frequency specific (because its duration is not infinite), the spectral differences between the stimulus with the gap and the one without are readily visible. We observe that the 2000-Hz tone has a broader bandwidth than the long duration tone. In this case, the additional frequencies may be audible to a listener and may provide a cue to the presence of the gap, rather than temporal interruption itself. If this were to happen in an experiment, the gap detection thresholds may not reflect temporal processing at all. The consequence of these spectral changes is that getting extremely frequency-specific measures for gap detection can be difficult.

Gap Detection: Psychophysical Findings

Gap detection is a fairly straightforward task— a listener is asked to determine which of two sounds has a brief temporal disruption. Gap detection experiments can provide a relatively rapid estimate of temporal processing abilities in the form of a single number representing temporal processing ability. As a result, a gap-detection experiment would be very appealing to include in a clinical test measuring temporal acuity. Yet, Plomp's initial experiments and those of other investigators have illustrated that the gap detection threshold depends on several stimulus characteristics, including the level and the bandwidth of sound. Thus, it is not straightforward to interpret gap detection from a clinical perspective—whether a listener can hear the frequencies present in the stimulus contributes substantially to whether a large or a small gap detection threshold is measured.

Level Effects

Plomp's original study demonstrated that gap detection thresholds for white noise were strongly dependent on stimulus level but only for low stimulus levels. Figure 5–5 shows data adapted from Plomp's experiment in which he measured gap detection thresholds at different sensation levels (defined as the sound level in dB above threshold). At very low stimulus levels, gap detection thresholds decreased (they improved) with increasing level. At 10 dB sensation level (SL), gap detection thresholds were around 20 ms and decreased to slightly less than 3 ms between 10 and 30 dB SL. Once the stimulus level reached about 30 dB SL, further increases in stimulus level were not associated with large increases in performance.

The effect of level on the gap detection threshold has clear implications for the ultimate utility of using gap detection as a clinical test of temporal acuity. A listener must

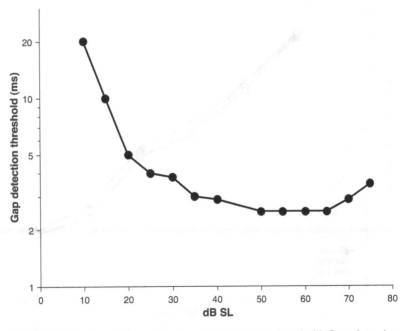

FIGURE 5–5. The effects of level on gap detection threshold. Gap detection thresholds (ms) are plotted as function of sensation level in dB. Adapted from Plomp (1964).

be presented with a stimulus at an adequate sensation level to achieve the lowest threshold possible. Thus, gap detection thresholds can be difficult to interpret when measured in listeners who have large amounts of hearing loss. If a patient were to have a high gap detection threshold, we have to ask, "Is the gap detection threshold high because the patient can't easily hear the stimulus? Or is it because of poor temporal processing?" This is a problem if this test were used diagnostically in isolation—a high gap detection threshold does not automatically imply poor temporal processing, particularly for an individual with hearing loss. More regarding the influence of SNHL will be discussed later in this chapter.

Bandwidth and Frequency Effects

The bandwidth of a stimulus also has a profound effect on the ability to detect a gap. In short, gap detection thresholds decrease (get better) as the bandwidth of a stimulus is increased. Across a large number of studies, we observe that gap detection thresholds depend greatly on stimulus bandwidth. Data from Eddins et al. (1992), who measured gap detection thresholds in high-pass filtered bands of noise with bandwidths ranging from 50 to 1600 Hz, are plotted in Figure 5–6. Eddins et al. also varied the high-frequency cutoff frequencies of the noises, and data for the different cutoff-frequencies are illustrated using different symbols. Eddins et al.'s experiment tested the effects of bandwidth and frequency region at the same time.

There are several notable features in the data presented in Figure 5–6. First, we clearly see that the gap detection threshold decreased with increasing bandwidth. The best (lowest) thresholds were achieved when the bandwidth of the stimulus was the widest. We also observe that the frequency region did not influence gap detection abilities. As a result, we can con-

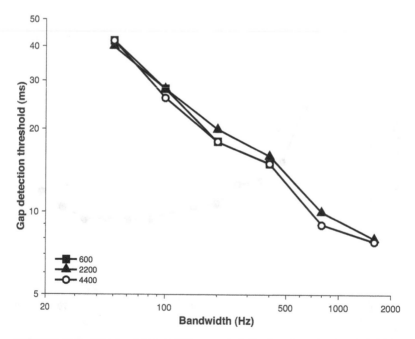

FIGURE 5–6. Effects of bandwidth on gap detection. Gap detection thresholds (ms) are plotted as function of stimulus bandwidth (Hz) for three different high-frequency cutoff frequencies. Adapted from Eddins et al. (1992)

clude that the bandwidth affects the measurement of the gap detection threshold, but not the frequency region.

We interpret the effects of stimulus bandwidth on gap detection as support for a hypothesis that, even for temporal processing, the ear can utilize information across many frequency bands. A similar finding was discussed in Chapter 3 in which we discussed the auditory representation of sound spectrum, but we now see that this ability can be applied to temporal processing. Although this interpretation may not immediately be obvious, consider the following: When we introduce a gap into the time course of a stimulus, all of the stimulus frequencies are stopped simultaneously. For a white noise stimulus that is fully audible, a temporal gap causes a temporal disruption down the full length of the basilar membrane. This effect is illustrated in Figure 5–7, which shows the output waveforms of multiple auditory filters plotted as a function of time for a

noise with a 10-ms temporal gap. This format is similar to a spectrogram, only each individual trace represents the output of a single auditory filter estimated from human psychophysical studies. Here, we can see that the gap is represented across the frequency range, as each auditory filter processes a signal that is turned on and turned off very quickly. All but the very low frequency filters (<250 Hz or so) represent the gap very well.

Considering the example illustrated in Figure 5–7, we can evaluate two possibilities for detecting the presence of the gap in a noise. In one of those possibilities, the auditory system could *listen* to the output of only one auditory filter, essentially *picking* one of the auditory filter outputs. On the other hand, *listening* across multiple auditory filters would be a viable alternative, and multiple auditory filters code the gap extremely well. If the ear always listened to the same auditory filter, or even switched which auditory filter was

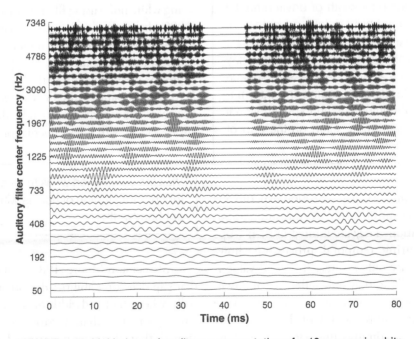

FIGURE 5–7. Multi-channel auditory representation of a 10-ms gap in white noise. Similar to a spectrogram, this plot represents the output of multiple auditory filters as a function of time.

used, regardless of stimulus bandwidth, gap detection thresholds would not change with increasing bandwidth. However, if the ear listened to more and more auditory filters as the bandwidth increased, gap detection thresholds would improve with increasing bandwidth, as there would be more and more opportunities to detect the gap. In this way, the improvement of gap detection thresholds with increasing bandwidth indicates that listeners can use many frequency regions to detect a gap.

Consider how the telephone, which only represents frequencies up to about 3500 Hz, or a hearing aid with a bandwidth of 6000 kHz, might impair the representation of temporal information present in speech, which has a bandwidth closer to 8000 Hz, and music, having a bandwidth of 14,000 Hz. In both cases, a listener is in an impoverished auditory environment. By not having access to the full bandwidth of environmental stimuli, the ability to take advantage of broadband temporal changes may be negatively impacted. Although we may not notice a large decrease in speech understanding, decoding the information in the impoverished speech signal may require more effort on the part of the listener.

In summary, gap detection experiments provide an intuitive way to measure temporal resolution. They are limited in their scope of measuring temporal processing, however, because only a single threshold value is obtained. Thus, they only reflect the ability to detect whether a stimulus is *on* or *off* and are not sensitive to the ability of the ear to code for different stimulus fluctuation rates. Furthermore, the thresholds themselves depend on the frequency span of the stimulus, and a

fully audible stimulus is needed to obtain the best gap detection thresholds.

Gap Detection in Fluctuating Sounds

The previous two sections discussed gap detection in steady stimuli, stimuli that do not have large amplitude variations over time. However, many sounds have inherent fluctuations that are also represented by the auditory system. Gap detection experiments that use these sounds help us to understand the representation of slowly fluctuating sounds by the ear. Although there are many types of sounds that contain slow fluctuations, here we discuss a specific class of sound: narrowband noise. Narrowband noises are filtered versions of white noise—they contain fewer frequencies, but they also have slower amplitude fluctuations.

Before we discuss the data on gap detection in narrow bands of noise, we must first understand the acoustic representation of these sounds. Figure 5–8 illustrates the effects of filtering white noise using filters with a very wide (1000-Hz bandwidth; left panel), a moderately narrow (200-Hz bandwidth; middle panel), and a narrow (50-Hz bandwidth; right panel) bandwidth. As the bandwidth of the noise decreases (left to right panels), the fluctuation rate also decreases. Thus, narrower bandwidth stimuli are associated with slower fluctuation rates.

Visit the companion website for an auditory demonstration of noises with different bandwidths.

Shailer and Moore (1985) demonstrated that gap detection abilities degraded substantially when the bandwidth of noise was very narrow and less than a critical band. They argued that these very narrow bandwidth sounds have robust fluctuations that can be easily confused with the gap. Figure 5–9

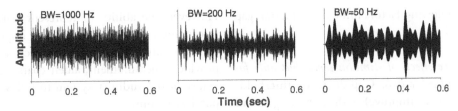

FIGURE 5–8. Effects of filtering noise on the waveform. Going from the left panel to the right panel, each waveform reflects a noise band with the same center frequency with a wide (1000 Hz), medium (200 Hz), and narrow (50 Hz) bandwidth, respectively.

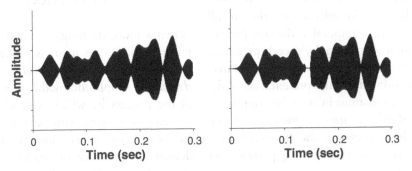

FIGURE 5–9. Illustration of a gap inserted into a fluctuating stimulus. The left panel shows a narrowband noise without a gap, whereas the right panel shows the same noise with a gap inserted at 130 ms into the stimulus.

illustrates this idea. The left panel shows the stimulus with its natural fluctuations, and the right panel illustrates that stimulus with a gap inserted. In this figure, the gap is inserted near one of the waveform valleys. One can see that if the gap, as in this case, is presented near or in one of the temporal valleys of the waveform, it would be difficult to detect, particularly in comparison to a gap inserted near a peak.

Glasberg and Moore (1992) explicitly tested whether gap detection was made more difficult by the presence of stimulus fluctuations. They used a cleverly designed stimulus, originally developed by Pumplin (1985), to determine whether the fluctuations make gap detection more difficult. This stimulus, called *low fluctuation noise (LFN)*, contains the same frequencies present in white noise, but undergoes an algorithm designed to reduce the fluctuations present in the stimulus. LFN

does not completely eliminate temporal fluctuations in a stimulus, but it greatly reduces them, particularly in comparison to natural narrow bands of noise with the same bandwidth. Glasberg and Moore showed that gap detection thresholds were much better in LFN than in narrowband noise, supporting the hypothesis that fluctuations can make gaps difficult to detect. Because listeners have difficulty detecting gaps in fluctuating sounds, we know that those fluctuations are robustly represented in the auditory system.

Gap Detection: Summary and Implications

Taken together, the ear can follow relatively quick changes in amplitude, as the gap detection threshold for white noise is 2 to 3 ms.

The following factors influence temporal gap detection:

- *Large effects of stimulus level, but only for low-level sounds.* Gap detection thresholds decrease (improve) with increasing sound level, but only for low-level sounds. Once a moderate level is reached, stimulus level has little effect on gap detection thresholds. Poor gap detection at low levels suggests a necessity to present stimuli well above auditory threshold in order to give the ear full access to the temporal variations present in stimuli. For example, speech presented near threshold, or even at 20 dB SL, may not provide sufficient representation of the temporal variations in everyday sounds.
- *Limited effects of stimulus frequency.* When possible to measure, the frequency of a stimulus does not affect gap detection threshold.
- *Large effects of stimulus bandwidth.* The wider the stimulus bandwidth, the better the gap detection threshold. The auditory system can use information across a wide frequency range to gather information, even temporal information. We can infer from this result that providing access to stimuli with the widest bandwidth possible is important for robust coding of acoustic temporal information.
- *Large effects of stimulus fluctuation.* Fluctuations in the stimulus are associated with poorer gap detection thresholds. This result indicates that the ear represents these fluctuations and may use these fluctuations to benefit perception. An example is the fluctuating masker benefit, in which the ear can *listen* in low-level temporal epochs to improve speech understanding and detection abilities.

Gap detection experiments may seem contrived and have no obvious application to our understanding of everyday listening.

However, the ability to represent temporal information in a stimulus is clearly important for communication, and gap detection tasks provide a measurement, albeit coarse, of the ability of the auditory system to follow temporal variations.

TEMPORAL RESOLUTION: AMPLITUDE MODULATION DETECTION

When a more thorough method of temporal resolution assessment is desired, we use a method based on *amplitude modulation detection*. Amplitude modulation is defined as the process by which a steady sound is turned into a sound with variable amplitude. In these types of experiments, the listener detects the presence of modulation that is imposed on a stimulus. Before psychoacoustic studies using this method are discussed, we review the acoustics of amplitude modulation.

Amplitude Modulation: Acoustics

An amplitude-modulated sound is described in two parts: the *envelope* (or *modulator*), the portion of the stimulus that slowly varies over time, and the *fine structure* (or *carrier*), the portion of the stimulus with rapid pressure fluctuations. One formula to generate an amplitude modulated stimulus, y, is given by the following equation:

$$y(t) = [1 + m \cdot \text{mod}(t)] \, \text{car}(t) \qquad \text{Eq. 5–1}$$

where m refers to the modulation depth, $\text{mod}(t)$ is the modulator, $\text{car}(t)$ is the carrier, and t is time. The modulator and carrier can be any type of stimulus, and in many psychoacoustic experiments, the modulator is a pure tone, and the carrier is either a pure tone or a noise. Note that the frequency of a stimulus can also be modulated, but in the context of this text, the term modulation always refers to *amplitude modulation*.

A special case referred to as *a sinusoidally amplitude modulated (SAM)* tone occurs when both the modulator and carrier are pure tones. For a SAM tone, Equation 5–1 becomes $y(t)=[1+m\sin(2\pi f_m t)]\sin(2\pi f_c t)$, where f_m and f_c are the frequencies of the modulator and the carrier, respectively.

The amount of modulation is controlled by the parameter, m, which ranges between 0 (unmodulated) and 1 (fully modulated). To facilitate an intuition of modulation, the top panels of Figure 5–10 illustrate the waveforms of a tone with three different sinusoidal modulators (*SAM tones*). The left panel shows an unmodulated tone, the middle panel shows a 20% modulated ($m = 0.2$) tone, and the right panel shows a fully (100%) modulated ($m = 1$) tone. In Figure 5–10, the fine structure is represented in the rapid pressure fluctuations and the envelope in the slow fluctuations. The

fine structure is the same across panels, but the degree of fluctuation in the envelope is reduced as we look from right to left in the figure. Even the unmodulated sound has an envelope, but it is flat over time, reflecting the steady nature of this sound.

Visit the companion website for an auditory demonstration of noise stimuli with different modulation depths.

Not surprisingly, the process of modulating sounds impacts the spectra of those sounds, which are plotted in the upper left-hand corners along with the waveforms in Figure 5–10. The spectra clearly demonstrate differences in comparison to that of the unmodulated sound, in the form of *side bands*. The modulation rate (f_m) determines the frequency of these side bands, and the modulation depth (m) determines the size of the side bands. The higher the modulation rate, the farther the sidebands occur from the carrier. Each sideband is exactly f_m Hz away from the carrier. The modulation depth determines the size of the side bands—the larger the modulation

m=0 (unmodulated)   **m=0.2 (20% modulated)**   **m=1 (100%modulated)**

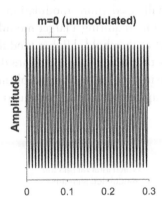 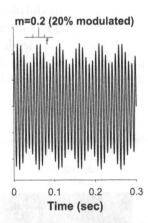 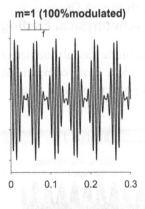

Time (sec)

FIGURE 5–10. Waveforms of three different SAM tones at different modulation depths. Going from left to right, the stimuli progress from no modulation (m=0), 20% modulation (m=0.2) and fully modulated (m=1). The small insets in the upper left-hand corners represent the spectra of the SAM tones.

depth, the greater the amplitude of the side bands. A 100% modulated stimulus will have both sidebands at 6 dB below the level of the carrier. Decreasing the modulation depth will decrease the size of the side bands. In many instances, the ear is very capable of hearing these frequency components as being separate from the carrier, particularly when they fall outside of the critical band. These stimuli can be heard as a *chord* or complex tone, rather than as a temporal pattern. Consequently, as with gap detection, these acoustic consequences can make it quite difficult to obtain frequency-specific measures of temporal processing using amplitude modulation detection. On the other hand, noise stimuli have an amplitude spectrum that is the same, regardless of whether the noise is modulated or not. Thus, it is common to use amplitude-modulated noise in amplitude-modulation detection experiments.

than gap detection. Viemeister (1979) was one of the first to use modulation detection and apply it to measure temporal resolution. Viemeister's listeners detected the presence of amplitude modulation on an otherwise steady stimulus, and he measured the ability to detect amplitude modulation as a function of the modulation rate. The modulation was sinusoidal, and the carrier was a white noise. He measured the *just detectable modulation depth* (m), which ranged between 0 (no modulation) and 1 (100% modulation). Viemeister asked "How much does a sound need to be modulated before the listener can tell it is modulated?" For illustration, Figure 5–11 shows how this task would be implemented using a 2I-2AFC paradigm. Here, a listener is presented with two intervals: one that contains a modulated stimulus and one that does not. The listener selects which of the two intervals contains the modulation.

> Visit the companion website for an auditory demonstration of the perceptual effect of modulation rate on tones and noises.

> Visit the companion website for an auditory-visual demonstration of an amplitude modulation detection experiment.

Modulation Detection: Psychophysical Findings

Amplitude modulation detection experiments provide a more comprehensive view of the temporal resolution of the auditory system

Listeners having difficulty detecting modulation will need more modulation to detect it, therefore requiring a larger modulation depth (*m*) at threshold. Higher modulation detection thresholds would indicate difficulties following the changes in amplitude over time, compared with lower modulation

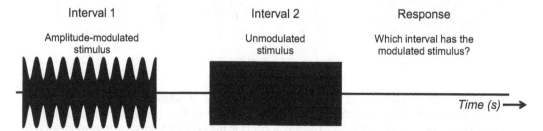

FIGURE 5–11. Illustration of an experimental trial for a modulation detection task. Here, the modulated stimulus has 50% amplitude modulation (a modulation depth of 0.5).

detection thresholds. We could also interpret this result to indicate that the modulation rates associated with high modulation detection thresholds are not well represented in the auditory system.

Viemeister named the plot that relates modulation detection threshold (*y*-axis; 20log*m*) to modulation rate (*x*-axis; *f*$_m$) *the temporal modulation transfer function, or the TMTF*. Figure 5–12 illustrates the TMTF and plots better thresholds at the top (low modulation detection thresholds) so that the function has the appearance of a low-pass filter. In Viemeister's experiment, listeners most easily detected modulation at relatively low modulation rates (<30 Hz). In these cases, very little modulation was needed for detection—about 5%! As the modulation rate increased, the task became more difficult, and listeners needed more modulation to detect

it. The poorest threshold was reached at a modulation rate of approximately 1000 Hz, but even here listeners still only needed about 40% modulation to detect it. If one considers the TMTF to be similar to a low-pass filter, the TMTF has a cutoff frequency of 55 to 65 Hz. Thus, modulation rates below about 55 Hz are well represented by the auditory system, and rates higher than that progressively become more poorly represented. Across the board, however, the ability to detect the presence of modulation is quite excellent.

Visit the companion website for an auditory demonstration of the TMTF.

Different ways of characterizing the features of the TMTF are illustrated in Figure 5–12, and each of these features describes a

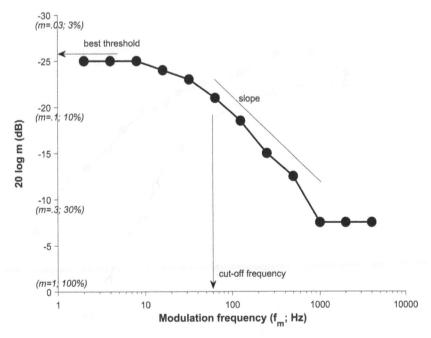

FIGURE 5–12. A temporal modulation transfer function (TMTF). Modulation detection thresholds in 20log(m), where m is the modulation depth, are plotted as a function of modulation frequency in Hz. The amount of modulation in percent is also shown. Better thresholds are shown at the top of the figure so that the function has the appearance of a low-pass filter. Different features of the TMTF are highlighted on the figure. Adapted from Viemeister (1979).

different characteristic of temporal resolution. (1) The *best threshold* achieved reflects a listener's overall ability to follow amplitude changes in the stimulus. (2) The *cutoff frequency* is related to the bandwidth of modulation rates represented well in the auditory system (e.g., the TMTF *bandwidth*). (3) The *slope* of the function indicates how much change in ability occurs across the different modulation rates. A low best threshold, a higher cutoff frequency, and a shallower filter slope would all be associated with superior temporal processing measures. The TMTF has been measured at different stimulus presentation levels, for different frequencies, and for different bandwidths, with the following results:

- *Large effects of stimulus level, but only for low-level sounds.* The TMTF was generally unaffected by stimulus level, except at very low levels where portions of the stimulus

may be inaudible (Viemeister, 1979). As with gap detection, this result indicates that stimulus levels need to be high enough to support good access to temporal information present in sounds.

- *Limited effects of stimulus frequency.* Although very few studies have measured TMTFs for frequency-specific stimuli, Kohlrausch et al. (2000) measured TMTFs for sinusoidal carriers. Frequency effects of temporal resolution were only interpretable at high frequencies due to the acoustic constraints discussed previously. At least for these high frequencies, they found no effect of frequency on the TMTF.

- *Large effects of stimulus bandwidth.* Generally, TMTF measurements are highly dependent on the bandwidth of the stimulus. Bacon and Viemeister (1985) showed this when they measured TMTFs for low-pass noises. Data adapted from their study

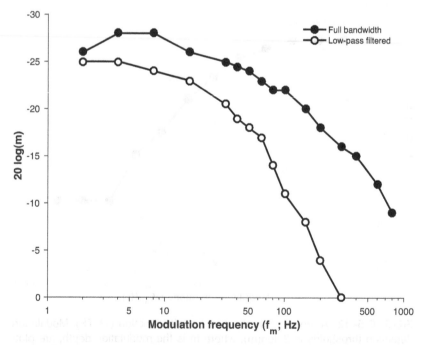

FIGURE 5–13. Effects of bandwidth on the TMTF. Modulation detection thresholds in 20log(m) are plotted as a function of modulation frequency in Hz for unfiltered (*filled circles*) and low-pass filtered (*unfilled circles*) stimuli. Adapted from Bacon and Viemeister (1985).

are illustrated in Figure 5–13. Here, the best threshold was poorer (worse), and the cutoff frequency was lower (worse) for the TMTF measured for the low-pass noise compared with the TMTF measured for the unfiltered noise. These results suggest that reducing the stimulus bandwidth limits the ability of the ear to use temporal information. Consequently, the bandwidth of the stimulus must be considered when interpreting TMTF data. As with gap detection, these effects demonstrate that the ear uses information across the frequency range of the stimulus to detect the presence of modulation.

TEMPORAL MASKING

Another class of experiments that measure the temporal resolution of the ear is ***temporal masking***. This approach to measuring temporal resolution is also sometimes referred to as ***forward masking***. Although we discussed forward masking in Chapter 3, here we look at the way this technique allows a measurement of temporal processing. Recall that in a forward masking experiment, the signal

and masker <u>do not</u> overlap in time. Typically, the signal is presented very close in time to the masker, and always is presented after the masker has been turned off. The first stimulus to arrive at the ear is the masker, which can be a noise or a tone or really any other stimulus. The second stimulus to arrive at the ear is usually a tone and has a short duration compared with the masker. In temporal masking experiments, the threshold of the signal in the presence of the masker is measured as a function of the time delay between the signal and the masker.

To refresh our memory, the stimulus sequence for a forward-masking experiment is illustrated in Figure 5–14, which shows a typical 2I–2AFC experiment in which one of two observation intervals contains a signal and both observation intervals contain a masker. To demonstrate how using two stimuli that do not overlap in time might allow a measurement of temporal processing, Figure 5–15 illustrates how the perceptual representation of the masker might decay and provide masking of a signal. This decay is illustrated by the dashed line. As the two stimuli are separated farther in time, the effect of the masker on

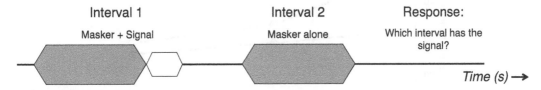

FIGURE 5–14. Schematic of the stimulus presentation sequence used in a 2I-2AFC task for forward masking.

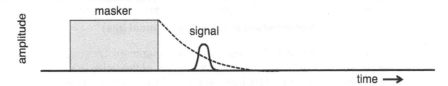

FIGURE 5–15. Schematic of the concept of forward masking. Temporal effects of masking are illustrated by a masker (*gray rectangle*) and a signal presented after a certain time delay. The dotted line shows the decay of the internal representation of the masker.

the signal should decrease, and the signal will become easier to detect. In a forward masking experiment, the level of the signal needed for detection is typically measured as the dependent variable. The experimental, independent variable is the time between the masker and the signal. Thus, the signal threshold is measured as a function of the time delay between the masker and signal. In some ways, this paradigm is very similar to Plomp's gap detection paradigm. However, rather than measuring the size of the just noticeable gap, we measure the threshold of a signal following a gap of a specified duration.

> Visit the companion website for an auditory-visual demonstration of a forward-masking experiment.

Forward masking occurs when the masker is high in intensity and has frequency components similar to the signal. The temporal relationship between the two sounds is also relevant, and forward masking decreases as the signal moves farther away from the masker in time. The decrease in detection threshold as the signal and masker are increasingly separated is the ***release from forward masking***. Figure 5–16 shows data taken from Plack and Oxenham (1998), who measured the signal detection threshold as a function of the delay between the masker and the signal. In their experiment, the signal and masker were both tones, and they measured forward masking at different stimulus levels. Figure 5–16 illustrates the effects of temporal separation, masker level, and the delay between the signal and masker have on the signal detection threshold.

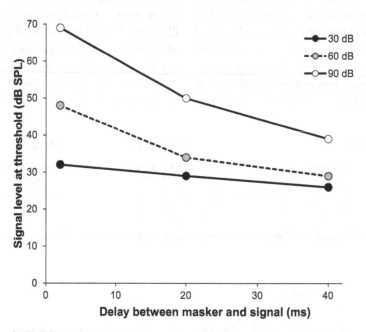

FIGURE 5–16. Data from forward a masking experiment. Detection thresholds in (dB SPL) are plotted as a function of the delay in ms between the masker (a 2-kHz tone) and signal (also a 2-kHz tone) for three different masker levels (30, 60, and 90 dB SPL). Adapted from Plack and Oxenham (1998).

Visit the companion website for an auditory demonstration of the effects of forward masking.

Figure 5–16 illustrates two major factors that are relevant to the amount of forward masking:

- *Temporal relationships.* The amount of masking decayed as signal and masker became farther apart. The closer the two sounds were in time, the greater the signal detection threshold and therefore, more masking. In all cases, we observe a release from forward masking as the masker and signal became more separated in time.
- *Level effects.* The release from forward masking *was higher for high-intensity signals than for low.* First, the greater the intensity of the forward masker, the more forward masking. Note that thresholds were higher across the board for the more intense maskers. Second, increasing the level of the forward masker also led to greater release from masking. This is observed in the greater decrease in thresholds with time for the higher masker levels than for the lower masker levels.
  - This finding has some interesting implications and suggests that the ear has mechanisms that support release from masking, particularly in situations where masking effects are large. Although a more intense masker produces more masking than low-level sounds, the ear provides some added release through nonlinear auditory processes.

Results from forward-masking experiments demonstrate that sounds that precede other sounds in time impact the perception of those occurring sounds. Given that many everyday sounds contain informative components that unfold over time (e.g., like speech), forward masking has strong implications for everyday listening. A listener who is very susceptible to forward masking, or who has an ear that does not release from forward masking quickly, is likely to experience difficulties understanding rapid speech, due to the temporal smearing of auditory representations.

COMPARISON OF TEMPORAL PROCESSING MEASURES

A variety of different techniques have been used to assess temporal resolution in the auditory system: gap detection, amplitude modulation detection, and forward masking. Because each technique has strengths and weaknesses, an experimenter or clinician can choose the method that best suits the particular application. Gap detection is an intuitive task, relatively easy to implement, and yields a single number to describe temporal acuity. Gap detection experiments can also be executed relatively quickly compared with more comprehensive methods of assessing temporal resolution because they generally yield a single number representing temporal resolution. Yet, gap detection experiments are fairly limited in their ability to broadly characterize temporal processing performance, as they only measure the ability to detect when a sound is interrupted.

On the other hand, the TMTF is comprehensive and results in multiple parameters that describe temporal acuity. Because temporal resolution is measured at multiple modulation rates, the TMTF provides a more complete picture of the temporal resolution of the ear. Further, the TMTF can be used to better pinpoint any sources of temporal processing difficulties because it contains more comprehensive information about temporal resolution than gap detection. However, measuring the TMTF is relatively time consuming and requires modulation detection thresholds to be measured at multiple modulation rates.

Finally, forward-masking experiments specifically evaluate the effects of one sound on another and provide a measure of temporal processing rather different from gap and amplitude-modulation detection. Such measures can be used to assess temporal representations between sounds, rather than within the same stimulus.

Despite the differences in these techniques, they effectively converge on the same conclusions:

- *Temporal acuity is poorer at low levels versus high.* The implication is that sufficient audibility is necessary to provide the ear with access to the temporal information in sounds.
- *Temporal acuity depends on stimulus bandwidth.* The wider the bandwidth, the better access the ear has to the temporal information in sound. Thus, filtering sounds will negatively impact the ear's ability to use temporal information.

Both findings have implications for listeners with sensorineural hearing loss who experience reduced audibility, and therefore an impoverished representation of sound level, and often a restricted audible bandwidth, particularly if they have a sloping or rising hearing loss. These issues are discussed in the hearing loss section of this chapter.

TEMPORAL INTEGRATION

The previous sections of this chapter focused on temporal resolution, or the ability of the auditory system to follow amplitude changes in a stimulus. Another well-known aspect of auditory temporal processing is that absolute thresholds of sounds depend on their dura-

tion. This process is referred to as *temporal integration* or *temporal summation*, defined as the ability of the ear to accumulate information over time to improve detection threshold.

The Critical Duration

Temporal integration experiments measure changes in auditory abilities as a function of the duration of a stimulus. Temporal integration has been demonstrated using a variety of experimental paradigms, including loudness (Zwislocki, 1969), intensity discrimination (Garner & Miller, 1944), and frequency discrimination (Moore, 1973). Broadly speaking, temporal integration follows a similar pattern for all tasks. Because detecting pure tones is so important for audiology, we review those data here as representative for temporal integration.

Here we review temporal integration for detecting pure tones. Watson and Gengel (1969) measured the threshold for detecting a pure tone as a function of its duration and frequency. Data adapted from their study are illustrated in Figure 5–17. To understand this figure, we first note that Watson and Gengel (1969) calculated thresholds relative to the average threshold obtained for durations of 512 and 1024 ms, which they defined to be 0 dB. In this way, they could easily observe the change in threshold produced by shortening the duration of the stimuli. Figure 5–17 shows the relative threshold as a function of the stimulus duration. Each curve represents data from a different signal frequency. In general, Figure 5–17 demonstrates a robust decrease in threshold as duration increases. Although the improvement of threshold with duration varied somewhat for the different signal frequencies, all frequencies demonstrated a clear pattern of improvement. Additionally, once the stimulus duration exceeded about 250 ms, large changes in threshold were not evident. The duration at which thresholds

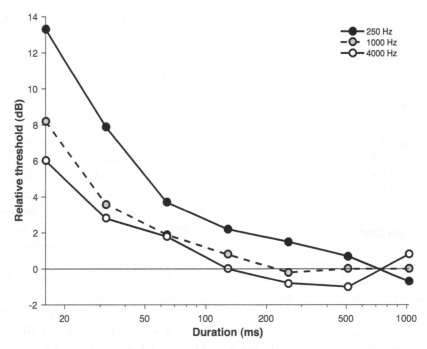

FIGURE 5–17. Data from a temporal integration experiment. Normalized thresholds of pure tone signals are plotted as a function of the stimulus duration. Thresholds are normalized to the 512- and 1024-ms thresholds averaged together. Adapted from Watson and Gengel (1969).

no longer increase has been referred to as the ***critical duration***. For a variety of psychophysical experiments, the critical duration has been estimated to be approximately 200 to 300 ms. The slopes of temporal integration also depended on frequency and were steeper for the lower frequencies. Thus, listeners benefitted more from increased duration of sounds at high frequencies compared with low frequencies.

> Visit the companion website for an auditory demonstration of temporal integration.

We should keep in mind that temporal integration does not imply that short-duration sounds are inaudible. Rather temporal integra-

tion indicates that thresholds for short-duration sounds are higher than for long-duration sounds. We have the ability to detect short-duration sounds and to discriminate between short-duration sounds, although these tasks will be more difficult if the sounds are short in duration. Essentially, our perception is at its optimal performance when perceiving stimuli with durations that exceed the critical duration.

Mechanisms of Temporal Integration

Two major hypotheses have been proposed that explain temporal integration, and they differ primarily in their assumptions about the time frame over which integration occurs (i.e., the ***time constant***). The first class of models assumes a *long time constant* (on the order of hundreds of milliseconds). These models were developed to explain a critical duration between 200 and 300 ms. However, a second class of models assumes a *short time constant* (e.g., 5 or 10 milliseconds). Both models can predict that performance improves with increasing duration and that beyond a certain duration, improvements are so small as to be negligible. They do, however, make different predictions under certain circumstances, as will be discussed here.

Energy Detection

A few variants of the long time constant integration models exist, which all propose some form of integration or accumulation process over time. A common implementation of this model is an **energy detector** (Green, 1960), which posits that the ear integrates the intensity over time, like the calculation of stimulus energy, up to the critical duration. Because temporal integration varies with frequency, the constant would also be different for different frequencies, and integration would only occur up to the critical duration.

The energy detector model follows the equation:

$$I \times t = k,$$

where I is the intensity of the stimulus at threshold, t, is the time of the stimulus in seconds, and k is a constant. A stimulus with a short duration will require a high intensity at threshold to maintain the constant, k, whereas a stimulus with a longer duration will require a lower intensity at threshold.

The Multiple Looks Hypothesis

Viemeister and Wakefield (1991) questioned the energy detector model and suggested that

perhaps temporal integration is not based on long-term intensity integration. They noted that the energy detector is not an *intelligent* model, as it simply integrates (or accumulates) sound intensity over time rather than *information*. They noted that any type of stimulus information, even if it comes from an interfering sound, would be accumulated into the energy detector. They proposed a more sophisticated model and hypothesized that, over time, the ear conducts a series of short *snapshots* that provide more opportunities to detect the stimulus. In this way, snapshots that do not contain information could be discarded.

They described the **multiple looks hypothesis**, which essentially states that increasing the duration of the stimulus provides multiple opportunities to detect the stimulus. This model is based on the integration of information, in which information from the shapshots (the *looks*) is combined, so that detection ability is better when the observations carry useful information. If the ear takes a series of snapshots of a stimulus over time, the ear can use information from the snapshots that help with the decision and discard the unhelpful snapshots. In this way, detection could occur for a long-duration sound presented at a much lower stimulus level than a brief sound because the ear has many looks at the stimulus. If the ear has only one or a few looks at a stimulus, the ear has a limited ability to combine information across the looks. So, the more snapshots provided to the auditory system via increased duration, the better the threshold (up to a point). This hypothesis and the energy detector both would lead to better thresholds as stimulus duration increased.

Viemeister and Wakefield (1991) asked "which model does a better job of describing temporal integration? The energy model, or the multiple looks model?" They designed a clever experiment to answer this question. They first measured the threshold for one and two pulsed tones but put a noise between the pulses. They proposed that the multiple looks model would *ignore* the noise (see the top panel of Figure 5–18): Two tones would be easier to detect than one and the size of the noise in between the tones would not matter. In contrast, the energy detector would *integrate* that noise into the perception and detecting two tones would be harder than one tone, particularly if the noise level was high (see the bottom panel of Figure 5–18). They measured thresholds for each individual pulse and the two pulses together at three intervening noise levels: 34-, 40-, or 46-dB spectrum level. Figure 5–19 plots the thresholds obtained for pulse 1 (filled, black circles), pulse 2 (filled, gray circles), and both tone pulses (open circles) as a function of the level of the noise. First, thresholds were better for two tone pulses than for one for all noise levels. Second, the intervening noise had only a small effect on the detection threshold, regardless of its level. Viemeister and Wakefield concluded

that the ear ignored the intervening noise and, therefore, there was support for the multiple looks model.

The multiple looks experiment is consistent with the idea that a signal can be sampled and stored in memory so that only the informative temporal looks can be used for the task at hand. One interpretation is that the auditory system conducts a form of intelligent processing in the way it integrates information over time. Such a mechanism would be very useful for everyday listening. In certain circumstances, the auditory system may be capable of discarding extraneous information.

Implications of Temporal Integration for Audiometric Testing

The concept of temporal integration is extremely important for audiological testing. When testing absolute thresholds in the

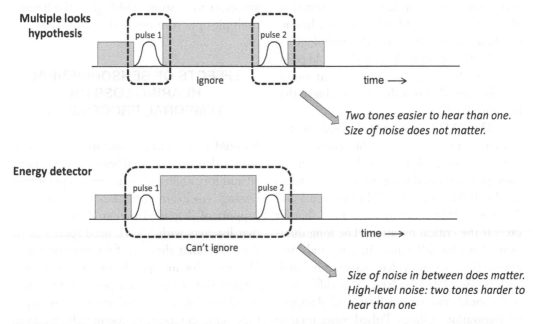

FIGURE 5–18. Illustration of the predictions for the multiple-looks versus energy models for Viemeister and Wakefield's (1991) experiment. The dashed areas illustrate the portions of the stimulus that would be used for a decision. The top panel, which shows the multiple looks hypothesis, only uses the time epochs around the pulses. The lower panel, which shows the energy detector, uses the entire time epoch.

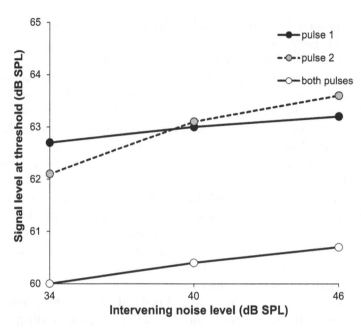

FIGURE 5–19. Data from the multiple-looks experiment. Thresholds for the detection of one tone pulse (*filled circles*) or two tone pulses (*unfilled circles*) plotted as a function of the intervening noise level. Adapted from Viemeister and Wakefield (1991).

audiogram, the audiologist is interested in obtaining the "lowest level sound the listener can hear." Under this goal, the audiologist is tasked with obtaining the best threshold possible. Thus, the audiologist must present sounds at a duration that is sufficient to achieve that best threshold.

The ASHA standards for audiometric assessment provide two possible stimulus presentation modes that are both based on the concept of temporal integration. Steady tones for threshold testing should be between 1 and 2 seconds (ASHA, 2005), a duration that far exceeds the critical duration. The long duration allows for differences in temporal integration that may be evident across individuals with hearing loss who have large differences in thresholds and potentially degraded temporal integration abilities. Pulsed tones used in obtaining the audiogram are also standardized at 200 ms (ASHA, 2005), a value very similar to the critical duration. Three pulsed tones are

sufficient for testing, which gives the listener multiple opportunities to detect the tone.

EFFECTS OF SENSORINEURAL HEARING LOSS ON TEMPORAL PROCESSING

It would be easy, but incorrect in many cases, to assume that sensorineural hearing loss degrades all auditory abilities, including temporal processing. An example that is often given in support of degraded temporal processing is that listeners with SNHL need speech to be slowed so that they can fully understand it. However, slowing speech may simply allow a listener time to process a poorly represented signal that has a degraded spectral and amplitude representation. Consequently, we must measure temporal processing directly before making inferences about temporal processing using speech stimuli.

The prevailing consensus is that when temporal processing is measured by gap detection and amplitude modulation detection, many listeners with sensorineural hearing loss do not have degraded temporal processing. In other cases, such as forward masking and temporal integration, SNHL indeed disrupts the temporal representation of sounds. The studies discussed in this section also have demonstrated huge variability in abilities within the group of listeners with sensorineural hearing loss. Thus, we should avoid making general, sweeping statements about the temporal processing abilities of listeners with sensorineural hearing loss. Such variability stresses the importance of making measurements in individual listeners.

Temporal Resolution in SNHL

The hallmark of hearing loss is elevated thresholds, which lead to a reduction in stimulus audibility in a frequency-dependent way. Hearing loss decreases the representation of sound level in the auditory system and in many cases alters the internal representation of stimulus bandwidth (i.e., hearing loss acts as a filter), particularly for sloping or rising losses. Thus, care must be taken when interpreting the results of temporal processing experiments, as experiments on temporal resolution (gap detection, TMTF, and forward masking) all, to some degree, illustrate level and bandwidth effects.

Recall that low stimulus levels and restricted stimulus bandwidths lead to elevated gap detection thresholds and poorer modulation detection thresholds. Stimulus level also impacts forward masking, and lower stimulus levels are associated with less release from forward masking. In order to interpret temporal processing measurements in listeners with hearing loss, then, we must consider stimulus audibility and the frequencies that

a person can hear. The experiments discussed here have gone to great lengths to address these two issues. Approaches include presenting stimuli at supra-threshold levels, equating sensation levels between two groups of listeners, and simulating hearing loss by presenting a threshold-equalizing noise to normal hearing listeners while they perform the tasks at hand.

Temporal Resolution and SNHL: Steady Sounds

Several studies have measured both gap detection and TMTFs in listeners with SNHL for steady sounds, such as white or relatively wide bands of noise. Fitzgibbons and Wightman (1982) measured gap detection thresholds within band-pass sounds presented at similar sensation levels (SLs). They found a large range of performance across the listeners in their study, and on average, gap detection thresholds were slightly elevated for listeners with SNHL relative to listeners with normal hearing. Florentine and Buus (1984) controlled for audibility by simulating hearing loss with a masking noise presented to the listeners with normal hearing during the task. They measured gap detection thresholds within noise stimuli presented at the same SPL. They found that the listeners with true sensorineural hearing loss and those with simulated hearing loss had higher gap detection thresholds than the listeners with normal hearing. From this result, Florentine and Buus concluded that the increase in thresholds associated with hearing loss caused the higher gap detection thresholds, not a true temporal processing pathology. Yet, Florentine and Buus also noted that some listeners with SNHL performed worse than the listeners with simulated hearing loss at the highest presentation levels. These listeners likely experienced true temporal processing deficits.

We can conclude from these studies that whereas many listeners with SNHL do not experience deficits in temporal processing when measured using gap detection, some listeners likely experience temporal processing deficits associated with SNHL. The audiogram has not been a reliable indicator of who may or may not experience such deficits.

Equating the stimuli used in studies that compare performance between groups of listeners with different hearing levels can be very difficult. Presenting sounds at equal sensation level sounds is appealing, but the internal representations of the sounds likely differ between two groups due to loss of cochlear nonlinearity. As a result, we may not be comparing *apples to apples*. Studies also frequently use noise masking to elevate thresholds of listeners with normal hearing. This experimental manipulation is considered to yield more valid comparisons between the two groups of listeners than equating sensation level, but also has limitations because the listeners with normal hearing must conduct perceptual measurements in the presence of an audible noise masker.

Bacon and Viemeister (1985) measured TMTFs in listeners with normal hearing and SNHL. When stimuli were broadband noises, the listeners with SNHL had higher modulation detection thresholds and a lower TMTF cutoff frequency than listeners with normal hearing. However, when Bacon and Viemeister low-pass filtered the stimuli, the TMTFs measured in listeners with normal hearing demonstrated the same trend—higher modulation detection thresholds and a lower TMTF cutoff frequency, suggesting that this result may have occurred due to portions of the broadband noise being inaudible to the listeners for SNHL. Other well-controlled

studies have confirmed that TMTFs are generally similar for listeners with normal hearing and those with hearing loss (Bacon & Gleitman, 1992; Moore et al., 1992). Although most studies come to this conclusion, there are studies that document small deficits in the ability to detect amplitude modulation in listeners with SNHL (Lamore et al., 1984).

Taken together, it is thought that sensorineural hearing loss does not yield large deficits in either gap detection or amplitude modulation detection when audibility is taken into account. Across the studies conducted, however, one hallmark is a wide range of performance by listeners with sensorineural hearing loss. Gap detection thresholds can be very elevated in some listeners with SNHL, suggesting that a small subset of listeners may have true deficits in temporal processing. Because these deficits can exist, we should not treat listeners with SNHL as a homogenous group in their perceptual abilities. We must consider that some listeners with SNHL experience temporal processing deficits, even if many do not.

Temporal Resolution and SNHL: Fluctuating Sounds

When stimuli contain slow fluctuations, such as narrowband noise, listeners with SNHL demonstrate significant deficits in gap detection compared with those with normal hearing (Glasberg & Moore, 1992; Glasberg et al., 1987). These differences can be attributed to a loss of compression in the ear with sensorineural hearing loss, which greatly alters the internal representation of fluctuating sounds for listeners with sensorineural hearing loss and leads to an elevated gap detection threshold.

Consider that sensorineural hearing loss is almost always associated with a loss of outer hair cells. Absent or damaged outer hair cells cause low-level sounds to be inaudible and contribute to a loss of the compressive nonlinearity within the cochlea. Loss of the compressive non-linearity changes the cochlear response and has a particularly profound effect on the representation of sounds that fluctuate over time. To illustrate these effects, Figure 5–20 provides a schematic of how loss of the compressive nonlinearity alters the shape of the internal psychological representation of a fluctuating waveform. The top panel of Figure 5–20 illustrates the representation of a fluctuating sound in an ear with the compressive nonlinearity intact (a typical ear), and the bottom panel depicts the same sound without the compressive nonlinearity (the ear with SNHL). By comparing the two panels, we observe that the waveform that has been passed through the compressive nonlinearity has reduced fluctuations compared with the waveform that has not been processed. We observe that compressed sound also has fewer temporal valleys in the waveform than the uncompressed sound. If we consider that

when listeners are asked to detect a gap, they may be confused between the naturally occurring valleys in the waveform and a gap placed into a sound by the experimenter. Thus, listeners who do not have the compressive nonlinearity may have greater difficulty determining if a gap is present, resulting in an elevated (larger) gap detection threshold.

In one way, we can think about this as an indication that the ear with SNHL provides a more faithful representation of the fluctuations present in sounds. This more faithful representation leads to an internal representation in which the stimulus envelope is exaggerated compared with someone with normal hearing. In fact, when audibility is carefully controlled for and sounds are presented at the same sensation levels, listeners with SNHL sometimes demonstrate better amplitude modulation detection thresholds than listeners with normal hearing, in certain circumstances (Bacon & Gleitman, 1992). This finding supports an

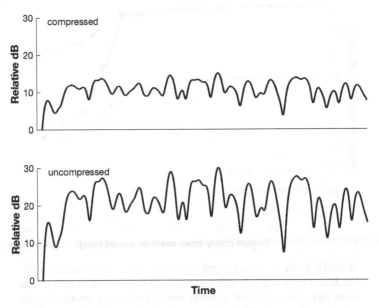

FIGURE 5–20. Two internal representations of a fluctuating envelope. The top panel illustrates the envelope of a waveform representative of an ear with a functioning compressive nonlinearity. The bottom panel illustrates the same envelope, but for an ear that has lost compressive nonlinearity.

interpretation that the representation of the envelope may be exaggerated in listeners with SNHL. We can envision that the exaggeration of stimulus envelope could alter the perception of envelope in everyday sounds and is not necessarily advantageous.

Forward Masking

Forward masking is highly impacted by the presence of hearing loss. Regarding masking in general, listeners with sensorineural hearing loss experience greater effects of masking and poorer frequency selectivity in both forward and simultaneous masking paradigms. Applied to temporal processing measures, we observe that listeners with SNHL experience a reduced release from forward masking—that is, the decay of a forward masker persists for

a longer period of time than for listeners with normal hearing. Figure 5–21 illustrates this result by plotting Glasberg et al.'s (1987) data obtained from a forward-masking experiment. Glasberg et al. measured the detection threshold of a brief 10-ms tone pulse presented at various temporal locations within and after a 200-ms band-limited noise masker. They measured performance for the listeners with SNHL at a high and audible level. They measured performance for listeners with normal hearing at two levels: the same sound pressure level (SPL) and the same sensation level (SL) as the listeners with SNHL.

Examining the data obtained at the same SPL (black, filled circles versus unfilled squares), we observe that detection thresholds were very similar for the two groups of listeners as long as the tone pulse was presented within the masker. However, for the presentations

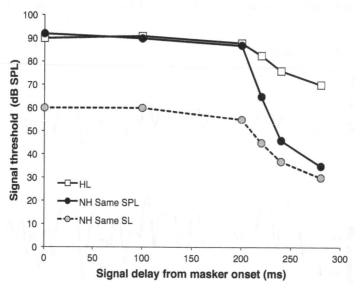

FIGURE 5–21. Forward masking effects for listeners with SNHL. Masked thresholds (dB SPL) are plotted as a function of the time delay between a 200-ms masker onset and signal onset. Thresholds from listeners with hearing impairment are plotted with unfilled squares. Data from normal-hearing listeners measured at the same SPL (*filled circles*) and same SL (*gray circles*) are also shown. Adapted from Glasberg et al. (1987).

occurring after cessation of the masker, we see a marked difference in thresholds between the two groups, where thresholds decreased much more rapidly with signal delay for the listeners with normal hearing than for those with sensorineural hearing loss. Thus, these listeners with sensorineural hearing loss experienced: (a) more forward masking and (b) less of a release from forward masking than those with normal hearing. The reduced release from forward masking suggests that the maskers and signals need to be separated farther in time from one another for the listener with SNHL to experience a return to absolute threshold.

Next, evaluating the data from the listeners with normal hearing, we see that thresholds were much lower for the same-SL conditions than the same-SPL conditions. Here, the release from forward masking over time was reduced compared with the same-SPL data measured in the same listeners. However, when we compare these data with the data from the listeners with SNHL, the masking release was still faster but only slightly. Presenting stimuli at the same sensation levels illustrates that forward-masking effects can be similar between two groups of listeners, although sensorineural hearing loss is still associated with a reduced release from forward masking.

The reduced release from forward masking has substantial implications for listeners with sensorineural hearing loss. Even when target stimuli are presented in a quiet environment, components of the target stimulus that precede other components can drastically influence the ability to extract information present throughout the duration of the target. For example, within a speech signal, a high-intensity vowel could, in theory, forward- mask a low-intensity consonant, causing difficulty for the listener with SNHL to identify that consonant. Slowing speech can also help with forward masking effects but is not always easily achievable.

Temporal Integration and SNHL

Recall that temporal integration is the ability to take advantage of increases in stimulus duration to improve perception. Not surprisingly, temporal integration is also impacted by SNHL. Listeners with SNHL have poorer temporal integration than listeners with normal hearing (Carlyon et al., 1990; Hall & Fernandes, 1983), and the data from Florentine et al. (1988) are shown here to illustrate this result. Florentine et al. measured thresholds for pure tones at a variety of stimulus durations and attempted to control for audibility and bandwidth using a noise masker to simulate hearing loss. Figure 5–22 plots their average data from listeners with normal hearing (solid line) and individual data from the listeners with sensorineural hearing loss. Because of the different degrees of hearing loss across these listeners, they normalized thresholds by setting the threshold for the 500-ms stimulus to 0 dB. For reference, functions with steeper slopes indicate greater amounts of temporal integration. All the listeners with sensorineural loss demonstrated thresholds that changed less with increasing duration (shallower slopes), indicative of a temporal integration deficit.

As we observe in Figure 5–22, listeners with sensorineural hearing loss achieved their lowest threshold at a duration somewhere between 200 and 500 ms. This value is very similar to the critical duration for listeners with normal hearing. However, a similar critical duration does not automatically imply typical temporal integration abilities, as we also observe that these listeners did not benefit from increasing the duration of the stimulus to the same degree as listeners with normal hearing. One conclusion, then, is that the duration of the stimulus matters much less for those with sensorineural hearing loss than it does for listeners with normal hearing. In

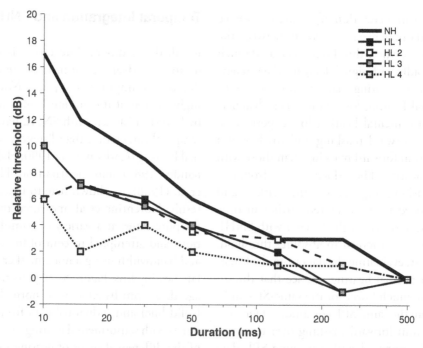

FIGURE 5–22. Temporal integration in listeners with SNHL. The threshold difference in dB between the measured signal threshold and the signal threshold for a 500-ms stimulus is plotted as a function of the signal duration. Data from individual listeners with SNHL are shown as squares with different shading, whereas average data from listeners with normal hearing are shown as the solid line. Adapted from Florentine et al. (1998).

general, these listeners do not benefit from the increased duration to the same degree as those with normal hearing.

Although temporal integration is often measured using detection, Buus et al. (1999) also measured temporal integration of loudness in listeners with SNHL. This approach allowed the investigators to measure temporal integration at supra-threshold levels. In this study, the amount of temporal integration varied widely across the listeners. However, in comparison to listeners with normal hearing, many of the listeners with hearing loss experienced reduced temporal integration for stimulus levels near thresholds, but similar or somewhat greater temporal integration when tested at high sound pressure levels.

Perceptual Consequences of Changes to Temporal Processing

Many listeners with SNHL do not have large distortions to their ability to follow temporal changes in a sound, when measured using gap and modulation detection. However, reduced recovery from forward masking and reduced temporal integration have implications for the perception of both speech and music, in quiet and noisy situations. Yet, as we have discussed previously, it can be difficult to link speech perception difficulties to a singular perceptual deficit, as perceptual changes associated with SNHL often do not occur in isolation. With regards to temporal processing, outer hair cell loss, which contributes to reduced temporal processing, is also associated with loudness recruitment and reduced frequency selectivity. With that, there is a general association between poorer temporal processing with increased speech perception difficulties, and it is well-established that slowing down speech improves understanding for listeners with SNHL.

Logically, it makes sense that someone with diminished temporal processing abilities would have poorer speech perception. Speech is a temporal signal that contains information in the high-and low-amplitude portions of the stimulus (i.e., the vowels and consonants). Within speech, the high-amplitude components have the potential to forward mask the low-amplitude ones. As such, an individual with a reduced release from forward masking might experience perceptual smearing between low-energy consonants and high-energy vowels. These changes to temporal processing would also affect speech understanding in fluctuating noise as they directly impact the ability to take advantage of dips in a fluctuating masker.

A few studies have been able to connect specific temporal processing measures with speech understanding. Gordon-Salant and Fitzgibbons (1993) associated elevated gap duration discrimination thresholds with lower speech perception scores, and they showed that these effects were prominent when speech was time distorted or reverberant. Festen and Plomp (1990) showed that listeners with SNHL had more difficulty understanding speech presented in a fluctuating background than would be predicted by elevated thresholds alone. Further, whereas listeners with normal hearing experienced lower thresholds in the fluctuating noise than in the steady noise, the listeners with SNHL did not (recall Figure 3–21). Dreschler and Plomp (1985) also showed that poor gap detection and forward masking abilities were associated with poorer speech perception in quiet and in noise, respectively. Tyler et al. (1980), who demon-strated poorer temporal integration in listeners with noise-induced hearing loss, also reported that listeners with poorer temporal integration had poorer speech perception scores than listeners with better temporal integration. Taken together, when temporal processing deficits are present, they lead to difficulty understanding speech in a variety of situations.

Summary of Temporal Processing in SNHL

Listeners with SNHL experience a variety of deficits in temporal processing, but not all measures of temporal processing demonstrate these deficits. For gap detection and amplitude modulation, listeners with SNHL in general do not experience deficits. Only a small subset of listeners with SNHL experience true temporal resolution deficits. Nevertheless, poor audibility and a reduced audible bandwidth prevent all listeners with SNHL from fully perceiving the temporal fluctuations in sound. On the other hand, forward-masking experiments illustrate poorer temporal processing in listeners with SNHL. Listeners experience a reduced release from forward masking, in which the representation of the masker persists for a greater period of time than for listeners with normal hearing. Finally, these listeners can commonly experience a reduction in temporal integration, but temporal integration when measured at high stimulus levels may be more similar to that measured in listeners with normal hearing.

AUDITORY NEUROPATHY SPECTRUM DISORDERS (ANSD) AND TEMPORAL PROCESSING

Auditory neuropathy spectrum disorders (ANSD) are characterized by intact outer hair cell function and a disruption to afferent neural transmission (Zeng et al., 1999). Audiometrically, these individuals present with a variety of audiometric configurations ranging from thresholds within normal limits to profound sensorineural hearing loss. There is no characteristic shape or hallmark to the audiogram, particularly in children. Poorer speech perception than would be predicted by the audiogram is an important characteristic of this disorder for many individuals.

Because ANSD is a rare disorder, there are relatively few psychoacoustic studies on listeners with ANSD. However, those studies compellingly report a connection between disrupted neural synchrony and psychoacoustic abilities that depend on that neural synchrony, primarily temporal processing. In one of the first studies available, Zeng et al. (1999) found that poor speech perception of individuals with auditory neuropathy was connected to a severe deficit related to specific temporal processing abilities. They measured temporal integration, gap detection, and amplitude modulation detection in a group of eight individuals with auditory neuropathy. Seven of the eight participants revealed typical temporal integration, but these individuals also demonstrated elevated thresholds in gap detection and amplitude modulation detection. For gap detection and the TMTF, many listeners demonstrated *severe deficits* in temporal processing. Correlation analyses indicated a connection between speech understanding and temporal processing abilities and no relationship between speech perception and audiometric thresholds. The absence of neural synchrony in these individuals is thought to lead to a *temporally smeared* representation of sounds, thus contributing to speech perception difficulties.

To confirm these hypotheses, Zeng et al. (2005) measured additional psychoacoustic abilities in 21 adults with ANSD. They included measures that were expected to be dependent on neural synchrony and others

that were not. They assessed loudness/intensity perception, temporal processing, pitch perception, masking, and binaural hearing. Their results demonstrated that the ANSD only affected perceptual abilities dependent on temporal processing, such as gap detection, amplitude modulation detection, and forward masking. Because these skills require a representation of temporal cues, it was not surprising that these skills were all negatively influenced by neuropathy. Note that this pattern of results differs from that observed for listeners with sensorineural hearing loss of presumed cochlear origin, who generally have robust gap detection and amplitude modulation detection thresholds. Again, the investigators concluded that the loss of neural synchrony associated with ANSD was responsible for the poor temporal processing abilities.

In modern clinical practice, a diagnosis of ANSD generally requires the audiogram, measures of speech perception (when possible, such as for adults), and physiological tests, such as otoacoustic emissions—a test of cochlear function—and the Auditory Brainstem Response, ABR—a test of the neural representation in the brain. However, the strong connection between temporal processing and ANSD suggests that clinical practice may benefit from the inclusion of psychoacoustic testing of temporal processing. A test of temporal processing could be less time consuming and less expensive than an ABR, particularly if rapid implementations of temporal processing measurement (Shen & Richards, 2013) are adopted clinically.

SUMMARY AND TAKE-HOME POINTS

Temporal processing measures relate to the ability of the ear to perceive a variety of temporal events in sound and fall into distinct categories: temporal resolution, temporal masking, and temporal integration. Temporal resolution experiments, such as gap detection and amplitude modulation detection, reflect the ability of the ear to represent the envelope of a stimulus. Temporal masking experiments are also used to measure the amount and duration of internal decay produced by a masker. Temporal integration experiments measure the ability of the ear to benefit from increasing the duration of the stimulus.

Sensorineural hearing loss impacts temporal masking and temporal integration, but many listeners with SNHL do not demonstrate deficits in temporal resolution when measured using gap detection or amplitude modulation detection. Some listeners, however, may experience true temporal resolution deficits, and there is considerable variability in temporal resolution measures in this group of listeners. Overall, the audiogram provides insufficient information to determine whether these deficits are present and the degree to which listeners experience temporal processing difficulties. This observation is particularly evident for some listeners with ANSD, who experience severe deficits in temporal processing.

The following points are key take-home messages of this chapter:

- Gap detection and the temporal modulation transfer function (TMTF) provide estimates of temporal resolution. The best thresholds require audible stimuli and broad bandwidth.
- Forward masking is commonly used to measure temporal masking. Listeners experience a release from forward masking as a signal is moved later in time from a masker.
- Temporal integration experiments demonstrate an improvement in detection thresholds with stimulus duration up to about 200 to 300 ms.
- For many listeners with sensorineural hearing loss, gap detection and TMTF measures are similar to those for normal hearing, as long as audibility is taken into account.

- SNHL leads to less of a release from forward masking and a decrease in temporal integration. These deficits can negatively impact speech perception and may require conversation partners to slow their speech.
- Individuals with ANSD experience significant disruption to temporal processing.

EXERCISES

1. Gap detection is often a component of an auditory processing disorder test battery, and one indicator of auditory processing disorder may be an elevated gap detection threshold. What must be considered in order to interpret whether this threshold is related to poor temporal processing?
2. Consider the following TMTFs measured in two listeners (Figure 5–23). Which listener has the best modulation detection threshold? Which one has the highest cutoff frequency? Can you conclude which listener has better or worse temporal processing? Discuss.
3. Studies have demonstrated that amplitude modulation rates below 16 Hz are the most important for speech intelligibility. Given this information, which listener in Exercise 5–2 will have the easiest time understanding speech? Explain.
4. Discuss the advantages and disadvantages of measuring temporal processing using gap detection versus the TMTF. In your answer include which of these methods might be more appropriate in a clinical setting?
5. Loudness is subject to temporal integration. Sketch data for loudness as a function of stimulus duration that you predict would be consistent with temporal integration.
6. The multiple looks experiment showed that thresholds decreased by 3 dB for the detection of two tone pulses compared with one. If the threshold for one tone

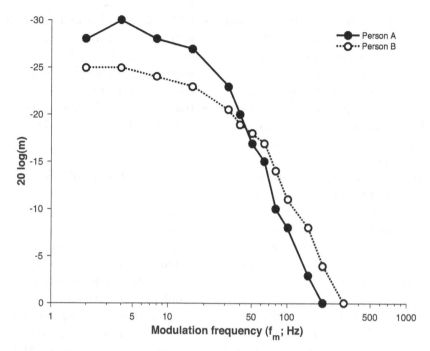

FIGURE 5–23. TMTFs for Exercise 5–2.

pulse was 50 dB SPL, sketch predicted thresholds for 1, 2, 4, and 8 tone pulses (all separated by about 20 ms).

7. ASHA suggests that three 200-ms tone pulses can be used to test thresholds. If your patient has normal hearing, would using more tone pulses improve his threshold? Discuss. What if your patient had a hearing loss?

8. ASHA suggests that three 200-ms tone pulses can be used to test threshold. Using your knowledge of temporal integration, would using three 100-ms tone pulses provide poorer thresholds? Discuss. Consider whether the frequency of the test tone matters and whether any expected changes in threshold are within test-retest reliability of the clinical adaptive procedure.

9. Using your knowledge of temporal integration, is there any benefit of presenting a steady tone of three seconds instead of one second when measuring an audiogram in a listener with sensorineural hearing loss?

10. Discuss how a reduced release from forward masking by listeners with hearing loss might make speech more difficult to understand, even if presented in quiet.

11. Discuss whether making sounds louder would be expected to improve the temporal representation of speech for listeners with sensorineural hearing loss.

12. Sketch a possible TMTF for an individual with normal hearing and one with ANSD who has audiometric thresholds within normal limits.

Visit the companion website for lab exercises.

REFERENCES

American Speech-Language-Hearing Association. (2005). *Guidelines for manual pure-tone threshold audiometry* [Guidelines]. https://www.asha.org/Policy

Bacon, S. P., & Gleitman, R. M. (1992). Modulation detection in subjects with relatively flat hearing loss. *Journal of Speech and Hearing Research, 35*(3), 642–653.

Bacon, S. P., & Viemeister, N. F. (1985). Temporal modulation transfer functions in normal-hearing and hearing-impaired listeners. *Audiology, 24*(2), 117–134.

Buus, S. R., Florentine, M., & Poulsen, T. (1999). Temporal integration of loudness in listeners with hearing losses of primarily cochlear origin. *Journal of the Acoustical Society of America, 105*(6), 3464–3480.

Carlyon, R. P., Buus, S. R., & Florentine, M. (1990). Temporal integration of trains of tone pulses by normal and by cochlearly impaired listeners. *Journal of the Acoustical Society of America, 87*(1), 260—268.

Dreschler, W. A., & Plomp, R. (1985). Relations between psychophysical data and speech perception for hearing-impaired subjects. II. *Journal of the Acoustical Society of America, 78*(4), 1261–1270.

Eddins, D. A., Hall, J. W., & Grose, J. H. (1992). The detection of temporal gaps as a function of frequency region and absolute noise bandwidth. *Journal of the Acoustical Society of America, 91*(2), 1069–1077.

Festen, J. M., & Plomp, R. (1990). Effects of fluctuating noise and interfering speech on the speech-reception threshold for impaired and normal hearing. *Journal of the Acoustical Society of America, 88*(4), 1725–1736.

Fitzgibbons, P. J., & Wightman, F. L. (1982). Gap detection in normal and hearing-impaired listeners. *Journal of the Acoustical Society of America, 72*(3), 761–765.

Florentine, M., & Buus, S. (1984). Temporal gap detection in sensorineural and simulated hearing impairments. *Journal of Speech and Hearing Research, 27*(3), 449–455.

Florentine, M., Fastl, H., & Buus, S. (1988). Temporal integration in normal hearing, cochlear impairment, and impairment simulated by masking. *Journal of the Acoustical Society of America, 84*(1), 195–203.

Garner, W. R., & Miller, G. A. (1944). Differential sensitivity to intensity as a function of the duration of the comparison tone. *Journal of Experimental Psychology, 34*(6), 450–463.

Glasberg, B. R., & Moore, B. C. J. (1992). Effects of envelope fluctuations on gap detection. *Hearing Research, 64*(1), 81–92.

Glasberg, B. R., Moore, B. C., & Bacon, S. P. (1987). Gap detection and masking in hearing-impaired and normal-hearing subjects. *Journal of the Acoustical Society of America, 81*(5), 1546–1556.

Gordon-Salant, S., & Fitzgibbons, P. J. (1993). Temporal factors and speech recognition performance in young and elderly listeners. *Journal of Speech, Language, and Hearing Research, 36*(6), 1276–1285.

Green, D. M. (1960). Auditory detection of a noise signal. *Journal of the Acoustical Society of America, 32*(1), 121–131.

Hall, J. W., Grose, J. H., Buss, E., & Hatch, D. R. (1998). Temporal analysis and stimulus fluctuation in listeners with normal and impaired hearing. *Journal of Speech, Language, and Hearing Research, 41*(2), 340–354.

Kohlrausch, A., Fassel, R., & Dau, T. (2000). The influence of carrier level and frequency on modulation and beat-detection thresholds for sinusoidal carriers. *Journal of the Acoustical Society of America, 108*(2), 723–734.

Lamore, P. J. J., Verweij, C., & Brocaar, M. P. (1984). Reliability of auditory function tests in severely hearing-impaired and deaf subjects. *Audiology, 23*(5), 453–466.

Moore, B. C. (1973). Frequency difference limens for short-duration tones. *Journal of the Acoustical Society of America, 54*(3), 610–619.

Moore, B. C. J., Shailer, M. J., & Schooneveldt, G. P. (1992). Temporal modulation transfer functions for band-limited noise in subjects with cochlear hearing loss. *British Journal of Audiology, 26*(4), 229–237.

Plack, C. J., & Oxenham, A. J. (1998). Basilar-membrane non-linearity and the growth of forward masking. *Journal of the Acoustical Society of America, 103*(3), 1598–1608.

Plomp, R. (1964). The rate of decay of auditory sensation. *Journal of the Acoustical Society of America, 36*(2), 277–282.

Pumplin, J. (1985). Low-noise noise. *Journal of the Acoustical Society of America, 78*(1), 100–104.

Shailer, M. J., & Moore, B. C. (1985). Detection of temporal gaps in bandlimited noise: Effects of variations in bandwidth and signal-to-masker ratio. *Journal of the Acoustical Society of America, 77*(2), 635–639.

Shen, Y., & Richards, V. M. (2013). Temporal modulation transfer function for efficient assessment of auditory temporal resolution. *Journal of the Acoustical Society of America, 133*(2), 1031—1042.

Tyler, R. S., Fernandes, M., & Wood, E. J. (1980). Masking, temporal integration and speech intelligibility in individuals with noise-induced hearing loss. In I. Taylor & A. Markides (Eds.), *Disorders of auditory function* (pp. 211–236). Academic Press.

Viemeister, N. F. (1979). Temporal modulation transfer functions based upon modulation thresholds. *Journal of the Acoustical Society of America, 66*(5), 1364–1380.

Viemeister, N. F., & Wakefield, G. H. (1991). Temporal integration and multiple looks. *Journal of the Acoustical Society of America, 90*(2), 858–865.

Watson, C. S., & Gengel, R. W. (1969). Signal duration and signal frequency in relation to auditory sensitivity. *Journal of the Acoustical Society of America, 46*(4B), 989–997.

Zeng, F. G., Oba, S., Garde, S., Sininger, Y., & Starr, A. (1999). Temporal and speech processing deficits in auditory neuropathy. *Neuroreport, 10*(16), 3429–3435.

Zeng, F. G., Kong, Y.Y., Michalewski, H. J. & Starr, A. (2005). Perceptual consequences of disrupted auditory nerve activity. *Journal of Neurophysiology, 93,* 3050–3063.

Zwislocki, J. J. (1969). Temporal summation of loudness: An analysis. *Journal of the Acoustical Society of America, 46*(2B), 431–441.

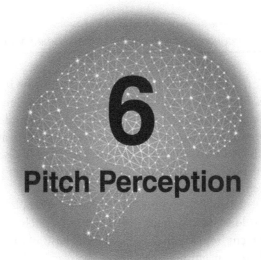

6

Pitch Perception

INTRODUCTION

The perception of pitch is an important part of everyday sound perception: From identifying a person's voice in a background to following the melody of a musical passage, perceiving pitch facilitates our communication and allows us to enjoy the sounds around us. *Pitch* is defined as the "attribute of auditory sensation in terms of which sounds may be ordered on a musical scale" (ANSI S1.1, 2013). This definition may appear somewhat vague, and it may be easier to think of pitch as the perceptual property of sounds that allows them to be ordered from *low* to *high*.

In many cases, pitch can be considered a perceptual correlate of frequency: Increases in frequency are often associated with increases in the perceived pitch. Yet, the terms frequency and pitch are not interchangeable—pitch is a perceptual attribute, whereas frequency is an acoustic property. It is misleading to substitute the word pitch when one means frequency and *vice versa*. Notably, as we will see in this chapter, factors other than frequency influence the pitch of sounds. Even more importantly, not all sounds have a pitch, even though all sounds have frequency content. This reason alone is compelling enough to avoid the common mistake of interchanging these two, rather different, terms.

Because pitch is a psychological perception (like loudness), we cannot measure it directly. Consequently, experiments employ measurement techniques like those used for loudness assessment. Matching and rating have historically often been used to quantify pitch. However, as we will see in this chapter, subjective assessments of pitch, particularly those adopting rating techniques, have been much less successful than when those same techniques are applied to loudness. Perhaps this is because pitch is different from loudness, as pitch does not really have a magnitude—a high pitch is not really bigger than a low pitch. Furthermore, the pitch of sounds contains more dimensions than just *high* or *low*. Rather, sounds have pitch strengths—they can be clear, strong pitches or they can be weak.

Over the years, many techniques have been used to study pitch perception and this chapter will focus on the following aspects:

- *The codes for pitch perception.* This section reviews the two possible codes for pitch perception—the place model, a spectral code for pitch, and the temporal model, a code for pitch based on temporal periodicities.
- *Pitch of pure tones.* Here, we review the experiments that have led to our understanding of whether the place model or temporal model codes for the pitch of pure tones, and we cover both scaling/rating procedures as well as frequency discrimination experiments.
- *Pitch of complex sounds.* Here, we review the experiments that have led to our understanding of whether the place model or temporal model codes for the pitch of complex sounds. We discuss the pitch of the missing fundamental, rating experiments, and fundamental frequency discrimination.

The perception of pitch has been of great interest to auditory scientists and musicians for centuries, so it may not be surprising that the study of pitch has historically been a cen-

tral question for the field of psychoacoustics. This chapter will review how experiments have contributed to our understanding of pitch and how sensorineural hearing loss affects pitch perception. We will discuss the following concepts, as they apply to pitch perception:

- Acoustics: Complex tones
- Theories of pitch perception and the physiological basis of pitch
  - The place code
  - The temporal code
- Pitch perception of pure tones
- Pitch perception of complex sounds
- Sensorineural hearing loss and pitch
- Importance of pitch perception in everyday listening, including for listeners with sensorineural hearing loss

ACOUSTICS: HARMONIC COMPLEX TONES

Many types of sounds in our environment have a pitch, including both pure tones and complex sounds. Pure tones are typically considered to have the purest and the strongest pitch, and we have extensively reviewed the acoustic characteristics of pure tones in Chapter 2. Complex sounds can also have pitch; the pitch of those sounds and the strength of their pitches depend on certain acoustic characteristics that are important to our understanding of pitch perception. Complex sounds can be noisy in nature, or they can be harmonic. Here, we focus specifically on harmonic stimuli, although it is worth noting that in certain circumstances, noises can also evoke a pitch, as is discussed later in this chapter. In order to fully understand how sounds evoke a pitch, we must first review the acoustics of those sounds.

Whereas a pure tone can be characterized by its amplitude and frequency, with the period (T) being easily determined by $1/f$, where f is the frequency of the pure tone, *complex tones*, on the other hand, consist of multiple tones. Complex tones containing frequencies that are related to each other by integer multiples are called *harmonic* sounds or *harmonic* tones. In many but not all stimuli, the lowest frequency of a complex tone is the *fundamental frequency (f₀)*. Importantly, the harmonics occur at integer multiples of the fundamental frequency. There are numerous examples of harmonic sounds in our daily lives, such as vowels and sounds typically generated by stringed, woodwind, and brass musical instruments.

The following equation characterizes the waveform of harmonic tones:

$$y = \sum_{n=1}^{N} a_n sin(2\pi n f_0 t + \theta_n),$$

where a_n refers to the amplitude of the nth tone or *harmonic*, f_0 refers to the fundamental frequency (in this type of sound, the lowest frequency in the stimulus), t refers to time, θ_n indicates the phase of the nth tone, and N indicates the total number of harmonics in the complex tone. Note that the Σ denotes a sum, and therefore this equation represents the sum of harmonics 1 to N.

All harmonic sounds contain certain common acoustic characteristics:

- *They are periodic.* Periodic sounds repeat over time. A pure, synthesized sound will repeat exactly; however, most natural sounds contain some variability such that each cycle of the period appears slightly different from the others.
- *The repetition rate is determined by the f₀.* The rate at which the stimulus repeats (the *repetition rate*) is determined by the fundamental frequency (f₀) and can be calculated by 1/f₀. We can also quantify the repetition

rate in terms of the period (T) of the complex sound.

To illustrate the nature of complex tones, the acoustics of a natural complex sound produced by a trumpet (middle-C; C4) are illustrated in Figure 6–1. The waveform shown in the left panel is a short snapshot of the full note. We see that this waveform is not that of a pure tone because the overall characteristic does not appear to be sinusoidal. Yet, we also observe a very consistent structure in the waveform that repeats over time: The repetition rate of the stimulus is 3.83 ms; there is a peak in the waveform occurring every 3.83 ms. Because the period of this sound is 3.83 ms, we can calculate the fundamental frequency of the stimulus to be 261 Hz (i.e., 1/0.00383s = 261 Hz).

We also easily see the representation of the fundamental frequency in the spectrum, plotted in the right panel of Figure 6–1. The peaks in the spectrum occur every 261 Hz. For example, the first four peaks occur at frequencies of 261, 522, 783, and 1044 Hz. The spectral representation contains information about the fundamental frequency in two different ways. The first is that the fundamental frequency is represented as the lowest frequency component in the spectrum. We see this in Figure 6–1 as a harmonic at the 261-Hz frequency. It is extremely common for natural sounds to contain a spectral peak that corresponds exactly to the f_0. However, the fundamental frequency is also represented by the relationship between the various harmonics. Note that the spectral peaks occur at multiples of the fundamental frequency (e.g., 261, 522, 783, and 1044 Hz), and as a result they all have a common frequency of 261 Hz. More generally, the f_0 of any sound is the greatest common frequency (GCF) among the harmonics.

When we use the GCF to calculate the fundamental frequency, we notice that removing the lowest frequency of the stimulus does

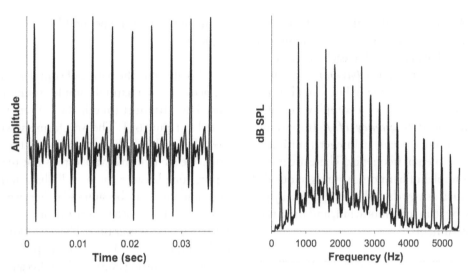

FIGURE 6–1. Waveform (*left panel*) and spectrum (*right panel*) of the musical note C4 (f_0 = 261 Hz) played by a trumpet.

not alter the fundamental frequency. For example, the harmonics of 522, 783, and 1044 still have a GCF of 261 Hz. The effects of removing low-frequency components from a complex tone are illustrated in Figure 6–2. This complex tone has a fundamental frequency of 200 Hz. The top panels illustrate the effects of removing low-frequency harmonics from the sound spectrum. The bottom panels show the waveforms of each of the corresponding sound spectra. As the top panels illustrate, removing the low-frequency harmonics does not alter the spacing between the other spectral components, keeping the GCF and, therefore, the f_0 intact. The bottom panels indicate that removing the harmonics does not change the repetition rate of the stimulus, although some of the waveform characteristics do change. For any stimulus, we can remove subsequent harmonics (e.g., the 1st, 2nd, 3rd, 4th, and so on) with the same results: The fundamental frequency will remain at 261 Hz until all harmonics are removed except the very last one. Note also that removing the odd harmonics will yield a different result: If 261, 783, 1305

Hz, and so forth, are removed, the remaining components will be 522, 1044, 1566 Hz, and so forth. This stimulus would have a fundamental frequency of 522 Hz.

This section has primarily focused on the representation of the fundamental frequency, as that is a primary determinant of the pitch of complex tones (Helmholtz, 1863). However, as we observed in Figure 6–1, each harmonic can have a different amplitude. Although the amplitudes of those harmonics have little to do with the pitch of the sound, they contribute to different attributes of the stimulus, primarily its loudness and timbre (the quality). The characteristics of the sound source (e.g., voice source at the glottis) and the filtering of that source (e.g., resonant cavities of the vocal tract) determine the amplitudes of the harmonics.

THEORIES OF PITCH PERCEPTION

There are two main theories underlying perception of pitch in the auditory system: the *place code* and the *temporal code*. Both mod-

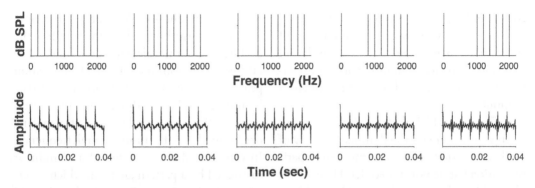

FIGURE 6–2. Illustration of the acoustic effect of removing low-frequency harmonics. Spectra (*top panels*) and waveforms (*lower panels*) are shown. Low-frequency harmonics are progressively removed from a complex tone, illustrated by moving from the left panels to the right panels.

els were originally developed to describe the phenomena that the frequency of a pure tone determines its pitch, and that the fundamental frequency of a complex tone determines its pitch. Each code has its roots in the acoustics of stimuli; the place code is based on a spectral representation, whereas the temporal code is based on a temporal representation of the sound. These theories come about because of the interchangeability between the frequency, or fundamental frequency, and the period of both simple and complex sounds. Essentially, the period and the f_0 are two different ways of describing the same acoustic property. Physiological evidence also supports these two codes, as we now know that the auditory system contains place and temporal representations of the frequency and fundamental frequency in the auditory periphery. Yet, a physiological representation does not automatically infer a psychological representation. Thus, we must discuss psychoacoustic data in light of the physiological data in order to fully understand the perception of pitch. This section reviews the physiological evidence for the two codes and then places them in a psychoacoustic context. Subsequent sections will then present evidence to support or refute these two codes in the formation of pitch.

The Place Code

The place code is effectively a spectral model that posits that frequency of a sound is coded in terms of the place of stimulation in the auditory pathway. This code is rooted in the idea that the ear functions as a Fourier analyzer, with different locations on the basilar membrane (or different neurons) responding to different frequencies. In its simplest form, the place of maximum stimulation determines the pitch (Helmholtz, 1863). In more complex versions, the pattern of excitation determines the pitch in terms of the multiple locations maximally stimulated by harmonics (Goldstein, 1973).

Helmholtz's version of the place code is elegant, simple, and straightforward to understand. He believed that the pitch of a stimulus was determined from the place of maximum excitation in the cochlea. A pure tone evoked a pitch because there was a location on the basilar membrane that coded for the frequency of that pure tone. Thus, because tones of different frequencies stimulated different basilar membrane locations, different pitches were perceived. In addition, he argued that a complex tone evoked a pitch at the fundamental frequency because the harmonic component corresponding to the fundamental frequency was associated with maximal stimulation of the basilar membrane. Any manipulation that shifted the location of maximum excitation would be expected to alter the pitch of a stimulus.

For years, Helmholtz's place theory of pitch perception was the dominant theory of pitch perception. However, modern experimentation has demonstrated that Helmholtz's ideas, although elegant, have not been able to explain all pitch phenomena. These failings will be discussed in subsequent sections in this chapter. Because of failures of his model, more complex variants of the place model have been developed to explain the pitch of complex sounds.

These complex variants of the place model have been referred to as ***harmonic template models*** and are based on the principles that the fundamental frequency of a sound is coded on the basilar membrane and can be derived from the locations of the traveling wave peaks distributed along the length of the cochlea (similar to calculating the fundamental frequency from the GCF). The excitation peaks occur at locations that correspond to the harmonics, and, as we discussed in the section on acoustics, those peaks occur at a spacing determined by the fundamental frequency. In this case, then, the pitch of a stimulus is calculated by a pattern analyzer, which determines the frequencies from the locations of maximum vibration and searches for the common frequency.

The two versions of the place code are illustrated in Figure 6–3, which shows a schematic of the envelope of the cochlear traveling wave for a pure tone (top panel) and for a complex tone (bottom panel). The frequency of the tone in the top panel can be coded from the place of maximum excitation à la Helmholtz (a simple place model). This model can effectively explain why pitch increases with

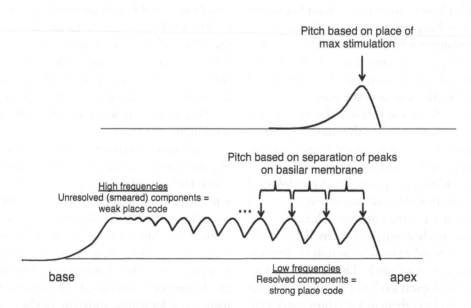

FIGURE 6–3. Schematic of the travelling wave envelope for a single tone (*top panel*) and a complex tone (*bottom panel*). The top panel illustrates a single place of maximum vibration. The bottom panel illustrates multiple places of high vibration and shows that low-frequency harmonics are resolved at the apex and high-frequency harmonics are unresolved at the base of the cochlea.

increasing stimulus frequency. Changing the frequency causes different basilar membrane locations to be associated with the peak excitation. The pitch of the complex stimulus, however, can be coded in multiple ways: (1) the location of the lowest-frequency (apical) component, as in Helmholtz's variant, and (2) the spacing between the places of maximum basilar membrane excitation, as in harmonic template models. Because the spacing between components decreases as frequency increases (as the place representation moves toward the base of the cochlea), the place code is a poor representation of the fundamental frequency at basal locations. When the excitation peaks associated with individual harmonics are not *resolved* (that is, they are smeared together), the place code indicates that the pitch of the stimulus should be difficult to determine or should be very weak. Although the place code is illustrated here using a cochlear representation, excitation patterns are commonly used to make psychoacoustic predictions.

The Temporal Code

Unlike the place code, which is a spectral representation, the temporal code postulates that the pitch of a stimulus is based on the temporal patterns of neural impulses evoked by that stimulus. Wever and Bray (1937) first proposed a physiological temporal code explanation for frequency coding and called their code the *volley theory*. Their theory stated that individual fibers could be synchronized to a waveform, even if they did not fire on every cycle. A group of fibers could then code for the frequency of sound via their pooled response. Through modern measurements, the volley theory has been refined and we now know that a temporal code for frequency is present in the auditory system (Tasaki, 1954) but is only available for frequencies below approximately 3000 to 5000 Hz in the mammalian ear. The temporal code begins at the level of the auditory nerve and requires responses of multiple auditory nerve fibers. The mechanism that codes the period of a stimulus is called *phase locking* and is defined as the propensity for auditory nerve fibers to fire at a particular phase of a low-frequency tone.

Phase locking is demonstrated in Figure 6–4, which illustrates the pattern of firing for multiple auditory nerve fibers in response to a single tone. The top panel of Figure 6–4 illustrates a periodic stimulating wave, whereas each of the bottom panels represents a potential firing pattern for a single auditory nerve fiber. Each of these fibers generates an action potential coincident with the peaks of the stimulus. However, due to refractory periods and other limiting factors, a single auditory nerve fiber cannot always fire at every peak in the waveform. For example, fiber 1 in Figure 6–4 fires during cycles 2, 4, 7, and 11. Other fibers, however, may fire during other cycles of the waveform. Perhaps a different fiber (fiber 2) fires during cycles 1, 4, 6, and 10. Another fiber might fire during cycles 1, 5, 8, and 11 and so on. Taken collectively, the firing pattern of multiple auditory nerve fibers provides a code for the period of a stimulus, as the temporal separation between spikes is always a multiple of the stimulus period. The temporal separation between the pooled spikes corresponds to the period.

A common way to represent the behavior of an auditory nerve fiber is to describe the firing patterns in the form of a period histogram. A period histogram represents the number of spikes, summed over many stimulus presentations, plotted as a function of the phase within a single period. To illustrate phase locking abilities measured physiologically, Figure 6–5 shows a period histogram measured in the auditory nerve of a squirrel monkey by Rose et al. (1971). Figure 6–5 illustrates the number of spikes generated for an auditory nerve fiber tuned to 1100 Hz and a stimulating

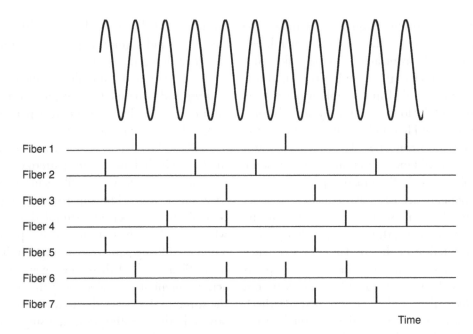

FIGURE 6–4. Illustration of phase locking to a pure tone. The top panel illustrates sine wave stimulation. The bottom panels illustrate firing of individual neurons, where each line represents an action potential (a spike). Note that neurons tend to fire at the peak of the sine wave, but not necessarily every cycle. Collectively, the nerve fibers code for the stimulus period.

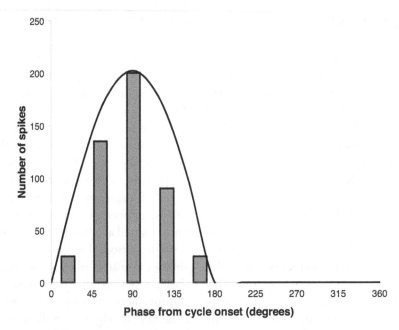

FIGURE 6–5. Period histogram of the squirrel monkey auditory nerve for a 1100-Hz tone. Adapted from Rose et al. (1971).

tone of 50 dB SPL. We observe that this fiber tends to generate the most spikes at the peak of the stimulus cycle (which is at 90° for a sine wave with 0° starting phase).

Numerous other investigators have measured phase locking abilities in the auditory nerve and have made the following observations:

- *Limited phase locking at high frequencies.* Phase locking to pure tones has been demonstrated to occur for stimulus frequencies up to approximately 3 to 5 kHz (Johnson, 1980) and depends on the species. The limiting factor in this case is the frequency of stimulation, and not the center frequency of the auditory nerve fibers themselves, as auditory nerve fibers are homogeneous—their properties do not vary based on the location of cochlear innervation.
- *Small, but measurable, dependence on intensity.* Phase locking to pure tones can be dependent on the intensity of the stimulus. The interval between spikes varies little with changing intensity (Rose et al., 1971). However, other measurements, such as those by Young and Sachs (1979), demonstrated that the synchronization of phase

locking across fibers increases with stimulus level.

The auditory nerve can also phase lock to the envelope of a stimulus. Although high-frequency auditory nerve fibers may not be able to phase lock to an individual harmonic within a complex stimulus, it can phase lock to the period of that complex stimulus (Joris & Yin, 1992). Figure 6–6 illustrates how this might work. The top panel illustrates a complex waveform with slow envelope fluctuations. Schematics of firing by two fibers are shown in the bottom panels. Here, the fibers fire in response to the peaks of the stimulus envelope, and not to the fast fluctuations of the stimulus. In this way, high-frequency auditory nerve fibers can code the fluctuation rate.

Taking these results together, we note that auditory nerve fibers may phase lock to pure tones, as long at the stimulus frequency is below 3 to 5 kHz. For pure tones, then, the temporal code is a relatively *low-frequency phenomenon*. For complex tones, however, the temporal code is present in both high-and low-frequency fibers. Although high frequency fibers will not phase lock to pure tones, they

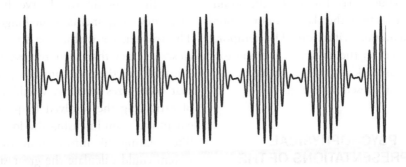

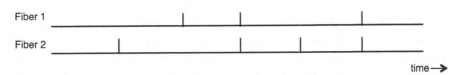

FIGURE 6–6. Illustration of phase locking to a complex stimulus.

can and do phase lock to slow fluctuations of complex stimuli (i.e., the envelope). Given that fundamental frequency is represented as individual harmonics but also in the repetition rate, both high-and low-frequency auditory nerve fibers can code for the fundamental frequency. Low-frequency fibers will phase lock to individual harmonic components, whereas high-frequency fibers will phase lock to the fluctuation rate of the envelope.

A focus of the field has been to determine which code best describes pitch perception, but both codes might work in concert. One possibility is a combination of the place and temporal codes. This *spectral-temporal code* is based on the idea that the temporal patterns in the auditory nerve form the code for the pitch, but these temporal patterns must align with the appropriate place in the cochlea (Loeb et al., 1983). This version of the code requires both place and temporal information to be appropriately aligned and synchronized. Distortions to either cochlear representation could lead to altered pitch.

In summary, auditory physiology provides two potential codes for representing the frequency and the fundamental frequency of a stimulus—the place and the temporal code. The place code is based on extracting stimulus frequencies from the place(s) of maximum basilar membrane vibration. The temporal code is based on the ability of the auditory nerve to phase lock as a representation of temporal patterns present in sounds.

PSYCHOPHYSICAL REPRESENTATIONS OF THE PLACE AND TEMPORAL CODE

As we have just discussed the physiological representation of stimulus frequency, we now turn to psychoacoustical representations. To demonstrate how the ear provides multiple representations for complex sounds from a psychoacoustical perspective, Figures 6–7 and 6–8 depict how the pitch of a stimulus might be generated for a 100-Hz harmonic tone. Figure 6–7 represents the place code in the form of the excitation pattern, whereas Figure 6–8 illustrates the temporal code by showing waveforms at the output of different auditory filters across the range of frequencies in the stimulus.

Figure 6–7 illustrates the place code. The top panel shows the spectrum of a harmonic stimulus with a 100-Hz fundamental frequency, which is passed through an auditory filter bank. The power at the output of each auditory filter is calculated, resulting in the excitation pattern. The excitation pattern in the bottom panel Figure 6–7 reveals the two possible place models: an excitation pattern peak at 100 Hz and a representation of the integer-multiple harmonics in the low frequencies. Note that the low-frequency harmonics are resolved, meaning that their peaks are represented in the excitation pattern. We can see the peaks at 100, 200, and 300 Hz and so on. However, these peaks reduce in size as harmonic frequency increases, due to the broadening of frequency selectivity with increasing frequency. At some point, around the 10th harmonic, we observe that the high frequency components are no longer resolved. The frequencies within the stimulus are so close together that their representations are smeared together. A complex place model that recognizes patterns would be capable of extracting the resolved frequencies present in the stimulus using the low-frequency filters. Using this information, the auditory system could calculate the greatest common frequency and determine the pitch.

The temporal model also uses the auditory filter bank but is based on the waveform output from those filters. Figure 6–8 illustrates how the temporal code might work. The top panel represents the waveform of the same sound illustrated in the top panel of Figure

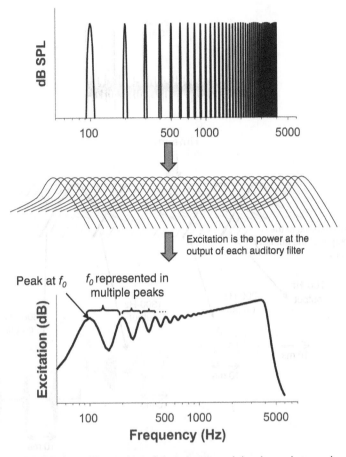

FIGURE 6–7. Illustration of the place model using a harmonic tone with a 100-Hz fundamental frequency. The spectrum is shown in the top panel, the auditory filter bank in the middle panel, and the excitation pattern in the bottom panel.

6–7. This stimulus is passed through the bank of auditory filters, shown in the middle panel, and the outputs of selected auditory filters are illustrated in the bottom panel of the figure, with frequencies ranging from low to high. For the filters centered at 100 Hz and 200 Hz, the outputs look nearly sinusoidal, illustrating that these filters pass a single harmonic. A temporal code based on consistent periodicities could represent these two frequencies easily—the auditory nerve can phase lock to these low frequencies. As the auditory filter frequency increases, however, interactions between components begin to occur and the

output waveforms no longer appear sinusoidal. The waveform outputs of the 1300- and 3000-Hz auditory filters contain multiple frequencies leading to modulated waveforms having both slow and fast fluctuations. A temporal code would have the ability to represent the slow fluctuations, as the auditory nerve would phase lock to the fundamental frequency. Note that these filtered waveforms repeat at the same rate as the 100-Hz tone, and their 10-ms periods are illustrated in Figure 6–8. Synchrony in the output waveforms across multiple auditory filters could provide a very robust code for the period (and therefore

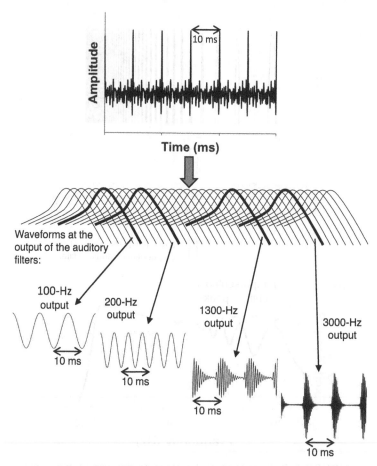

FIGURE 6–8. Illustration of the temporal model using a harmonic tone with a 100-Hz fundamental frequency. The waveform shown in the top panel and the auditory filter bank in the middle panel. Waveforms at the outputs of four auditory filters are shown, and the 10-ms periodicity is illustrated on each output waveform.

the pitch) of a sound. Psychophysical models capture the temporal synchrony across frequency bands in the form of across-frequency *autocorrelation*, which determines the periodicities present in the stimulus and captures whether those periodicities are coherent across frequency.

As we have discussed, a physiological representation of a temporal code for frequency does not automatically imply that this information is used at higher levels of the auditory

system to create a pitch, although it is probable. Coupling behavioral measurements with physiological provides more powerful arguments to support of one model over the other for pitch perception, or perhaps the operation of both. After all, physiological measures do not assess hearing and must be interpreted under measurements of perception.

The primary questions addressed by the studies on pitch perception are "Which mechanism is responsible for pitch perception?" and "Is that mechanism the same for pure and complex tones?" So far, it has not been straightforward to deduce which mechanism is dominant, and all mechanisms likely work together to varied degrees. The codes can operate simultaneously and in parallel, and it can be very difficult to determine whether one code dominates over another. Furthermore, if one code is disrupted, say through hearing loss or another factor, another code may remain to provide a pitch perception.

PITCH OF PURE TONES

Subjective Measures

The earliest work on pitch perception consisted of connecting scientific observations with acoustics. Musicians, physicists, and otologists understood that there was a strong relationship between the acoustic quantity of frequency and the psychological quantity of pitch and that increases in frequency were associated with increases in pitch. This knowledge formed the beginning of our understanding of the relationship between pitch and stimulus frequency and led to models of pitch perception that are still accepted by modern scientists.

However, the early observations did not allow the measurement of pitch for two reasons. First, as with loudness, we cannot measure the pitch of a pure tone—we can only measure the pitch of that tone relative to another tone. Second, to measure the relationship between the pitch of one tone and that of another tone, we need a reference stimulus and a measurement scale. In the 1930s, S. S. Stevens, a pioneer in the study of loudness perception, also paved the way for measurement of pitch. He applied his methodologies to pitch, although, as we will see, with less success. Although we can be rather critical of

many of Stevens' methodologies and assumptions, there is no doubt that his investigations laid the groundwork for our understanding of pitch perception.

Effects of Frequency

Stevens et al. (1937) employed a *magnitude production* technique to determine the relationship between the pitch of a pure tone and its frequency. In this seminal study, Stevens et al. presented a reference tone to listeners and asked them to adjust the frequency of another tone so that its pitch was estimated to be 1/2 that of the reference. In this way, they measured the relationship between the pitch of one sound and another. Stevens et al. then assigned the number of 1000 to the 1000-Hz tone, and called the unit of pitch the *mel*, where 1000 mels is defined as the pitch associated with a 1000-Hz tone. The mel scale can be interpreted in the following way: 500 mels corresponds to a pitch ½ that of 1000 Hz and 2000 mels would be a pitch twice that of the pitch at 1000 Hz. Figure 6–9 illustrates the relationship between frequency and pitch in mels.

The data in Figure 6–9 show several important findings:

- *Increases in frequency were associated with increases in pitch.* There was a clear, monotonic relationship between frequency and pitch, in which increasing the frequency also increased the pitch.
- *The relationship between frequency and pitch was not linear.* The relationship between the pitch of the sound in mels and frequency was different above and below 1000 Hz. For frequencies below 1000 Hz, there was a mostly linear relationship between the pitch in mels and frequency: A 500-Hz tone had a pitch of approximately 500 mels and a 100-Hz tone had a pitch of approximately 100 mels. On the other hand, for frequencies

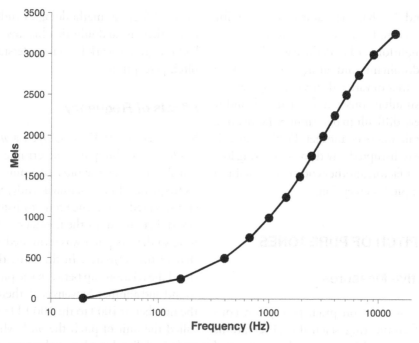

FIGURE 6–9. Mels vs. frequency (Hz). Adapted from Beranek (1949).

above 1000 Hz, the pitch in mels tended to be lower than the frequency of the test tone, and the higher the frequency the greater this discrepancy.

> Visit the companion website for an auditory demonstration of magnitude production of pitch.

Criticisms of the mel scale are many, ranging from bias in experimental techniques to wide variability within and across listeners with normal hearing to the fact that it does not correspond to the musical scale and its associated perceptions. In fact, if we conceptually consider the implications of applying subjective scaling procedures to a perception like pitch, further questions arise. Unlike loudness, pitch does not have a *magnitude*, and the mel scale ignores pitch strength (the

degree to which a pitch is clear and strong) and pitch chroma (the perception of similarities of octaves), which are also important aspects of the pitch percept. The data relating the mel to frequency are suspect and potentially problematic. As a consequence, the mel is rarely used in the psychophysical literature, although it is still used in the field of speech perception and by acoustic engineers. However, the experimental result that increasing frequency leads to increasing pitch is important and has been replicated numerous times. The difference in the shape of this function at low vs. high frequencies is also repeatable and suggests different physiological mechanisms responsible for the perception of pitch of sounds of low versus high frequencies.

Pitch Strength

Although the mel scale was an attempt at quantifying the pitch of a stimulus, it does not provide a description of the clearness of the pitch, or whether the sound can be used in a melody. We have all heard sounds with very clear pitches—like those generated by a clarinet or a trombone—and weak pitches —like noises or a whisper. High-frequency pure tones do not evoke a clear, strong pitch. Illustrating this very compelling result, Ward (1954) asked listeners to adjust the frequency of a higher-frequency tone so that it was an octave above a reference tone. When the higher-frequency tones were greater than about 4000 Hz, the matches became highly variable. Later, Attneave and Olson (1971) demonstrated that pure tones at frequencies above 5 kHz do not produce a clear sense of melody, even when their frequencies are organized in a way that one would expect a melody. Attneave and Olson (1971) state, "Something changes rather dramatically at this level [5000 Hz]; phenomenally it is identifiable as a loss of musical quality, whatever that may be" (p. 163). Semal and Demany (1990) measured the upper limit of *musical pitch* and found that it was approximately 4.7 kHz. Thus, it is likely not a coincidence that the highest note on a piano has a fundamental frequency of 4186 Hz. These observations support the idea that pure tones at high frequencies do not evoke a clear, strong pitch, unlike pure tones at low frequencies. High-frequency pure tones can even be perceived as unpleasant, rather than melodic.

The data described here point to an aspect of pitch that is not present in the perception of loudness—sounds can also have a weak or a strong pitch. This dimension is referred to as **pitch strength**. Pitch strength is typically quantified using magnitude estimation techniques, in which the listener rates the pitch strength of a sound. We consider high-frequency pure tones to have low pitch strength, whereas low-frequency pure tones have high pitch strength.

Effects of Intensity

The pitch of a stimulus is dependent not only on its frequency, but also on its intensity, though pitch shifts with intensity are not nearly as large as pitch shifts with frequency. Stevens (1935) made some of the earliest measurements of pitch under conditions of various intensities and demonstrated large changes in pitch with changes in intensity, as high as shifts of 15% to 20%. Using some modifications to Stevens' method, Morgan et al. (1951) found much smaller changes in pitch with intensity than Stevens. They employed a matching procedure in which listeners adjusted the frequency of a test tone so that its pitch matched that of a reference tone. The reference stimulus was always set at 100 dB SPL (indeed this must have been loud!), and the test tones were set to levels lower than that. They conducted their experiment at many different frequencies, three of which are shown in Figure 6–10. Their median data are plotted as the percent change in frequency between the test tone (the lower-level stimulus) and the reference tone (the higher-level stimulus) for the two sounds to have the same pitch.

Morgan et al.'s data illustrate that the relationship between the pitch of a tone and its intensity depends on the frequency of the sound being tested:

- *Low frequency*—as the intensity of a stimulus increased, the pitch of a low-frequency tone (shown as the black, filled circles) decreased.
- *Mid frequency*—as the intensity of a stimulus increased, the pitch of a mid-frequency pure tone (e.g., 500 to 2000 Hz; shown as the unfilled circles) changed very little.
- *High frequency*—as the intensity of a stimulus increased, the pitch of a high-frequency pure tone (shown as the gray, filled circles) increased.

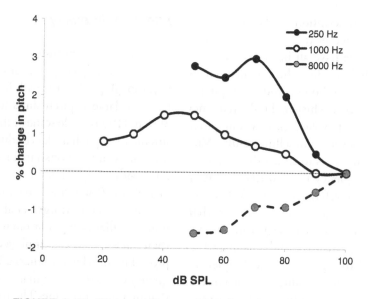

FIGURE 6–10. Pitch matches as a function of intensity. Median percent change in pitch is plotted as a function of stimulus intensity for pure tones presented at three frequencies. Adapted from Morgan et al. (1951).

Thus, although pitch changes with increasing intensity, it does so in a fairly complex way. We generally assume that pitch shifts with intensity are small, though the variability across listeners can be rather large.

Frequency Discrimination

Subjective measures of pitch can be valuable and inform our understanding of how sounds are assigned a pitch and the factors that affect that perception. Accompanying measures, such as just noticeable differences, can complement the subjective measures of pitch described previously. Due to the problematic nature of subjective pitch measurements, most modern experimental evaluations of pitch perception involve discrimination experiments. Techniques adopted in frequency discrimination experiments usually involve standard psychophysical procedures, such as 2-interval, 2-alternative-forced choice (2I–2AFC) and adaptive staircase threshold estimating procedures. A typical *frequency discrimination* task requires a listener to hear two (or more) sounds with differing frequencies and to select the sound with the (often) higher (or different) frequency. To illustrate how this might be implemented in an experiment, Figure 6–11 shows an experimental trial for a frequency-discrimination experiment, where the experimenters ask, "What is the smallest frequency difference necessary to tell that two sounds have a different pitch?" Although the frequency of the stimulus is manipulated, listeners are asked which of the two intervals contains the stimulus with the higher pitch.

Visit the companion website for an auditory visual demonstration of a frequency discrimination experiment.

Several investigators have evaluated frequency discrimination, but Wier et al. (1977) conducted one of the most comprehensive studies. They evaluated frequency discrimination for many different frequencies and many different stimulus levels. In their experiments, they measured the *frequency difference limen (FDL)*, otherwise known as the just noticeable frequency difference (Δf in Hz) between two tones. Data adapted from their study are illustrated in Figure 6–12, which plots the FDL

in hertz as a function of frequency for three different stimulus levels.

Taken together, the data illustrate three primary findings:

- *Exceptional sensitivity.* The frequency-discrimination data shown in Figure 6–12 indicate that humans have an exquisite ability to tell when two tones have different frequencies. At a moderate stimulus level (e.g., 40 dB sensation level), the FDL at

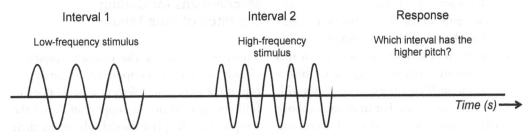

FIGURE 6–11. Illustration of an experimental trial in a frequency-discrimination experiment.

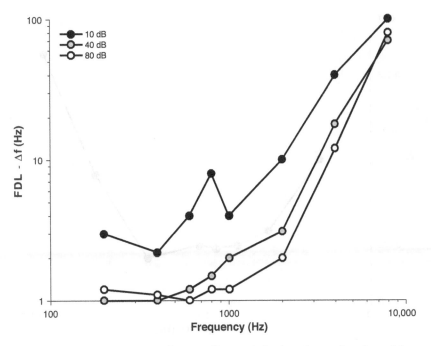

FIGURE 6–12. Frequency difference limens (Δf) plotted as a function of frequency in Hz. Different functions represent data collected from different stimulus levels. Adapted from Wier et al. (1977).

1000 Hz was roughly 2 Hz. Thus, we can hear a change in frequency approximately 2/1000ths of the reference frequency, or 0.2%!

- *Increasing FDL with frequency.* Most strikingly, the FDL increased as the frequency of the reference tone increased. Thus, in absolute frequency, it was more difficult for the listeners to discriminate between pure tones of different frequencies when the frequency was high. In relative terms, however, the relationship is more complicated. To illustrate this, Figure 6–13 plots the data in terms of the Weber fraction, which is $\Delta f/f$ when applied to a frequency discrimination task. Plotting the data in this way indicates that for frequencies below 1500 Hz, the Weber fraction decreases with increasing frequency. For frequencies above 2000 Hz, the ratio increases with increasing frequency.

- *Better FDLs at higher levels.* Referring to Figure 6–12, we observe that thresholds decreased (got better) as the intensity of the stimulus increased. Notably, the change in the FDL with level was also much larger for the low frequencies than the high ones. For example, between 10 and 80 dB SPL, thresholds decreased by about a factor of 4 at 800 Hz but only by a factor of 1.25 at 8000 Hz.

Mechanisms for Coding the Pitch of Pure Tones

Thus, we return to the primary question: Which mechanism is responsible for pitch perception of pure tones? Wier et al. had hoped to find strong evidence in support of either the temporal or the place model. However, their data, by themselves, did not provide strong

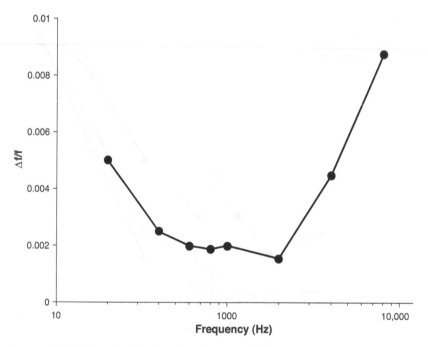

FIGURE 6–13. Weber fractions for frequency discrimination ($\Delta f/f$) plotted as a function of tone frequency measured at 40 dB SL. Adapted from Wier et al. (1977).

support for either the place or the temporal model, but they too identified different trends for low versus high frequencies in the form of the frequency and level effects just mentioned. Thus, their data do implicate two models at work for pitch perception. Further support of two codes operating for frequency discrimination can be found in Zeng et al.'s (2005) test of perceptual abilities in listeners with auditory neuropathy spectrum disorders (ANSD). Their listeners with ANSD had high (worse) FDLs at low frequencies but not high frequencies. Because ANSD is thought to influence temporal synchrony, such results provide evidence for a temporal code at low frequencies.

We can also look to another frequency discrimination experiment, conducted by Henning (1966), to provide additional input into this question as it relates to frequency discrimination. Henning measured frequency discrimination for multiple frequencies, just like Wier et al. However, on every trial, Henning randomly varied the intensity of the sound presented in each observation interval. Henning's manipulation would keep the temporal code intact because random variations in intensity do not affect the degree of phase locking. However, random variations would disrupt the place model, because increasing the intensity of a tone changes the pitch of the tone. Henning found that at low frequencies, the intensity variation did not affect the FDL. However, at high frequencies, the FDL was much worse under the intensity variation. Henning concluded that the place code was supported at high frequencies and the temporal code was supported at the low frequencies.

Across the studies we have discussed, we see a major trend: Pitch perception of pure tones seems to follow a different pattern at low frequencies versus high frequencies. It follows, then, that a different mechanism may be responsible for coding pitch at higher frequencies, above about 3 kHz, versus lower frequencies, below about 1 kHz, although the

breakpoint frequency is somewhat variable, depending on the experiment. Let us first consider the evidence in this vein:

- Mels and frequency are in rough correspondence below 1000 Hz but not above.
- The pitch strength of high-frequency tones is much weaker than for low-frequency tones.
- Morgan et al.'s intensity data indicated a lowering of pitch with increasing intensity at low frequencies but an increasing pitch with increasing intensity at high frequencies.
- The increasingly poor proportion ($\Delta f/f$) needed for frequency discrimination at high frequencies.
- The greater effects of level on the FDL at low frequencies compared with high frequencies.
- An influence of intensity variation on the FDL at high frequencies but not low.
- ANSD affects FDLs at low frequencies but not high.

Recall that the place code is a spectrally based code and is based on the place/s of excitation represented in the cochlea. On the other hand, the temporal code is based on the pattern/s of neural firing and is related to the representation of the period of a stimulus via neural synchrony. These two codes should lead to different patterns of pitch perception, particularly with respect to behavior at high and low frequencies.

Evidence in Support of the Place Code

We first consider the place code. The place code is likely the only code available for pitch perception of pure tones at high frequencies. Physiological data indicate that the temporal model is not in operation at high frequencies due to the lack of auditory nerve phase locking to high-frequency pure tones. Perceptual experimental evidence across a variety of studies also supports this conclusion: (1) The place code is consistent with the increasing pitch with increasing intensity. Recall that increasing the intensity of a stimulus leads to a basal shift in the peak of the traveling wave. This peak shift could lead to an increase in pitch with increasing intensity. However, it should be noted that the perceived shift in pitch is generally much less than that predicted by the shift in the traveling wave peak that occurs when the intensity of a tone is increased (McFadden, 1986); (2) Excitation pattern modeling of frequency discrimination data also supports the place code (Wier et al., 1977), as does (3) the effects of intensity variation on the FDLs as measured by Henning, and 4) the lack of an influence of ANSD on high-frequencies FDLs. On the whole, the place code is supported as coding pitch perception at frequencies above 3 to 5 kHz.

Evidence in Support of the Temporal Code

Next, we consider the temporal code as a potential mechanism for pitch perception of pure tones at low frequencies. Some data sets are encouraging for the temporal code, but not all data are in robust support. The strong perceptions of pitch of low-frequency tones, in contrast to the weak perceptions at high frequencies, suggest that the same code is not responsible for pitch perception in both low and high frequencies. Given that we just concluded that the place model is supported for the pitch of high-frequency tones, perhaps the temporal code is more active for low-frequency tones. Notably, FDLs are not correlated with measures of frequency selectivity- providing an indication of a failure of the place model (Moore & Peters, 1992). The drastic elevation of FDLs at low frequencies for individuals with ANSD provides some strong support for the temporal code. However, there are some issues

with a temporal account of pitch perception at low frequencies. The finding that low-frequency FDLs depend on stimulus level appears to contradict a purely temporal code, and the lowering of pitch with increasing intensity also poses some problems for a purely temporal interpretation. The degree or rate of phase locking does not depend on intensity; rather it is the synchrony across channels.

Summary: Place Versus Temporal Code

Overall, it seems clear that the place code is responsible for coding the pitch percept of pure tones at high frequencies. For low frequencies, however, the conclusions are less clear. The temporal code explains some of the findings, but not all experimental data are consistent with a pure temporal code. Given that the patterns of data are so different for pitch perception between high and low frequencies, we are driven to conclude that the place code is not exclusively responsible for both. Thus, we typically believe that the temporal code has a role to play in the perception of pitch of pure tones in the low frequencies, although further investigations are clearly necessary to fully flesh out the two possibilities. However, it is likely that both codes are in operation for low-frequency sounds to some degree and that the pitch of sounds is determined by a combination of both models, or the model that provides the most robust representation for the task at hand. As Chris Plack states in his book (Plack, 2018) "After all, if both sets of information are available to the auditory system, why not use both?" (p. 122).

PITCH OF COMPLEX SOUNDS

Observations of the pitch of complex sounds have been conducted over many centuries. Helmholtz, though not the first to make these observations, had a clear impact on the theories of pitch perception. A particularly notable observation from his time is that a complex tone produced a pitch that was similar to a tone with a frequency that matched the fundamental frequency of the complex tone. Consider the trumpet note (C4) illustrated in Figure 6–1. In general, someone would hear the pitch of this note as corresponding to middle C. Any instrument playing a note with the same fundamental frequency (261 Hz in this case), would also be perceived as having the same pitch. From observations such as these, we know that the pitch of a complex, harmonic sound is determined by the fundamental frequency.

Using observations like this one, Helmholtz theorized that the pitch of the sound was determined by the place of maximum excitation within the cochlea, and that location must be stimulated by the component corresponding to the fundamental frequency. The simple version of place model was a reasonable explanation for this perception at the time, as his complex tones all contained energy at the fundamental frequency. However, in 1843, Seebeck constructed a siren that produced a harmonic complex that was missing the component corresponding to the fundamental frequency. He observed that the pitch of this sound also matched to the fundamental frequency, despite the absence of that particular component in the stimulus. At the time, Helmholtz discounted Seebeck's observations, and although other investigators did continue to investigate Seebeck's result, little traction was gained on alternate theories of pitch perception until 1940 when Schouten revisited Seebeck's observations.

So, if Helmholtz's model wasn't correct, what model was? Could a temporal explanation explain the pitch of complex sounds? Over the years, several explanations have emerged. Given that both place and temporal codes are present in the auditory system and that both of these codes are present at a single frequency and across frequency (see Figures 6–7 and 6–8), it has been difficult to establish the main code responsible for the perception of pitch of complex sounds.

Pitch of the Missing Fundamental

In 1940, Schouten observed that Helmholtz's version of the place model could not account for the pitch of a complex sound when the harmonic associated with the fundamental frequency was removed (Schouten, 1940). Schouten dubbed this phenomenon the *residue pitch*, also sometimes called the *pitch of the missing fundamental*. One hypothesis explaining the residue pitch was related to Helmholtz's theory: The residue pitch occurred because distortion in the cochlea yielded a traveling wave representation at the location corresponding to the fundamental frequency. However, Licklider demonstrated that a residue pitch still was perceivable even when a low-frequency noise was added that would have masked any representation of that component (Licklider, 1954). This put the nail in the coffin on the distortion hypothesis and confirmed that Helmholtz's theory of pitch perception was incomplete and insufficient.

> Visit the companion website for an auditory demonstration of the pitch of the missing fundamental.

To address the mechanisms responsible for pitch perception, let us examine experiments that have followed those of Seebeck and Schouten to determine whether place or temporal models provide the best explanation for the perception of the missing fundamental. Given the presence of phase locking in the auditory nerve, it seemed distinctly possible that a temporal code for pitch might provide an explanation for the pitch of the missing fundamental.

Ritsma's (1967) seminal findings expanded on Schouten's work and showed that the residue pitch occurs even when <u>many low-frequency harmonics were removed</u>! This work advanced our understanding of the pitch of the missing fundamental and demonstrated that many components could be absent from the stimulus and still produce a residue pitch. Over a series of systematic investigations, Ritsma demonstrated that the residue pitch generally only occurs up to removal of about the 10th harmonic. Removing more harmonics than that causes the pitch of the stimulus to change. The frequency region over which the pitch does not change when harmonics are removed is called the ***existence region*** of the residue pitch. Data from Houtsma and Smurzynski (1990) are shown in Figure 6–14 to illustrate the existence region. They generated a series of complex sounds and asked listeners to identify the melodic interval (e.g., a musical third or a fifth). They then progressively removed the low-frequency harmonics and measured the percent correct identifica-

tion as a function of lowest harmonic present in the stimulus. Figure 6–14 illustrates, very strongly, that listeners began to have difficulty identifying the melodic intervals once about 9 or 10 harmonics were removed. However, even when many harmonics were missing, the scores obtained by Houtsma and Smurzynski were above guessing (50%).

The residue pitch is an astonishing phenomenon, and we probably experience it every day without being aware of it. The telephone does not represent frequencies below about 300 Hz, yet we do not notice difficulties in perceiving the pitch of adult voices that have fundamental frequencies below 300 Hz. Certain musical instruments also do not represent lowest harmonics very well, but we still perceive melodies and notes produced by those instruments. Audio engineers have been able to capitalize on the pitch of missing fundamental to generate the perception of low-frequency fundamental frequencies that are beyond the capability of their equipment to reproduce, and we benefit from this

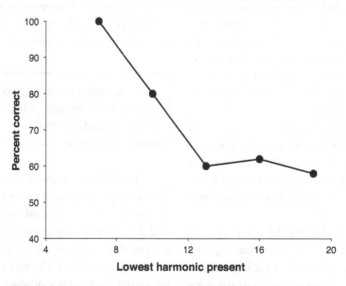

FIGURE 6–14. Data illustrating the existence region for pitch perception. Percent correct melodic interval identification is plotted as a function of the lowest harmonic present in the stimulus. Adapted from Houtsma and Smurzynski (1990).

when we listen to music over our mobile devices.

The Code for the Residue Pitch

The residue pitch effectively renders Helmholtz's view of pitch perception for complex tones obsolete and leaves two possibilities for pitch perception of complex tones. The variant of the place model, the harmonic template model, would require stimulus components to be resolved to extract the pitch of a sound. The existence region of the residue pitch supports this model. Recall that when a complex stimulus is presented, only the low-numbered harmonics have a robust representation in the excitation pattern (see Figure 6–7). Note that Figure 6–7 shows that only harmonics 1 to 8 or 10 have visible peaks in the excitation pattern, and this number does not vary much with fundamental frequency. When harmonics 1 to 10 are removed from the excitation pattern, only the high-frequency smeared portion of the excitation pattern remains. This stimulus, then, would not evoke a pitch based on the place code, and the findings on the residue pitch are consistent with this interpretation.

However, Houtsma and Smurzynski noted that performance on their melodic interval identification task was never at the level of guessing, even when about 20 harmonics were removed from the stimulus! Thus, these sounds must evoke a pitch, albeit a weak one. Thus, there must be some other code for pitch that allowed people to perform that task. The temporal code is a distinct possibility.

A Temporal Code for Complex Pitch Perception

Burns and Viemeister (1976) demonstrated strong support for a temporal code by using noises to evoke a pitch. They measured whether amplitude modulated noises, with modulation rates selected to correspond to musical notes, could be put together to form a melody. These stimuli contained no spectral cues, ensuring that the mechanism for coding pitch was temporally based. They then constructed several common melodies using these stimuli and found that all of their listeners were able to identify the melodies 100% of the time, using only temporal information present in the sounds.

However, data from Fastl and Stoll (1979) indicate that even though a temporal code is present in the auditory system, it does not yield strong pitches like the place code. Fastl and Stoll (1979) measured the pitch strength of a variety of different sounds and used a pure tone as the reference. All stimuli were designed to evoke a pitch matching a 250-Hz pure tone, which was assigned a pitch strength of 100. Their listeners rated the strength of the pitch of the test sounds in comparison to the pitch strength of that tone. A subset of their data is shown here in Figure 6–15 for illustration, which shows the pitch strengths of various sounds plotted in order from high to low. The spectra associated with each sound are also shown, except for the amplitude modulated noise, for which the waveform is plotted. The pure tone had the strongest pitch of all, the complex tones all had pitch strength ratings greater than 60, and the noisy stimuli were assigned pitch strengths close to zero. The amplitude modulated noises were assigned very low pitch strengths, despite their fluctuating nature. Their results demonstrate that low-frequency pure tones are generally associated with the highest pitch strength and that the pitch strength decreases as the acoustics of the stimulus become more like a noise and less like a tone. Note that white noise was assigned a rating of 0, suggesting that it did not evoke a pitch. Together, there is evidence for a temporal code in pitch perception, but the temporal code likely yields very weak pitches.

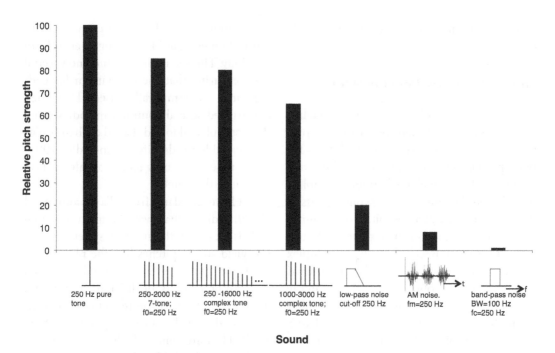

FIGURE 6–15. Pitch strength measured for different stimuli. Adapted from Fastl and Stoll (1979).

> Visit the companion website for an auditory demonstration of sounds with different pitch strengths.

f_0 Discrimination

As with pitch perception of pure tones, discrimination experiments can allow additional, rigorous tests of the place and temporal models. Discrimination experiments have provided considerable information about the perception of pitch of pure tones, and this is no different for complex tones. Rather than evaluating frequency discrimination, however, these experiments focus on the ability to discriminate between two sounds with different fundamental frequencies (f_0s) and they measure the ***fundamental frequency difference limen (F_0DL)***. The harmonics of the sound

can all be present or can be removed as Ritsma did in his experiments on the subjective experience of pitch.

> Visit the companion website for an auditory-visual demonstration of a fundamental-frequency discrimination experiment.

In one test of pitch perception models, Houstma and Smurzynski (1990) measured the F_0DL as a function of the lowest harmonic number present in the stimulus for a complex stimulus with a 200-Hz f_0. Their data are shown in Figure 6–16, which shows that as long as the low-frequency harmonics were present, fundamental frequency discrimination was excellent: The F_0DL was less than 1% of the fundamental frequency (Houtsma & Smurzynski, 1990). Removing the low-frequency harmonics led to

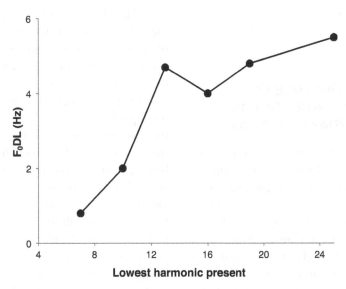

FIGURE 6–16. Data illustrating the existence region for pitch perception. The JND for f_0 (F_0DL) in Hz is plotted as a function of lowest harmonic present in the stimulus. Adapted from Houtsma and Smurzynski (1990).

greater and greater difficulties discriminating between two sounds with different f_0s. A general trend was that as long as the harmonic stimuli contained harmonics 1 to 10, f_0 discrimination was very good, but became worse after more harmonics were removed. Although the F_0DL was larger when some of the harmonics were removed, it was still very low at about 2.5% of the fundamental frequency.

Houstma and Smurzynski's data again provide support for the two models working in concert. When low frequency harmonics are resolved, f_0 discrimination is very good, suggesting a place mechanism. Here, the pitch can be extracted from the resolved components. Once harmonics are no longer resolved, f_0 discrimination becomes more difficult, and the pitch is extracted from the temporal waveform. There would be no possible way for the ear to represent the pitch on a place-based frequency-extraction process when harmonics are not resolved.

Comparison With Pitch Perception of Pure Tones

Taking the results for both pure tones and complex tones, there is compelling evidence in support of both place and temporal mechanisms of pitch perception in the human auditory system. For pure tones, the place code is predominant for high frequencies and the temporal code dominates for low frequencies, but the place code is also likely in operation for low frequencies as well. These two codes are also working in concert for pitch perception of complex sounds. Across-frequency representations and resolvability of harmonic components are important to yield clear and strong pitches. We also see support for both place and temporal codes when low-frequency harmonics are available, whereas the temporal code operates when harmonic components are not resolved. It should not be surprising, then, that models of pitch perception that use both place and temporal codes are the most successful (de Cheveigne, 2005).

IMPORTANCE OF PITCH PERCEPTION IN EVERYDAY LISTENING

Pitch plays a very important role for the perception of speech and music—we use pitch to identify voices, perceive emotion and intonation in speech, and hear melodies in music. Pitch perception is also important for our ability to represent and understand speech in the presence of background sounds. The ability to represent and follow a melody is important for perceiving music and allows a trained ear to listen in on a single instrument playing within an orchestra. This same process also likely influences our ability to focus on a single talker in a room, essentially inhibiting the other talkers to improve understanding.

The ability to use differences in fundamental frequency to improve understanding of speech has been conducted using several studies, ranging from sentences and words to *synthetic vowel* stimuli. Brokx and Nooteboom (1982) demonstrated that speech intelligibility for sentences improves with an increasing f_0 difference between speech and a speech interferer. These benefits generalize to benefits from perceiving speech from different talkers and are particularly beneficial at low signal-to-noise ratios (SNRs). Data from Brungart (2001) illustrate this robust benefit in Figure 6–17. In this study, listeners were presented with a speech signal having the following framework: "Ready <call-sign> go to <color> <number> now." There were eight possible call signs, four colors, and eight numbers. A listener was presented with two sentences, from either the same talker, or different talkers of the same sex, or different talkers of different sex. The target sentence always

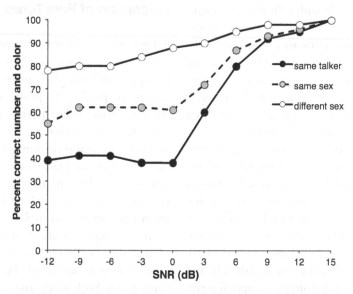

FIGURE 6–17. Percent correct for identifying both the color and number plotted as a function of the SNR in dB for different target + masker configurations. Target and masker sentences were spoken by the same talker, different talkers but the same sex, and different talkers with different sexes. Adapted from Brungart (2001).

had the call sign "baron," whereas the masker sentence had a different call sign. Listeners identified the color and number spoken in the target sentence. Figure 6–17 illustrates the percent correct for identifying both the color and number, plotted as a function of SNR for the three different talker configurations.

Figure 6–17 shows a robust benefit from two primary factors: increasing the SNR and increasing the difference between the target and masker voice characteristics. The benefits of presenting the talker with a background voice of a different sex were huge—at low SNRs performance increased by 40 percentage points! The largest effects were evident at the low SNRs, where performance was worst. The lack of benefit at the highest SNRs either may be due to ceiling effects, as performance cannot be better than 100%, or may reflect that the mechanism responsible for the release from masking is no longer necessary due to the ease of the task.

Using speech as an experimental stimulus has high ecological validity, as these are sounds that humans use and hear daily. However, natural speech stimuli can carry many other variations that might contribute to the benefits measured in this experiment. For example, although female voices have different fundamental frequencies than male voices, their speech has different formant frequencies and may also have temporal differences that facilitate the ability to separate sounds of interest from background sounds. Thus, interpreting data across multiple and different approaches allows better assessment of the mechanisms responsible for perception of natural stimuli.

In an experiment that bridges speech perception and auditory perception, a double-vowel task has also illustrated that listeners benefit from f_0 differences in speech-like stimuli. In this type of experiment, a listener is presented with two simultaneous harmonic sounds, having formants modeled after natural vowel sounds. The two synthetic vowels can have the same or different fundamental frequencies, and a listener identifies the two vowels in the double-vowel pair. Data obtained from Summerfield and Assmann (1991) are shown in Figure 6–18, to illustrate the benefits to speech understanding that can be provided by a simple difference in f_0 between two sounds. Summerfield and Assmann manipulated their frequency differences in the form of semitones, which are twelfths of an octave, the equivalent of adjacent keys on the piano. They showed that small differences in fundamental frequency were associated with improvements of 20 to 30 percentage points on the double-vowel task. Figure 6–18 shows that performance improved drastically for f_0 differences less than one half of a semitone.

Thus, we observe that this trend of benefits afforded by f_0 differences is also present for vowel perception. Even double-vowel experiments have their limitations, however. In some cases, the f_0 benefits may be attributed to a representation of the temporal interactions between the vowel sounds, which is why using all forms of stimuli (speech, synthetic speech, and complex sounds) are important to fully understand the mechanisms responsible for the representation of pitch and its use in everyday listening.

The studies described here both illustrate the importance of pitch perception in our ability to separate a target sound from a background. Given that much of everyday communication occurs in complex environments with many competing signals, robust pitch perception mechanisms are important to facilitate effective communication. Deficits in pitch perception are likely to lead to deficits in the ability to understand speech in the presence of background noise, particularly when that background noise is also speech. As we discuss next, sensorineural hearing loss nega-

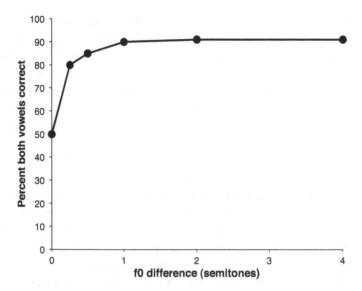

FIGURE 6–18. Percent correct double vowel identification plotted as a function of the f_0 difference between the two vowels in semitones. Adapted from Summerfield and Assmann (1991).

tively influences pitch perception and therefore contributes to difficulty communicating in complex environments.

PITCH PERCEPTION IN LISTENERS WITH SNHL

Listeners with sensorineural hearing loss experience disruptions in their perception of pitch. These disruptions come from alterations to both the place and temporal codes. We know that listeners with SNHL have disruptions to the place code, particularly in the form of reduced frequency selectivity. Consequently, to the extent that the place code is responsible for the pitch of sounds, disruptions to pitch perception are expected. Further, we can measure whether alterations to the place code occur in listeners with SNHL loss, using our tools to measure frequency selectivity. Broadening of frequency selectivity would impact the ability of listeners with SNHL to select

resolved harmonic peaks, thereby impacting pitch perception. Psychophysical experiments also have demonstrated disruption to the temporal code in listeners with hearing loss (Hopkins & Moore, 2011), suggesting that SNHL may alter both the place and temporal codes for pitch.

Subjective Measures

Pitch perception in listeners with sensorineural hearing loss is often poorer than for listeners with normal hearing, but as with other auditory phenomena, considerable variability exists across listeners. Because SNHL influences the perception of pitch, it can lead to *diplacusis*, or the perception of hearing the same tone at a different pitch in each ear. Another way to think of diplacusis is that a single tone is heard as two tones with different pitches, one in each ear. Diplacusis can be measured by asking a listener to adjust the frequency of a tone in one ear so that its pitch matches a tone in the other ear. Listeners with normal hearing have also been demonstrated to have diplacusis, with pitch discrepancies of about 1% to 2% across the ears (Albers & Wilson, 1968). Yet, the magnitude and prevalence of diplacusis is higher in listeners with sensorineural hearing loss. Diplacusis can be quite pronounced in listeners with asymmetrical and severe-to-profound hearing losses.

Yet, although diplacusis occurs in a small set of individuals, subjective studies of pitch perception, especially those that have used pitch-matching techniques, find that most listeners with SNHL do not experience vastly different pitches than listeners with normal hearing. That is, when a pure tone is presented to them, most listeners do not hear the *wrong pitch*. However, studies do demonstrate greater variability in the perception and weaker pitch perceptions in general (Leek & Summers, 2001). Burns and Turner (1986) measured pitch shifts with intensity, and found that some of their listeners with SNHL also experienced greater pitch shifts with intensity than listeners with normal hearing.

Frequency and f_0 Discrimination

Evaluating models of pitch perception, as mentioned earlier, is often conducted using discrimination experiments. Studies have demonstrated that listeners with SNHL experience abnormally large frequency discrimination thresholds for pure tones (FDLs; Moore & Peters, 1992; Tyler et al., 1983). However, these studies also document a wide range of performance abilities when it comes to frequency discrimination. FDLs can be nearly normal in some listeners, but severely elevated in others. Further, neither the audiogram nor frequency selectivity measures correlated with FDLs. The lack of correlation is particularly

problematic for place models of pitch perception, which would predict that poor frequency selectivity should elevate FDLs. The results from this work provide support for the involvement of the temporal code in the pitch perception of pure tones.

Numerous studies have also evaluated f_0 discrimination in listeners with SNHL. In one of these experiments, Moore and Peters (1992) tested a fairly comprehensive set of conditions to broadly characterize f_0 discrimination abilities in this population, and they used particular stimulus constructions designed to address the place code only, the temporal code only, and both the place and temporal codes. Moore and Peters found that, on average, sensorineural hearing loss elevated the F_0DL for all of their experimental conditions. Given that they selected stimuli to address both place and temporal codes, they concluded that deficits to both pitch codes are present in this population. However, as we have seen before, Moore and Peters also noted considerable variability across the listeners in the study, with some SNHL listeners having typical performance and others performing much worse than the listeners with normal hearing. They argued that some listeners may lose place cues to pitch, requiring them to rely more on the temporal code, and other listeners may lose temporal cues, requiring them to rely more on the place code. Taken as a whole, they suggested that both place and temporal cues can be important for pitch perception and that both codes can be impacted by SNHL.

Historically, the effects of SNHL on pitch perception have often been attributed to deficits in the place model of pitch perception. This interpretation has been widely influenced by the view that phase locking does not depend strongly on level or with SNHL (Harrison & Evans; 1979). However, modern psychophysical research suggests that there must be some deficit in the temporal code for listeners with SNHL. Behavioral experimental evidence strongly supports the idea that listeners with SNHL have an altered representa-tion of the temporal code (Hopkins & Moore, 2011). More recent physiological experiments, such as that by Heinz et al. (2010), also find that across-frequency representations of neural synchrony are disrupted in the impaired auditory nerve. Consequently, the poor pitch perception of listeners with sensorineural hearing loss may be due to temporal code distortion, although further investigation is needed.

Summary of Pitch Perception in Listeners with SNHL

Regardless, we see that pitch perception in listeners with SNHL can be disrupted in a variety of ways. Disruptions to the place code can occur because of poor frequency selectivity or an altered representation of the place of maximal stimulation on the basilar membrane. Distortions to the temporal code may also contribute to poor perception of pitch by listeners with SNHL. Asymmetries in pitch representations across the ears can also be problematic, leading to diplacusis, and sloping or rising SNHL could cause the pitch code to be contradictory at high versus low frequencies. In all, these deficits can have a great impact on the appreciation of music and in the perception of speech.

Perceptual Consequences of Changes to Pitch Perception

Deficits in pitch perception can lead to several problems for listeners with sensorineural hearing loss. Pitch provides an important cue for the understanding of speech in complex environments, and so it is not surprising that

deficits in pitch perception can degrade this ability. Listeners with sensorineural hearing loss demonstrate difficulty using pitch cues to segregate sounds from a background. For example, Arehart et al. (1997) showed that the ability to identify two synthetic vowels with different fundamental frequencies was negatively impacted by sensorineural hearing loss. The differences were small under quiet conditions but became much larger when the synthetic vowels were presented in a background noise. Summers and Leek (1998) measured deficits in f_0 discrimination abilities in listeners with SNHL and linked these deficits to difficulty discriminating between speech samples presented at different f_0s. Lorenzi et al. (2006) and Strelcyk and Dau (2009) noted that deficits in the perception of temporal fine structure were also connected to poor speech perception. Overall, poor pitch perception has a strong and detrimental effect on the ability to communicate in complex environments.

Pitch perception also facilitates voice identification, intonation perception, and the perception of emotional state. Alterations to pitch perception could undermine one's ability to gather this important information contained in speech. Diplacusis would be particularly problematic for the perception of pitch in music and can impact the ability of listeners to benefit from two ears if pitch perception differs substantially between the ears. When listeners have difficulty representing the pitch of sounds, we expect a variety of difficulties that are related to communication, and these difficulties are not exclusive to speech understanding.

SUMMARY AND TAKE-HOME POINTS

Two distinct models have been proposed to explain the perception of pitch: the place model and the temporal model. These two codes likely work in concert to produce the perception of pitch. For pure tones, the temporal model is likely the strongest for low-frequency sounds and the place model for high-frequency sounds. On the other hand, the temporal code likely operates in high-frequency regions when representing the pitch of complex sounds, and both codes code for sounds when harmonics are resolved. The perception of pitch is of great importance to facilitate listening in complex environments. Unfortunately for listeners with SNHL, disruptions to pitch perception are commonly associated with cochlear hearing loss.

The following points are key take-home messages of this chapter:

- The auditory system contains two codes of pitch perception: the place code and the temporal code:
  - The place code of pitch perception states that a pitch of a stimulus is determined from the locations stimulated by the frequencies contained in a sound on the basilar membrane.
  - The temporal code of pitch perception states that the pitch of a stimulus is calculated from the pattern of neural firing.
- Pitch perception of pure tones is determined primarily by the temporal code for frequencies below about 1 to 2 kHz and by the place code for frequencies above about 3 kHz.
- Pitch perception of complex sounds is determined primarily by both codes when harmonics are resolved and by the temporal code when harmonics are not resolved. For everyday listening, both codes likely work together to provide robust pitch percepts.
- Pitch perception plays a key role in the ability to separate a target sound from a background, particularly when both target and background are speech.

- Sensorineural hearing loss disrupts both the place and the temporal code, leading to poor pitch perception in listeners with sensorineural hearing loss. Disruptions to either code are associated with deficits in everyday listening.

EXERCISES

1. Determine the frequency of a pitch match for the following sounds. Also indicate whether the pitch is strong, weak, or nonexistent.
   a. A harmonic stimulus with components at 200, 400, 600, 800, 1000, and 1200 Hz
   b. A harmonic stimulus with components at 600, 800, 1000, and 1200 Hz
   c. A noise modulated at 150 Hz
   d. White noise
2. Describe how the place code works for pure tones. Can the place code work at high frequencies, low frequencies, or both?
3. Describe how the temporal code works for pure tones. Can the temporal code work at high frequencies, low frequencies, or both?
4. Using a sketch of traveling waves on the basilar membrane, illustrate how the place model can account for the pitch perception of a harmonic complex with a fundamental frequency of 100 Hz.
5. Using the same sketch in #4 as a baseline, illustrate how the place model can code for a residue pitch if the first three harmonics are missing. You may sketch a new illustration if necessary.
6. In your own words, explain the temporal theory for encoding the pitch of a harmonic complex with a fundamental frequency of 100 Hz. How might this theory explain the pitch of a harmonic complex that does not contain energy at

100 Hz but has a 100-Hz fundamental frequency?

7. You have a patient with a 50 dB SNHL at 1000 Hz and above. If the place model accounted wholly for pitch perception, what should happen to his pitch perception at 2000 Hz? If the temporal model accounted wholly for pitch perception, what should happen to his pitch perception at 2000 Hz? In your answer, discuss the pitch of the sound as well as the pitch strength of the sound. Assume that a 2000-Hz pure tone is presented at an audible level.

8. Tinnitus evaluation often includes pitch matching as a part of the procedures. Given everything that you have learned about pitch so far, consider the following:

    a. If your patient pitch matched his tinnitus to 1000 Hz, do you think that this is a valid measure? Discuss.

    b. Would your answer in (a) change if your patient had a sensorineural hearing loss at 1000 Hz?

    c. If your patient pitch matched his tinnitus to 8000 Hz, do you think that this is a valid measure? Discuss.

9. Harmony comes to your clinic complaining about difficulty understanding speech in the presence of other background talkers. You measure her hearing and find that her hearing levels are within normal limits. Given that she also complains about some deficits in her music perception, you suspect that she might have a deficit in her pitch perception. Consider the methodologies discussed in this chapter and discuss which method might be the best to measure whether poor pitch perception is the source of her difficulty. Discuss.

10. A variety of hearing aid algorithms have been developed to help listeners with hearing loss better understand speech. One of these technologies is a frequency-lowering hearing aid, which essentially takes high-frequency sounds that are inaudible and transposes (lowers) the frequencies so that they can be presented in a region of usable hearing. Considering what you have learned about pitch perception, what are your predictions on the pitch of sounds if they are processed by a frequency-lowering aid? Using the information you have just provided, address whether you would recommend a frequency-lowering aid to a musician. Consider:

    a. if pitch is based on a place code

    b. if pitch is based on a temporal code

11. As discussed in Chapter 5, ANSD is a disorder that primarily affects temporal processing. People with ANSD have good frequency discrimination at high frequencies but not at low frequencies. Using your knowledge of the models of pitch perception, describe why this would be the case.

Visit the companion website for lab exercises.

REFERENCES

Albers, G. D., & Wilson, W. H. (1968). Diplacusis: III. Clinical Diplacusimetry. *Archives of Otolaryngology*, *87*(6), 607–614.

American National Standards Institute ANSI. SI.1. (2013). USA standard acoustic terminology.

Arehart, K. H., King, C. A., & McLean-Mudgett, K. S. (1997). Role of fundamental frequency differences in the perceptual separation of competing vowel sounds by listeners with normal hearing and listeners with hearing loss. *Journal of Speech, Language, and Hearing Research*, *40*(6), 1434–1444.

Attneave, F., & Olson, R. K. (1971). Pitch as a medium: A new approach to psychophysical scaling. *American Journal of Psychology*, *84*(2), 147–166.

Beranek, L. L. (1949). *Acoustic measurements*. McGraw-Hill.

Brokx, J. P. L., & Nooteboom, S. G. (1982). Intonation and the perceptual separation of simultaneous voices. *Journal of Phonetics, 10*(1), 23–36.

Brungart, D. S. (2001). Informational and energetic masking effects in the perception of two simultaneous talkers. *Journal of the Acoustical Society of America, 109*(3), 1101–1109.

Burns, E. M., & Turner, C. (1986). Pure-tone pitch anomalies. II. Pitch-intensity effects and diplacusis in impaired ears. *Journal of the Acoustical Society of America, 79*(5), 1530–1540.

Burns, E. M., & Viemeister, N. F. (1976). Nonspectral pitch. *Journal of the Acoustical Society of America, 60*(4), 863–869.

De Cheveigne, A. (2005). Pitch perception models. In C. Plack & A. J. Oxenham. (Eds.), *Pitch* (pp. 169–233). Springer.

Fastl, H., & Stoll, G. (1979). Scaling of pitch strength. *Hearing Research, 1*(4), 293–301.

Goldstein, J. L. (1973). An optimum processor theory for the central formation of the pitch of complex tones. *Journal of the Acoustical Society of America, 54*, 1496–1516.

Harrison, R. V., & Evans, E. F. (1979). Some aspects of temporal coding by single cochlear fibres from regions of cochlear hair cell degeneration in the guinea pig. *European Archives of Oto-Rhino-Laryngology, 224*(1), 71–78.

Heinz, M. G., Swaminathan, J., Boley, J. D., & Kale, S. (2010). Across-fiber coding of temporal fine structure: Effects of noise-induced hearing loss on auditory-nerve responses. In E.A. Lopez-Poveda, A. R. Palmer, & R. Meddis (Eds.), *The neurophysiological bases of auditory perception* (pp. 621–660). Springer.

Helmholtz, H. (1863/1954). *On the sensations of tone.* English translation published in 1954 by Dover Publications. (First German edition, *on the Sensations of tone as a Physiological Basis for the Theory of Music*, published in 1863.)

Henning, G. B. (1966). Frequency discrimination of random-amplitude tones. *Journal of the Acoustical Society of America, 39*(2), 336–339.

Hopkins, K., & Moore, B. C. (2011). The effects of age and cochlear hearing loss on temporal fine structure sensitivity, frequency selectivity, and speech reception in noise. *Journal of the Acoustical Society of America, 130*(1), 334–349.

Houtsma, A. J., & Smurzynski, J. (1990). Pitch identification and discrimination for complex tones with many harmonics. *Journal of the Acoustical Society of America, 87*(1), 304–310.

Johnson, D. H. (1980). The relationship between spike rate and synchrony in responses of auditory-nerve fibers to single tones. *Journal of the Acoustical Society of America, 68*(4), 1115–1122.

Joris, P. X., & Yin, T. C. (1992). Responses to amplitude-modulated tones in the auditory nerve of the cat. *Journal of the Acoustical Society of America, 91*(1), 215–232.

Leek, M. R., & Summers, V. (2001). Pitch strength and pitch dominance of iterated rippled noises in hearing-impaired listeners. *Journal of the Acoustical Society of America, 109*(6), 2944–2954.

Licklider, J. C. R. (1954). "Periodicity" pitch and "place" pitch. *Journal of the Acoustical Society of America, 26*(5), 945–945.

Loeb, G. E., White, M. W., & Merzenich, M. M. (1983). Spatial cross-correlation. *Biological Cybernetics, 47*(3), 149–163.

Lorenzi, C., Gilbert, G., Carn, H., Garnier, S., & Moore, B. C. (2006). Speech perception problems of the hearing impaired reflect inability to use temporal fine structure. *Proceedings of the National Academy of Sciences, 103*(49), 18866–18869.

McFadden, D. (1986). The curious half-octave shift: Evidence for a basalward migration of the traveling wave envelope with increasing intensity. In R. J. Salvi, D. Henderson, R. P. Hamernik, & V. Colletti (Eds.), *Basic and applied aspects of noise-induced hearing loss* (pp. 295–312). Springer.

Moore, B. C., & Peters, R. W. (1992). Pitch discrimination and phase sensitivity in young and elderly subjects and its relationship to frequency selectivity. *Journal of the Acoustical Society of America, 91*(5), 2881–2893.

Morgan, C. T., Garner, W. R., & Galambos, R. (1951). Pitch and intensity. *Journal of the Acoustical Society of America, 23*(6), 658–663.

Plack, C. J. (2018). *The sense of hearing* (3rd ed.). Routledge.

Ritsma, R. J. (1967). Frequencies dominant in the perception of the pitch of complex sounds. *Journal of the Acoustical Society of America, 42*(1), 191–198.

Rose, J. E., Hind, J. E., Anderson, D. J., & Brugge, J. F. (1971). Some effects of stimulus intensity on response of auditory nerve fibers in the squirrel monkey. *Journal of Neurophysiology, 34*(4), 685–699.

Schouten, J. F. (1940). The residue, a new component in subjective sound analysis. *Proceedings of the Koninklijke Nederlandse Akademie van Wetenschappen, 43*, 356–365.

Seebeck, A. (1843). Ueber die Sirene. *Annals of Physics and Chemistry, 60*, 449–481.

Semal, C., & Demany, L. (1990). The upper limit of "musical" pitch. *Music Perception: An Interdisciplinary Journal, 8*(2), 165–175.

Stevens, S. S. (1935). The relation of pitch to intensity. *Journal of the Acoustical Society of America, 6*(3), 150–154.

Stevens, S. S., Volkmann, J., & Newman, E. B. (1937). A scale for the measurement of the psychological magnitude pitch. *Journal of the Acoustical Society of America, 8*(3), 185–190.

Strelcyk, O., & Dau, T. (2009). Relations between frequency selectivity, temporal fine-structure processing, and speech reception in impaired hearing. *Journal of the Acoustical Society of America, 125*(5), 3328–3345.

Summerfield, Q., & Assmann, P. F. (1991). Perception of concurrent vowels: Effects of harmonic misalignment and pitch-period asynchrony. *Journal of the Acoustical Society of America, 89*(3), 1364–1377.

Summers, V., & Leek, M. R. (1998). f_0 processing and the separation of competing speech signals by listeners with normal hearing and with hearing loss. *Journal of Speech, Language, and Hearing Research, 41*(6), 1294–1306.

Tasaki, I. (1954). Nerve impulses in individual auditory nerve fibers of guinea pig. *Journal of Neurophysiology, 17*(2), 97–122.

Tyler, R. S., Wood, E. J., & Fernandes, M. (1983). Frequency resolution and discrimination of constant and dynamic tones in normal and hearing-impaired listeners. *Journal of the Acoustical Society of America, 74*(4), 1190–1199.

Ward, W. D. (1954). Subjective musical pitch. *Journal of the Acoustical Society of America, 26*(3), 369–380.

Wever, E. G., & Bray, C. W. (1937). The perception of low tones and the resonance-volley theory. *Journal of Psychology, 3*(1), 101–114.

Wier, C. C., Jesteadt, W., & Green, D. M. (1977). Frequency discrimination as a function of frequency and sensation level. *Journal of the Acoustical Society of America, 61*(1), 178–184.

Young, E. D., & Sachs, M. B. (1979). Representation of steady-state vowels in the temporal aspects of the discharge patterns of populations of auditory-nerve fibers. *Journal of the Acoustical Society of America, 66*(5), 1381–1403.

Zeng, F. G., Kong, Y.Y., Michalewski, H. J. & Starr, A. (2005). Perceptual consequences of disrupted auditory nerve activity. *Journal of Neurophysiology, 93*, 3050–3063.

7

Hearing With Two Ears

LEARNING OBJECTIVES

Upon completing this chapter, students will be able to:

- Discuss the benefits of hearing with two ears
- Evaluate the roles of interaural time differences (ITD) and interaural level differences (ILD) in sound localization
- Describe the different binaural mechanisms responsible for reducing the effects of noise on perception
- Assess the effects of hearing loss on binaural perception
- Relate deficits to binaural hearing to everyday listening

INTRODUCTION

Up to this point, we have discussed the perception of acoustic information that is represented by a single ear. In fact, many of the experiments discussed presented sounds to a single ear of the listener, and they therefore tested *monaural hearing*. Yet, a critical component of everyday listening is using two ears —our experiences in the natural environment would be drastically altered if we had only one ear. We also know that people who have monaural hearing loss experience great difficulties in communication compared with those who have *binaural hearing* (hearing with two ears). Further, the location of our ears, which are separated in space on the horizontal plane, causes each of our ears to receive different signals in natural environments.

Binaural hearing provides advantages in a multitude of ways, and this chapter is organized in a way that allows us to discuss the advantages of binaural hearing from multiple perspectives. We will discuss the following aspects of binaural hearing:

- *Binaural summation.* In this section, we review the literature on the advantages of having two ears on sound detection, sound discrimination, and speech understanding.
- *Localization and lateralization.* Acoustic cues and neural mechanisms both have roles in our ability to find the location of sound sources in a three-dimensional (3D)

space. In this section, we discuss the roles of time delays between the two ears, level differences between the two ears, and the function of the pinnae to facilitate sound localization.

- *Binaural unmasking.* Both acoustic and neural mechanisms work to cancel background noise from our auditory perception. In this section, we will review the variety of experiments that have led to our understanding of the role that two ears play in the reduction of the effects of masking noise on perception.

We have already reviewed some of the basic data on hearing with two ears in Chapter 2 in the threshold differences observed between the MAP and MAF functions. MAF thresholds can be 10 to 15 dB better than MAP thresholds. However, these data do not allow a definitive assessment on the hearing advantages that are specific to having two ears. In particular, free-field measurements cannot easily disambiguate the contributions of true binaural phenomena from acoustic interactions between the sound field and the body. Thus, this chapter reviews both free-field experiments as well as experiments conducted over headphones.

We cover the following key topics regarding binaural hearing:

- Binaural advantages in detecting and discriminating between sounds
- Principles of sound localization (binaural hearing in the free field)
  - Acoustic considerations
  - The Duplex Theory of sound localization
  - The physiological basis of binaural hearing
  - Sound localization: Perception
- Lateralization (studies conducted over headphones)
- Binaural unmasking
- Effects of SNHL on binaural abilities

BINAURAL ADVANTAGES TO DETECTION AND DISCRIMINATION

If asked whether two ears are better than one, most people would answer with an emphatic yes! Almost a century of psychoacoustical work has demonstrated small, but consistent, benefits on detection, discrimination, and identification when two of the same sounds are presented to two ears (*binaural*) versus one ear (*monaural*). These psychoacoustic experiments require presenting sounds over headphones, as free-field measures do not allow presenting identical stimuli to each ear. This is the only way to quantify the benefit provided by having a second, but independent, sample of the same stimulus. Note that these conditions are commonly referred to as **monotic** (one ear) and **diotic** (each ear receives an identical stimulus), respectively, and any time the ears receive different sounds, a **dichotic** stimulus results.

Psychoacoustic experiments that use headphones provide a unique opportunity to test the advantages of having two ears over one, as each ear can be stimulated independently from the other. Investigators have used this approach to assess whether detection and discrimination thresholds are better when tested using two ears versus one ear. When we measure the advantage provided by two ears, we are measuring **binaural summation** abilities.

Many of the early psychoacoustic studies demonstrated small benefits of binaural hearing on the threshold for detection or discrimination of sounds across various tasks. Results across the various types of studies that have been conducted are listed in Table 7–1. The table is not an exhaustive review of the extensive work that has been conducted on this subject but is intended to provide a broad overview of the advantages of the binaural system on detection, discrimination, and identification. Roughly speaking, Table 7–1 illustrates that the binaural advantage is small, consis-

TABLE 7–1. Amount of Binaural Advantage Measured in a Variety of Tasks

Task	Binaural Advantage	Investigators
Loudness Summation of Tones	Almost doubling of loudness	Algom, Rubin, and Cohen-Raz (1989)
Loudness Summation of Noise	Doubling of loudness	Marks (1980)
Absolute Threshold of Noise	2 to 3 dB	Pollack (1948)
Absolute Threshold of Tones	2 to 3 dB	Shaw, Newman, and Hirsh (1947)
Threshold in Noise	0 to 2 dB	Hirsh (1948)
Intensity Discrimination	~60%	Jesteadt and Wier (1977)
Frequency Discrimination	~60%	Jesteadt and Wier (1977)
Speech (Speech Recognition Threshold)	~2.5 dB	Shaw et al. (1947)

tent, and very similar across the different tasks. Reaction time experiments to pure tones have also demonstrated a small and consistent binaural advantage (about 4 ms; Simon, 1967).

Although variability across listeners can also be present, and benefits of binaural hearing can range from less than 1 dB to over 10 dB depending on the task and listener, no matter the approach (detection, discrimination, or identification), there is a consistent benefit afforded to the listener who is listening with two ears versus one. Binaural summation depends strongly on the degree of symmetrical hearing between the ears. Even small asymmetries in absolute threshold between the ears reduce the amount of binaural summation observed.

That said, a small improvement in detection threshold can be intensified by higher levels in the auditory system, particularly when we consider the four levels of perception. A small difference in detection threshold can manifest into a large change in performance at the identification level. For example, a change of 1 dB in the speech recognition threshold can be associated with a change of 15 to 20 percentage points on a speech identification

task (Duquesnoy, 1983). Thus, we should not underestimate the potential benefit of binaural summation on our ability to communicate.

SOUND LOCALIZATION IN THE HORIZONTAL PLANE

A primary function of having two ears is the ability to determine a sound's location in space, a process called localization. Humans are best at localizing in the horizontal plane (e.g., left versus right), primarily because that is where the acoustic cues are strongest due to the separation of our ears. Here, we discuss how the acoustical environment provides a situation in which the two ears each receive a different signal that depends on the location of sound. We then review how that acoustic information is utilized by binaural mechanisms in the auditory system.

Acoustics

The binaural representation of sound is primarily generated by the interaction between the head and the acoustic field. The signal received by each ear is determined by the characteristics of the acoustic field, the size of the head, and the location of the sound of interest with respect to the head. We also listen in a three-dimensional space, and so the location of sounds is specified in terms of *azimuth* and *elevation*. The azimuth of sound is represented by the angle on a spherical coordinate system representing the horizontal plane. For reference, 0° is the azimuth of the center of the head (i.e., the nose), 90° is the azimuth of the right ear, and –90° is the azimuth of the left ear. The elevation of sound is represented by the angle on the median plane (the plane that divides the body into left and right halves). A sound directly to the right has 90° azimuth and 0° elevation, whereas a sound directly above has 0° azimuth and 90° elevation.

The most relevant binaural cues to the human listener lie in the horizontal plane and differ only in their azimuth (e.g., left versus right). This is true as our ears are only separated from each other on the horizontal dimension; they are in the same location with respect to elevation (neither ear is higher than the other) and they are in the same location with respect to the front/back plane (neither ear is closer to the front of our bodies than the other). If we assume that the head is a sphere and has no pinnae, the acoustic cues across the ears would provide information about only azimuthal location. However, we should note that our pinnae are asymmetric in both elevation and front/back, and they (along with our bodies) alter sound in subtle ways that influence our binaural auditory perception. The effects of the pinnae are discussed in another section of this chapter.

To fully understand the mechanisms responsible for hearing with two ears, we must first discuss the relationship between the *wavelength* of sound (the distance sound travels in a single cycle) and the size of the human head. Any object within a sound field may disrupt that sound field, and the relationship between the wavelength of sound and the size of that object is of critical importance.

When a sound wave encounters an object, one or more of these events will occur:

1. The sound wave may reflect off the object,
2. The sound wave may diffract around the object, or
3. The sound may be absorbed by the object.

For the purposes of this course, we assume that the sound absorption by the head is negligible. Thus, we need only be concerned with whether sound reflects off the head or diffracts about the head. The degree to which these two events occur will determine the characteristics of the signals that are received by each ear.

Whether a sound is reflected or diffracted is determined by its wavelength and the size of the object encountered. The smaller the ratio between wavelength and object size, the greater the reflected sound energy. The wavelength of sound (λ) is determined by the frequency of sound and the speed of sound, $\lambda = v/f$, where v is the speed of sound and f is the frequency of sound in Hz. The speed of sound is roughly constant, and is approximately 340 m/s. Thus, we observe that the wavelength of sound is inversely proportional to its frequency: Low-frequency sounds have long wavelengths and high-frequency sounds have short wavelengths. Thus, high-frequency sounds are more likely to reflect from objects whereas low-frequency sounds are more likely to diffract around objects. Sounds with intermediate wavelengths will be reflected and diffracted.

Duplex Theory of Sound Localization

Lord Rayleigh (aka John William Strutt [1877]) first proposed the idea that the ability to localize sound was driven by two primary acoustic cues: the difference in level of a sound between the two ears (*interaural level difference; ILD*) and the difference in arrival time of a sound between two ears (*interaural time difference; ITD*). Rayleigh suggested that ILDs were used for high-frequency sound localization and ITDs were used for low-frequency sound localization. The two acoustic effects are illustrated in Figure 7–1, which shows how reflection and diffraction alter the acoustic signal received by each ear. The top panel of Figure 7–1 shows a sound with a short wavelength, whereas the bottom panel shows a sound with a long wavelength with respect to the size of the head. Here, the sound field is illustrated by the icon of a speaker on the right side of the body, and the curved lines emanating from that speaker indicate the peaks of the sound wave. The wavelength is the distance between the curved lines.

Interaural Level Differences (ILDs)

In the top panel of Figure 7–1, the sound source is a tone with a wavelength much smaller than the diameter of the human head (e.g., 5000 Hz, which has a wavelength of about 0.07 m, or 2.6 inches). Because the wavelength is smaller than the head, some portion of this sound reflects off the head. When a sound is to the right of a listener, the reflection reduces the sound energy that arrives at the left ear. Consequently, the intensity of the sound reaching the right ear will be much higher than the intensity of the sound reaching the left ear. The reduction in intensity at the ear distant from the source is called *head shadow*. The head shadow is greatest when the sound is to one side of the head. As a sound moves around the head from the left ear to the center of the head, the degree of head shadow will decrease. A sound directly in front of a listener will not yield a head shadow, and sound intensity at both ears will be the same.

As a result, the level difference (in dB) between the two ears, *the interaural level difference (ILD)* varies as a function of frequency and location of the sound source. Feddersen et al. (1957) measured ILDs as a function of the azimuthal angle and frequency using human listeners. They placed a small microphone in

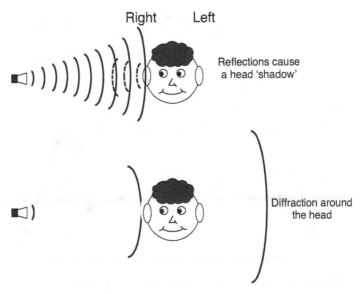

FIGURE 7–1. Illustration of the effects of a spherical body (e.g., a head) on a sound field. The top panel illustrates a high-frequency sound and the bottom panel illustrates a low-frequency sound. In both cases, the sound is depicted as being to the right of the listener.

their ears and measured the sound levels for a variety of sounds. Their measurements are shown in Figure 7–2, which plots the ILD in dB as a function of the angle between the center of the head and the sound. A sound directly in front is presented at 0°, whereas a sound directly to the side is presented at 90°. The different functions indicate measurements made for different tone frequencies. Figure 7–2 illustrates the following trends:

- For all frequencies tested, the ILD was 0 dB when the sound source was directly in front or in back of the listener.
- The ILD was greatest when the sound source was 90° to the side of the listener.
- The size of the ILD increased as frequency increased. The ILD can be as large as 20 dB for high frequencies (>4000 Hz), particularly for sounds located to one side of the body.

Feddersen et al.'s results demonstrate that ILDs become increasingly available to the ear as the frequency increases and as the sound approaches one side of the body.

Interaural Time Differences (ITDs)

In contrast to high-frequency sounds, low-frequency sounds, such as those with wavelengths longer than the diameter of the head, do not produce a large head shadow. The bottom panel of Figure 7–1 illustrates this case where the sound source is a low-frequency tone (e.g., 600 Hz, which has a wavelength of 0.57 m, or 18.7 inches). For very low-frequency sounds, reflections of the sound from the head are negligible and thus, there is no head shadow. In a sense, the head is invisible to the sound field. Rather, sound diffraction is the dominant acoustic effect. Because the two ears are separated in space, there is a delay between the time the sound arrives at the right ear compared with the left.

Feddersen et al. also measured the time delay between the two ears as a function of the location between the listener and the speaker.

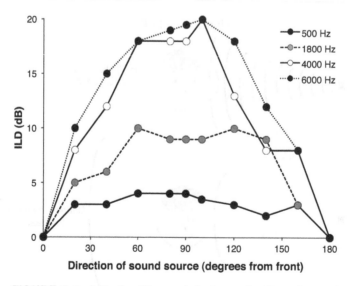

FIGURE 7–2. ILDs (in dB) are plotted as a function of sound location with respect to a human listener, where 0° is front and center. Each function represents an ILD measurement for a different frequency. Adapted from Feddersen et al. (1957).

Figure 7–3, which is adapted from Feddersen et al.'s data, shows the general pattern of time delay versus azimuthal angle. As with the head shadow effect, the time delay between the two ears was greatest for a sound source to the left or the right of the body. These *interaural time differences (ITDs)* were very small, even at the maximum ITD; the maximum ITD was about 0.66 ms or 660 μs.

Because the speed of sound does not vary with frequency, the time for a sound to travel from one ear to another does not depend on frequency. Consequently, both high-frequency and low-frequency sounds will produce an ITD of a fixed amount. However, the *availability* of this information to the ear does depend on frequency. A fixed delay corresponds to a different number of cycles for a low-frequency sound than for a high-frequency sound. For example, a 200-Hz tone presented directly to the right side of the body does not complete a full cycle in the 660 μs needed to reach the left ear, as its period is 5 ms. On the other hand, a 5000-Hz tone has

a period of 200 μs, and when presented to the right side of the body, cycles more than three times in 660 μs. Because of this phenomenon, we must consider the relationship between the ITD, which does not depend on frequency, and the *interaural phase difference (IPD),* which does vary with frequency. We can calculate the IPD for any given frequency from the following equation: 360° (660 μs/T), where T is the period of the stimulus.

Consider our two frequencies again and a sound presented to one side of the body. This location is associated with the largest ITD possible: 660 μs. For illustrative purposes, consider three different frequencies: 380 Hz, 1520 Hz, and 3040 Hz. Figure 7–4 plots two versions of tones at each of these frequencies, one with a 0° starting phase and a second with an ITD of 660 μs, as if the sound were received by the opposite ear 660 μs later. At 380-Hz (shown in the top panel), which has a period of 2.4 ms, 660 μs corresponds to ¼ of a single cycle, or a relative phase difference (IPD) between the two sounds of 90°. Here,

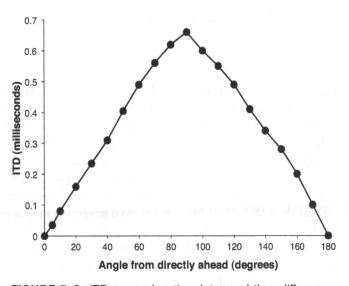

FIGURE 7–3. ITD versus location. Interaural time differences in milliseconds are plotted a function of sound's location with respect to a human listener, where 0° is front and center. Adapted from Feddersen et al. (1957).

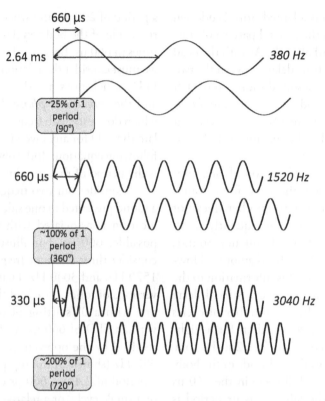

FIGURE 7–4. Illustration of the relationship between IPD and ITD for three frequencies (380, 1520, and 3040 Hz). Each set of waves shows one signal with a 0° starting phase, and a second signal delayed by 660 μs. The time delay imposes a greater phase delay as frequency increases.

at any given time, the signal received by one of the ears is always 90° phase shifted compared to the other ear. For this frequency, there is *unambiguous* information about the phase difference between the ears. More specifically, there is no other location on the horizontal plane that can produce that same IPD—all other azimuthal angles will yield phase differences that are smaller than 90°. 1520 Hz (illustrated in the middle panel) has a period of 660 μs, the same as the maximum ITD across ears. For this sound, the IPD is 360°, or also 0°! In this case, a listener could not differentiate whether the sound is presented to one side or to the front of the body, and therefore the ITD is *ambiguous*. Lastly, 3040

Hz has a period of 330 μs, or ½ of the ITD. This corresponds to an IPD of 720°, which is also equivalent to 360° and 0°. Here, there are three potential azimuthal locations that are associated with this IPD. Thus, we can see that for sounds above about 1500 Hz, phase differences across the ears provide *ambiguous* information about location on the horizontal plane. As a result, the ITD is realistically only available at frequencies below about 1500 Hz.

In summary, the duplex theory of sound localization is primarily based on the availability of acoustic cues to sound location. For high frequencies, the ILD is dominant and for low frequencies, the ITD is dominant. ILDs are only available at high frequencies due to head shadow, and ITDs are only available at low frequencies due to phase ambiguities.

The Cone of Confusion

Again, assuming a spherical, pinnae-less head, there would be a 3D conical surface extending out of each ear that represents the same ITD on the surface (Mills, 1972). Figure 7–5 illustrates this surface, which is called the *cone of confusion*, and it should be thought of as extending infinitely into space. Because the ITD is a relative feature of sound (i.e., it is a difference, not an absolute), sounds originating from a variety of locations could be perceived as being in the same location. The location of any sound on the cone of confusion could be confused with all other sound locations on that surface.

The cone of confusion is important because, without head movements, listeners cannot determine whether sounds are above or below them or whether they are in the front or in the back. Listeners would be able to tell if a sound was on the left or the right. However, the cone of confusion only exists if the head is held stationary. Head movements can easily resolve ambiguities and allow for improved localization, which are important as the cone of confusion illustrates one type of acoustic uncertainty present in our environment. The asymmetrical and curved shape of the pinnae also assists to resolve the cone of confusion.

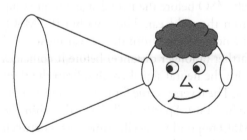

FIGURE 7–5. Illustration of the cone of confusion for a specific ITD. All points on that conical surface have the same ITD.

Sound Localization in the Horizontal Plane: Physiological Basis

To give a sense of the complex circuitry involved in the binaural processing that underlies sound localization, a brief overview of binaural auditory physiology is provided here. A schematic illustrating the binaural connections in the brainstem is shown in Figure 7–6. Binaural auditory interactions begin at the level of the brainstem in the superior olivary complex (SOC), a collection of brainstem nuclei. The left and right portions of the brain each contain components of the SOC, with the left and right SOCs receiving input from both ipsilateral (the same side of the body) and contralateral (the opposite side of the body) cochlear nuclei. Within each SOC are two nuclei with primary roles in binaural hearing: the lateral superior olive (LSO) and the medial superior olive (MSO). The LSO provides codes for ILDs, whereas the MSO codes for ITDs.

Coding for ILDs consists of both excitatory and inhibitory connections (Brownell et al., 1979), and the neural connections to the LSO are illustrated in Figure 7–6. An excitatory neural connection, shown by the solid line, exists between the cochlear nucleus and the ipsilateral (same side) LSO, whereas an inhibitory connection, shown by the dashed line, exists between the cochlear nucleus and the contralateral (opposite side) LSO. To illustrate how this might work, consider a sound located on the left side of the body with a large ILD. Because of head shadow, this sound has a high intensity on the left side of the body and a low intensity on the right and will produce the following pattern:

- The high-intensity sound on the left side will be associated with a large degree of excitation to the left LSO and a large degree of inhibition to the right LSO. This is illustrated by the thick solid lines for the excitatory

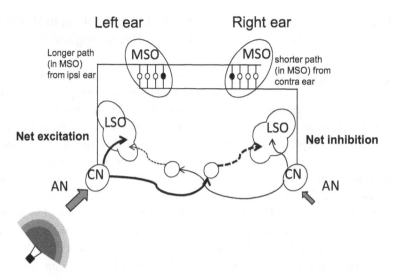

FIGURE 7–6. Schematic of the binaural connections in the superior olivary complex for a sound presented to one side of the body. AN—auditory nerve; CN—cochlear nucleus; LSO—lateral superior olive; MSO—medial superior olive. ILD processing in the LSO is illustrated with solid lines indicating excitatory connections and dashed lines indicating inhibitory connections. The weight of the line indicates the strength of the connection. Within the MSO, the cells receiving coincident input are illustrated by the black ovals.

connections and thick dashed lines for the inhibitory connections.

- The low-intensity sound on the right side will be associated with a small degree of excitation to the right LSO and a small degree of inhibition to the left LSO. This is illustrated by the thin solid lines for the excitatory connections and thin dashed lines for the inhibitory connections.

Together, the left LSO will have net excitation (strong excitation and weak inhibition) and the right LSO will have net inhibition (strong inhibition and weak excitation), providing a physiological cue that a sound is on the left side of the body.

These connections for the MSO are also shown in Figure 7–6. The MSO also receives input from the cochlear nucleus, but it functions as a delay line and coincidence detector (Jeffress, 1948), which is a mechanism for aligning and detecting the neural tempo-ral patterns across the ears. In this example, the left MSO will receive signals from the left cochlear nucleus sooner than it receives signals from the right cochlear nucleus, as it takes longer for the neural signal to reach the contralateral MSO. This effect is illustrated by the black cells responding in the MSO. For example, when sound arrives at the left ear before it arrives at the right ear, the neural signal originating from the left ear arrives at the left MSO before the neural signal originating from the right ear. Then, within the MSO, the neural signal from the left ear must travel farther (a longer distance) before it coincides with the neural signal coming from the right ear. The reverse is true for the cells active in the right MSO. Specific cells located within the MSO respond to specific time delays between the right and left ears.

Together, the LSO and MSO code for ILDs and ITDs, respectively, in the auditory system. They must receive appropriate level and temporal cues to properly represent spatial cues. Consequently, disruptions to auditory nerve input can lead to difficulties representing the appropriate environmental ILD or ITDs. Note also that the LSO and MSO are the first auditory nuclei to receive input from the two ears, but they are not the only binaural nuclei in the auditory system, and other auditory centers also contain binaural representations.

Sound Localization in the Horizontal Plane: Perception

Stevens and Newman (1936) made some of the earliest measurements of the localization of pure tones. As we have discussed, interactions between the head and the sound field are frequency dependent, and their study was among the first to test sound localization abilities in a frequency-specific manner. Stevens and Newman measured sound localization abilities in

the free field with a speaker placed 12 feet away from the listeners. The speaker was in one of 13 different positions on the right side of the listener, ranging from 0° (directly in front) to 180° (directly behind). A pure-tone sound was played from the speaker, and the listener indicated where the speaker was located. Stevens and Newman measured the errors (in degrees) in sound localization and obtained the results plotted in Figure 7–7.

Interestingly, the size of the errors was roughly constant for frequencies up to about 1000 Hz, but in the range of 2000 to 4000 Hz, the size of the errors increased considerably. The errors then decreased again for the very high frequencies. These data support Rayleigh's duplex theory that ITDs and ILDs operate in different frequency regions, with low-frequency localization driven by ITDs and high-frequency localization driven by ILDs. Neither acoustic cue is particularly strong in this frequency range, which explains

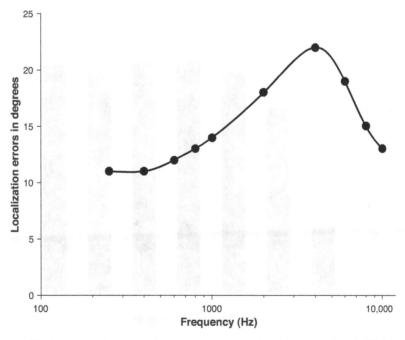

FIGURE 7–7. Sound localization errors for pure tones. Sound localization errors in degrees are plotted as a function of tone frequency (Hz) measured in the free field. Adapted from Stevens and Newman (1936).

the greater errors between 2000 and 4000 Hz. Stevens and Newman also calculated the errors in degrees as a function of the location of the speaker, collapsed across all of the frequencies tested. Figure 7–8 shows that they found the lowest error rates when the speaker was located in the front of the body (0°). Performance was considerably poorer and fairly equal when the speaker was in all other positions tested (between 15° and 90°). Their work indicates that good sound localization abilities are only achievable when our face is pointed toward the sound.

Mills (1958) took a somewhat different approach to measuring the ability to localize sounds and measured the just detectable angle between two sounds. This quantity is commonly called the ***minimum audible angle (MAA)*** today. Mills placed a speaker at a specific location (e.g., 0° in front or 90° to the side) and measured how far the speaker must be moved (in degrees) before the listener was

able to determine that the speaker was in a different location. Mills measured the MAA as a function of frequency and location of the sound source, and data adapted from his experiment are plotted in Figure 7–9. This Figure illustrates the MAA plotted as a function of frequency for three different reference speaker locations (in front, 0°, and 30° and 60° to the right side).

The curve obtained at 0° (in front of the listener) demonstrates that for low-frequency sounds the MAA was incredibly small, about 1°. However, the outstanding sound localization abilities only occurred for the low-frequency tones. Once the signal frequency exceeded about 1000 Hz, sound localization became relatively poor, being two to four times worse at about 2000 Hz. As Mills moved the reference location of the speaker, the MAA also increased. At the 30° reference location, localization for all frequencies was poorer by a factor of two or more than at 0°. Localiza-

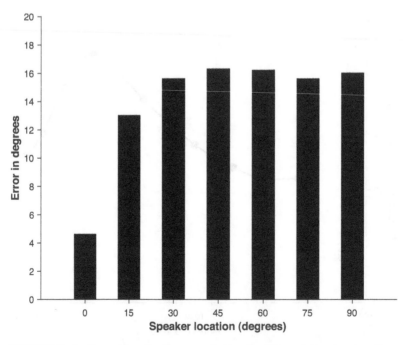

FIGURE 7–8. Sound localization errors as a function of speaker location. Adapted from Stevens and Newman (1936).

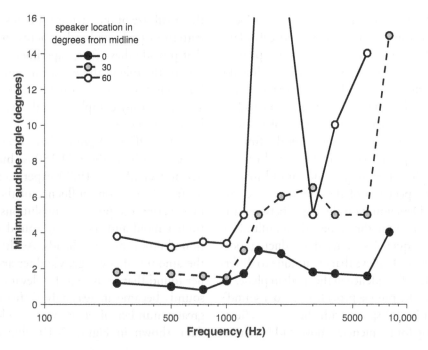

FIGURE 7–9. Minimum audible angle. The minimum audible angle (degrees) is plotted as a function of tone frequency. Each function represents a different reference spatial location with respect to the head, where 0° is front and center. Adapted from Mills (1958).

tion again degraded with increasing frequency and was poor for all frequencies above about 1000 Hz. For the 60° location, performance was so poor at some frequencies that Mills was unable to measure the MAA. In summary, we see similar results from Mills as we observed from Stevens and Newman. Sound localization is best when sounds are in front of the body. Further, sound localization abilities are very good at low and high frequencies, and worse for mid-frequencies.

Such results can also be explained using the duplex theory of sound localization. First, sound localization is best for low and high frequencies, suggesting that the acoustic cue to a sound's location is not robust in the mid-frequencies. These results provide supporting evidence that a different cue is used to localize sounds in the low frequencies (the ITD) compared with the high frequencies (the ILD).

Localization performance also degrades substantially when listeners are asked to localize sounds away from midline. Feddersen et al.'s (1957) data illustrate why this might happen, as their data show that ILD does not change much between 45° and 135°. These functions demonstrate a plateau in this range. In this case, moving the speaker does not produce a different ILD, making it difficult for listeners to use ILDs alone to precisely perceive sound location. As a result, orienting our heads to the sound source is necessary for good sound localization.

SOUND LOCALIZATION IN THE MEDIAN PLANE

Although the previous review has discussed how ITDs and ILDs provide information about sound localization in the horizontal plane, humans also have an ability to localize sounds in the median (or vertical) plane (e.g., elevation). These abilities are primarily influenced by the pinnae, which alter the characteristics of sound in a way that depends on the angle of incidence, thereby providing information about the elevation of a sound source and whether a sound is in the front or back. The pinnae contain ridges and cavities that modify incoming sound and ultimately alter the spectrum of the sound received by the ear. Depending on the angle between the sound source and the pinnae, the amplitude of specific frequencies is altered, producing spectral peaks and valleys that are unique to different angles of incidence in the median plane. In this way, the pinnae provide cues to a sound's location in 3D space, with the largest effects occurring for frequencies above 4 kHz (due to

the small size of the cavities). Because it is the pattern of peaks and valleys across frequency that provide these cues, experimental evaluation of the role of the pinnae in sound localization is only possible using complex sounds, and specifically complex sounds that contain high frequencies.

The effects of pinnae have been known since as early as the mid-1800s, but Gardner and Gardner's (1973) experiment demonstrated the strong influence of the pinnae by covering the pinnae convolutions using a rubber mold and measuring sound localization abilities for noise bands. As they varied the amount of coverage, Gardner and Gardner found that localizing the elevation of the sounds became increasingly difficult and a greater number of errors were made. Their data, shown in Figure 7–10, illustrate the

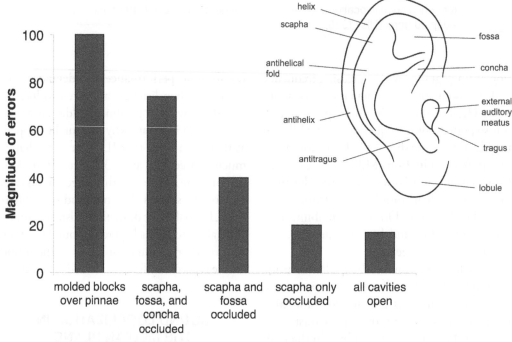

Extent of pinnae cavity occlusion

FIGURE 7–10. Magnitude of sound localization errors under different degrees of pinna occlusion. A schematic of the pinna is also illustrated for reference. Data adapted from Gardner and Gardner (1973), and image adapted from rendix alextian/Shutterstock.com.

magnitude of errors for sound localization in elevation as the ridges and convolutions of the pinnae were covered. They found that increasing amounts of pinnae occlusion led to poorer and poorer sound localization in elevation.

Gardner and Gardner also measured localization in elevation for noise bands with different cutoff frequencies and illustrated that pinnae influenced sound localization most in the high frequencies, but they had negligible effects at low frequencies. This result is consistent with the notion that pinnae cues are spectral in nature and result in a complex pattern of ILDs across the two ears.

Earlier, we discussed that the cone of confusion reflects an equal-ITD contour. However, ILDs are also very similar along the cone of confusion. Consequently, the pinnae can provide a mechanism to reduce the ambiguities associated with the cone of confusion, as the pinnae provide spectral cues that vary depending on the elevation of a sound source. However, the pinnae will not resolve the cone of confusion for low-frequency sounds, as their spectral alterations occur only in the high frequency regions. We should also note that the asymmetrical shape of the pinnae provides information about whether a sound is in the front or the back of a listener, although front-back errors are very common unless there is movement of the sound source or head.

LATERALIZATION

Stevens and Newman (1936) and Mills (1958) both measured sound localization using the free field. Although using the free field has some advantages over using headphones, such as having better real-world validity, some theories and ideas can only be tested using headphones for stimulation. Presenting sounds over headphones, however, does not always yield a perception of sounds being *outside* of the body, and the sounds are perceived instead

as being 'inside' the head. We refer to these experiments as *lateralization* experiments, as the experience of the listener is not one of sound localization.

However, presenting sounds over headphones does have benefits. For example, these methods provide the only way to manipulate one acoustic cue (such as ITD) without manipulating the other (ILD). Furthermore, the natural environment includes interactions between sound and the body, and these effects are eliminated with headphone presentation. Using headphones also allows psychophysical measurements in the absence of reverberation, which is a consequence of almost all natural environments except the anechoic chamber. Although one may argue that these experiments are artificial, they have greatly advanced our understanding of how the ear represents ITDs and ILDs. The discrimination experiments that have evaluated the perception of these two important cues independently from one another are discussed here.

ITD/IPD Discrimination

One advantage of using headphones pertains particularly to the ability to represent the IPD separately from the ITD. Manipulating the interaural phase without manipulating the interaural time delay is not easily done in the free field but is very straightforward when testing over headphones. In one of these experiments, Yost (1974) measured the just noticeable *interaural phase difference (IPD)* as a function of stimulus frequency and reference IPD. He was able to manipulate the IPD of the stimulus, but he used a 0-ms ITD in which stimuli to the left and right ear were presented simultaneously. This allowed Yost to directly test whether the ear is able to access the phase difference, independent of the time difference, across ears. Yost's data were also collected at a 0-dB ILD, and any perception of the ILD would have been constant across all experimental conditions. To simulate midline, listeners discriminated between a 0° reference IPD and an IPD of Δθ in degrees. To simulate other locations, he tested three other reference IPDs: 45°, 90°, and 180°. Figure 7–11 illustrates the just noticeable IPD as a function of frequency obtained from different reference IPDs. Yost's data showed small JNDs for IPD when the frequency was low and smaller JNDs for the reference angles closest to midline.

> Visit the companion website for an auditory-visual demonstration of an IPD discrimination experiment.

We see from this figure:

• *A constant just noticeable IPD at low frequencies.* The JND for IPD was about 3° when the sound was simulated to be at the front (the 0° condition). The JND for IPD

was fairly constant for frequencies below 1000 Hz.

• *Poorer performance at reference IPDs different from 0°.* Simulating sounds at different spatial locations led to higher just noticeable IPDs. This finding follows the same results we obtained in the free-field sound localization experiments, with midline performance being the best.

Although Yost's experiment was conducted using headphones, his results are entirely consistent with those obtained in the free field. They support the conclusion that the auditory system does not have robust access to interaural phase differences at frequencies greater than about 1000 Hz. His results also indicate that the best performance occurs when the head is pointed toward the sound source. Other IPD discrimination studies have also demonstrated that:

• *The JND for IPD varies with stimulus level.* Zwislocki and Feldman (1956) demon-

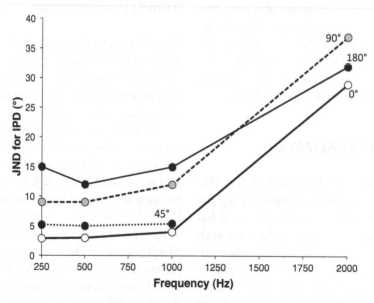

FIGURE 7–11. JND for IPD versus frequency. The just noticeable interaural phase difference (IPD; in degrees) is plotted as a function of frequency. Each function indicates a different reference IPD. Adapted from Yost (1974).

strated that the sensitivity to IPDs was poor at low levels. However, for levels above about 30 dB SL or so, sensitivity was fairly constant.

- *ITDs and IPDs are available in high-frequency regions for complex sounds.* Although Yost measured the JND for IPDs to be difficult to detect at high frequencies, we must consider that Yost measured this for pure tones. If complex stimuli are used, and ITDs are imposed upon the stimulus envelope, then the ear is capable of using interaural time differences present in the envelope (Henning, 1980).

ILD Discrimination

Yost and Dye (1988) conducted a similar experiment to that of Yost but measured the just noticeable ILD in an ILD discrimination experiment for tones of various frequencies.

Yost and Dye conducted these experiments with a fixed IPD/ITD of 0°/0 ms, and they measured the just noticeable ILD (in dB) as a function of reference ILD: 0 dB (simulating midline), 9 dB, and 15 dB. Note that because of the dependency of ILD and frequency, the ILDs of 9 and 15 dB could be associated with a variety of locations. However, neither of these ILDs would occur for a sound near the front of the body (see Figure 7–2).

> Visit the companion website for an auditory-visual demonstration of an ILD discrimination experiment.

Figure 7–12 plots data adapted from Yost and Dye and shows the just noticeable ILD plotted as a function of stimulus frequency and for the three different reference ILDs. Yost and Dye's data illustrate some striking results:

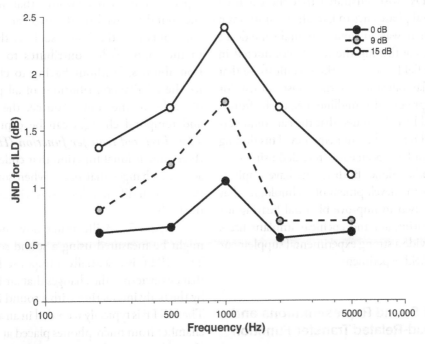

FIGURE 7–12. JND for ILD versus frequency. The just noticeable interaural level difference (ILD) is plotted as a function of frequency. Each function indicates a different reference ILD. Adapted from Yost and Dye (1988).

- *ILD discrimination was good at both low and high frequencies.* Even though ILDs are not robustly present in the environment at low frequencies, the ear possesses an ability to represent them. However, the elevation of the JND at 1000 Hz is noteworthy and suggests a poorer representation of the ILD in the mid-frequency range.

- *ILD discrimination ability decreased as the reference ILD increased.* Following the same trends observed in all previous studies, the ability to detect changes in the ILD decreased as the reference ILD increased. Again, this is evidence that using interaural level cues is more difficult when sounds are at the side of the body.

These psychoacoustic experiments using headphones provide a strong complement to the results obtained in the free field. However, by *overriding* the natural acoustic cues, psychoacoustic experiments illustrate some important aspects of auditory processing of ITDs and ILDs. Yost illustrated that the ear used interaural phase cues to lateralize sounds even when there was no environmental time delay. Further confirming the results conducted in the free field, these experiments illustrate that sound lateralization is the most robust for sounds presented at midline (i.e., to the front). Yost and Dye illustrated that the ear could perceive ILDs regardless of frequency. This finding could not have been easily revealed using free-field studies alone. Both results have implications for the development of technologies that may be used to improve binaural hearing for both hearing aid and cochlear implant users and provide a strong experimental supplement to free-field experiments.

Virtual Sound Representations and the Head-Related Transfer Function

Although experiments using pure tones and headphones have advanced our understanding in binaural auditory processing, they do not test sound localization. The experiments discussed above led to perceptions of the sounds as *inside the head*. The reasons for this are generally related to the simplification of sounds that is common to psychoacoustic experiments. These sounds do not contain natural filtering produced by the pinnae or interactions between the sound field and the body. They also often contain incongruent cues to the true location of the sound source. For example, in the natural environment, a sound with a 0-ms ITD always has a 0-dB ILD, but headphone experiments can present ITD/ILD combinations that could never occur in the environment. Yet, if natural acoustic interactions are considered, sound manipulations can produce an externalized experience even when headphones are used. Applications of this work are currently being used for video gaming, music, military applications, and even medical rehabilitation.

The pinnae and head are not the only aspects of human anatomy that influence the sound received by the two ears, and any component of the body, such as the torso, in the sound field contributes to localization abilities. Without having to characterize the relative contributions of all potential obstacles to the sound source, the spectral and temporal changes can be captured by a ***head-related transfer function (HRTF)***, a three-dimensional function that codes for the acoustic changes that occur when sounds are presented at different locations with respect to the body.

Figure 7–13 illustrates how an HRTF might be measured using a sound source, S. The HRTF is essentially a response function that characterizes the changes that are imposed by the body interacting with a sound in space. The HRTF is typically recorded in an anechoic chamber from microphones placed at each ear (for either a human or a manikin), and the HRTF is measured by presenting S at multiple sound locations in the 3D space.

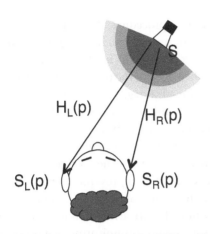

FIGURE 7–13. Illustration of HRTF measurement. S represents the sound source, whereas $S_R(p)$ and $S_L(p)$ represent the stimulus recorded at the right and left ears, respectively, for each point in space, p. $H_R(p)$ and $H_L(p)$ represent the head-related transfer functions for each ear for that same spatial location.

$H_R(p)$ and $H_L(p)$ are the transfer functions for the right and left ears, respectively, at each point, p, in space. Once an HRTF is recorded, sounds can be passed through the HRTF for presentation over headphones to a listener. Sound will then be perceived as external to the body, despite the headphone presentation. Interestingly, for localization in the horizontal plane, a listener-specific HRTF is not necessary. Wenzel et al. (1993) compared sound localization abilities for people listening over headphones using their own HRTF and an HRTF measured using different people. They found that localization in the horizontal plane was generally unaffected by the specific HRTF. However, listeners performed better at localizing in the other two planes when they were presented sounds from their own HRTF. It appeared that the pinnae cues were most relevant. Consequently, depending on the application, a specific HRTF may or may not be important. For example, listening to a concert over headphones may not require an individualized HRTF. However, video games in which targets may come from above or below could be associated with a better immersive experience using an individualized HRTF.

Visit the companion website to listen to sounds processed through a HRTF at different spatial locations.

BINAURAL UNMASKING

Sound localization indeed is a primary function of the auditory system, but perhaps more important for the daily life of modern people is the ability of the binaural system to functionally reduce the effects of noise on listening. We saw earlier in this chapter that having two ears can assist a person when detecting sounds in noise, but the effect was an improvement of 3 dB or less. A characteristic of these binaural summation studies is the diotic presentation of sound. Essentially, these experiments mimicked a situation where a signal and noise are originating from the same location in front of the body (i.e., they had a 0-ms ITD and a 0-dB ILD). However, in the section on sound localization, we saw that the perception of different locations requires different signals presented to each ear. Such cases reflect *dichotic* presentation of sound. The *diotic* situation is rarely encountered in daily life, as each ear commonly receives different signals, even if only slightly different between the two ears. For dichotic sounds, our binaural system plays an important role in allowing us to better detect (or understand) a signal when it is not co-located with a noise. As described in the previous sections, experimenters have made measurements both in the free field and over headphones. Many of the experiments have also used speech, rather than tones or complex sounds.

Binaural Unmasking in the Free Field

Many investigators have been interested in the auditory mechanisms for understanding speech in noise. The ability to understand speech or detect a signal has been measured in free-field environments, with the signal and masker originating at different locations. Detection is much better when a masker and signal are in different locations. For free-field listening, aside from binaural summation, there are two primary binaural effects that reduce the effects of the masker: the better-ear advantage and binaural squelch. These effects are most commonly measured using speech and are discussed here.

Better-ear advantage—In most environmental listening situations, one of the two ears receives a sound mixture with a higher signal-to-noise ratio (SNR) than the other. Acoustic head shadow causes the SNR at the two ears to be different, unless the rare condition occurs when the signal and masker are in the same location (e.g., like someone standing in front of a stereo speaker). In this way, typical everyday listening generates a *better ear* for listening. Consider a situation where a person is looking at a talker (the signal), but a noise source (such as a fan) is on their right side. Head shadow will attenuate the high-frequency components of the noise on the left side of the body, but the level of the talker will be the same at the two ears. In this way, the right ear receives a lower (poorer) SNR than the ear on the left.

Experiments that quantify the better-ear advantage are often conducted using headphones but with recordings obtained from the free-field environment, as ear-specific measures are necessary to quantify the better-ear advantage. Recordings are made at each ear and then played over the right and left earphones separately. Thresholds (or identification scores) for each ear are then obtained. The *better-ear effect* is then calculated by subtracting the performance scores between the two ears. The better-ear effect then indicates how much better performance is at the better ear compared to the other ear. Following

this type of procedure, Bronkhorst and Plomp (1988) measured *speech-recognition thresholds (SRTs*—the dB level at which words are identified 50% of the time) and found a 10-dB better-ear advantage when the target was to the front (0°) and the noise was to the right (90°) versus noise at the front. A 10-dB improvement in SRT can be a huge advantage to a listener, particularly one with hearing loss. In some cases, this improvement and can correspond to an increase of >75 percentage points for word identification (Duquesnoy, 1983). For someone communicating in a noisy environment, this effect alone could be the difference between participating in a conversation or not.

For individuals with normal hearing, the driver of the better-ear effect is primarily acoustic: The ear with the better SNR is the one that will lead to superior performance. However, the better-ear effect is measured perceptually, and therefore it is influenced by perceptual and physiological factors. For example, if someone has SNHL in one ear, speech perception in the ear with better thresholds may be superior to speech perception in the ear with poorer thresholds, even if that ear has a better SNR. Whether a listener has good hearing or some SNHL, anyone can take advantage of the better-ear effect by strategically placing their body and using head movements to influence the SNR at both ears.

Binaural squelch—Binaural squelch, first defined by Koenig (1950) is the advantage provided by the ability to supplement performance of the ear with the better SNR with the ear with the poorer SNR. This effect is contrasted with the better ear advantage in Figure 7–14 for illustration. Binaural squelch is determined by first measuring performance in the ear with the better SNR and then performance in the binaural hearing condition. Squelch is then calculated by subtracting the threshold obtained for the binaural condition

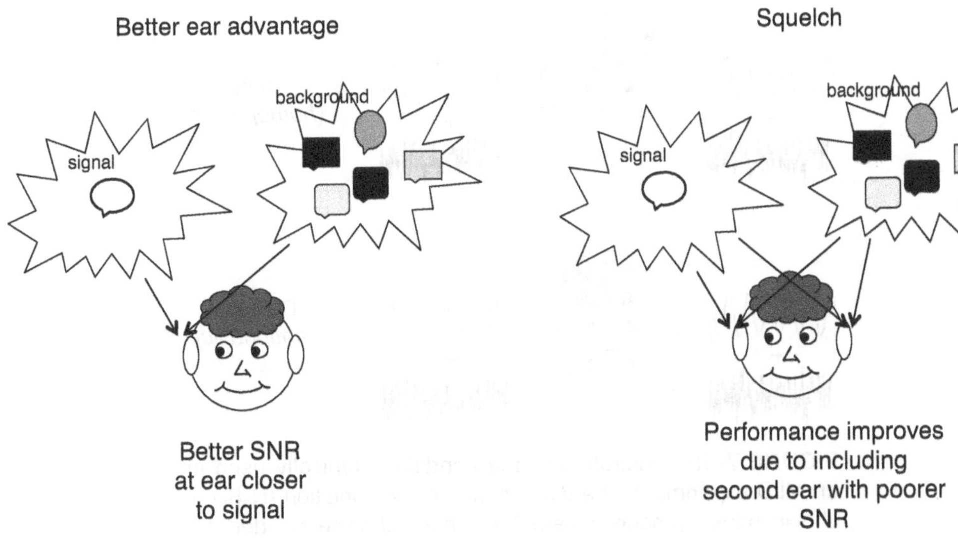

Better ear advantage · Squelch

FIGURE 7–14. Illustration of better ear advantage (*left panel*) versus binaural squelch (*right panel*).

from the threshold obtained for the ear with the better SNR. In this way, binaural squelch characterizes the benefits from including the ear with the poorer SNR. Generally speaking, the binaural squelch effect is considered to be fairly small for listeners with normal hearing but does improve the SRT by about 3 to 5 dB (Bronkhorst & Plomp, 1988). The binaural squelch effect is not a purely acoustic phenomenon and demonstrates that the ear utilizes even the more poorly represented signal to improve perception.

Both types of experiments also illustrate the benefits of having two ears. In monaural hearing, the single ear is always *the better ear* regardless of the SNR at that ear. Importantly, however, binaural squelch illustrates how both ears function together to further reduce the effects of noise on speech perception.

The Binaural Masking Level Difference

Another set of compelling experiments demonstrating the strength of the binaural audi-

tory system is the ***binaural masking level difference (BMLD or MLD)***. In 1948, Licklider measured speech intelligibility for a particular dichotic speech stimulus. In his experiment, the same speech signal was presented to the left and right ears. In one condition, the speech signal was *homophasic* (identical at the two ears) and in the other the speech signal was inverted at one of the ears (*antiphasic*). A homophasic noise stimulus was presented simultaneously with the speech in both conditions. An example of this type of experiment is illustrated using a pure tone in Figure 7–15, to allow better visualization of the phase inversion for the signal but not the noise in the antiphasic/dichotic case.

The top panel of Figure 7–15 illustrates the homophasic condition, in which the signal and noise are identical at both ears. The bottom panel represents the antiphasic condition, which has the signal inverted at one of the ears. Notice the face in bottom panel is smiling—he is receiving a benefit in performance from this condition compared with his twin in the top panel. In particular, Licklider found that word identification was 20 percentage

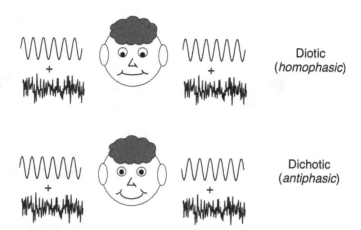

FIGURE 7–15. Illustration of the conditions typically used in an MLD experiment. The diotic homophasic condition (N_0S_0) is shown in the top panel, where the signal and noise are identical in the ears. In the dichotic antiphasic (N_0S_π) condition shown in the bottom panel, the noise is identical between the ears, but the signal phase is inverted in one ear compared to the other.

points better in the antiphasic condition compared with the homophasic condition. The difference in scores was most pronounced at low SNRs and essentially vanished at SNRs greater than 4 dB. Licklider noted that when the speech is out of phase compared with the noise (the antiphasic condition), "the speech literally jumps out of the noise-filled center of the head . . . and is immediately more intelligible." (Licklider, 1948). Such findings indicate a large release from masking by a simple inversion of the phase of the signal stimulus. These results were compelling, both in the amounts of benefits provided to a listener and in the perceptual experience provided by the experimental manipulations. The binaural system provided robust benefits to communication and functioned best at low SNRs.

> Visit the companion website for an auditory visual demonstration of a BMLD experiment and an auditory demonstration of the BMLD.

Psychophysical studies evaluating detection of pure tones have been able to more closely evaluate the frequency-specific nature of the masking benefit. Because phase differences are manipulated, we expect benefits to be the most pronounced for low-frequency stimuli. The largest release from masking is obtained from the two conditions mentioned above: a homophasic condition (signal and noise are the same at both ears; also known as N_0S_0) and an antiphasic condition (the noise is the same at both ears, but signal is inverted at one ear compared with the other; commonly referred to as N_0S_π). The subscripts refer to the phase relationships across the ears. Recall that π radians is the equivalent of a 180° phase shift (an inverted signal). In order to calculate the BMLD (which is sometimes shortened to MLD), the threshold obtained in the N_0S_π-condition is subtracted from the threshold obtained in the N_0S_0-condition. This quantity reflects the amount of release from masking, in dB, provided by the phase shift.

Hirsh (1948) made the first measurements of the MLD using pure tones, and his data have been replicated and clarified in numerous studies. Summary MLD data obtained by Durlach and Colburn (1978) from a variety of MLD experiments are reported in Figure 7–16. Across these experiments, the MLD varied with frequency. It was largest for low frequencies, and as large as 15 to 20 dB for frequencies at or below 500 Hz. For frequencies greater than 500 Hz, the MLD gradually decreased with increasing frequency and then asymptoted at about 3 dB at 2000 Hz and above. Large MLDs at low frequencies have also been observed for homophasic signals and antiphasic noise ($N_\pi S_0$ is about 13 dB) and monaural signals and homophasic noise ($N_0 S_m$ thresholds are about 9 dB lower than $N_m S_m$). The $N_0 S_m$ configuration illustrates a striking binaural release from masking: A signal + noise in a single ear (monaural) yields a threshold that is 9 dB higher than a monaural signal presented with a binaural, diotic noise.

Intuitively, we might expect that adding noise would increase the masking, but rather our binaural auditory system is able to take advantage of the correlated noise between the two ears and enhance performance.

Robust release from masking depends heavily on the amount of interaural correlation of the masking noise. Robinson and Jeffress (1963) demonstrated this by varying the amount of correlation of the noise between two ears. They found a systematic increase in the release from masking as the correlation of the noise between the ears progressively decreased. Noise highly correlated between the ears (e.g., identical noises to the two ears) led to the largest masking effects, whereas uncorrelated noise between the ears afforded the largest release from masking. Their results have formed the foundation for modern models of binaural hearing, which use interaural correlation as the basis for determining binaural benefit.

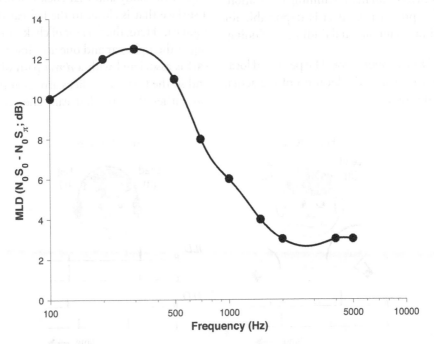

FIGURE 7–16. Data from a masking level difference (MLD) experiment. Masking level differences in dB are plotted as a function of tone frequency. Adapted from Durlach and Colburn (1978).

The Precedence Effect

The amazing aspects of binaural hearing do not end with binaural unmasking studies. The ear also contains mechanisms that work to reduce the influence of room reverberation. Rooms produce a complex acoustic field that consists of a direct path of sound from the source to the ear and multiple reflected paths because sound is reflected from surfaces and objects. These multiple sound paths produce a great deal of noise in the acoustic signal, yet we normally do not notice these sound reflections, nor do they drastically affect our judgments of sound location. Wallach et al. (1949), who coined the term the ***precedence effect***, demonstrated that sound localization is based on the acoustic cues associated with the sound that arrives first at the ears. That the reflections do not alter the perceived sound location of the source implies that the first arriving sound takes *precedence* over the reflections of that sound in determining its location.

The precedence effect is responsible for several important binaural findings, including:

- *Localization dominance.* The perceived location is at or near the location of the actual sound source.

- *Fusion.* The originating sound and its reflections are fused into the perception of a single sound.
- *Echo suppression.* The precedence effect suppresses the perception of the echoes caused by reflections.

Wallach et al. developed a paradigm to evaluate the precedence effect that is still in use today. Wallach et al. measured the precedence effect under ITD manipulations, but ILDs have also been tested. Their general paradigm is illustrated in Figure 7–17, which also shows how these experiments can be conducted in the free field (anechoic chamber) or over headphones. To simulate reflections, the experimenter can manipulate the delay between a source sound and a reflection as well as the direction of the reflection. The left panel, which illustrates a free-field experiment, shows a simulated scenario in which a click originates from a speaker at the right side of the body and that click is reflected off a surface that is closer to the left ear than the right ear. Here, the first set of clicks (one arriving at the right ear and one arriving at the left ear) is associated with a *direct* path of sound, and so the first set of clicks arrives at the right ear earlier than the left ear. The second set

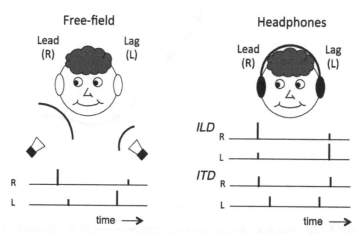

FIGURE 7–17. Schematics of the different stimulus configurations that can be used to measure the precedence effect.

of clicks would be associated with a *reflected* path of sound, and so the reflection arrives at the left ear before the right. If headphones are used, an experimenter can independently manipulate the ITD and ILD, as shown in the right panel.

Using this technique, experimenters have measured sound localization abilities and the echo threshold (the delay at which the echo [the second set of clicks in an experiment] is just noticeable). Localization based on the first set of clicks would indicate a sound to the right. Sound localization based on the echo would indicate a source near the left ear. Results indicate that location of the sound is associated with the direction of the first sound, not the reflection (*localization dominance*). Investigators have also shown that as long as the echo delay is short (on the order of milliseconds), the ear will fuse the two sets of clicks and hear only a single sound (*echo fusion*). Further, if the two sounds are fused, listeners are unable to localize/lateralize the lagging sound (*echo suppression*).

The precedence effect is a powerful process of the ear to reduce the impact that sound reflections have on perception and is extremely important for our hearing in enclosed spaces. Without it, we likely would experience greater masking effects when communicating in rooms. The precedence effect can also be exploited in algorithms used to enhance signals presented across speakers.

IMPACT OF SENSORINEURAL HEARING LOSS ON BINAURAL HEARING

Sensorineural hearing loss can have a drastic effect on binaural hearing, and several factors must be considered when evaluating the effects of sensorineural hearing loss on binaural hearing. Here, we will only consider cases in which a listener has residual hearing in both ears, as a listener with profound unilateral hearing loss has no binaural hearing. Most studies have been conducted using listeners with bilateral, symmetrical sensorineural hearing loss, but small asymmetries in hearing across the ears can disrupt binaural hearing abilities.

One important factor is the consideration of audibility. Even if listeners with hearing loss have symmetrical hearing loss, acoustic effects can render certain components of sound inaudible. Head shadow effects are of particular concern, due to their importance at high frequencies, and they may interact with the common high-frequency sloping hearing loss configuration. Listeners with hearing loss are compromised in their abilities to use ILDs simply from the interaction between the acoustic environment and the hearing loss. Surely listeners cannot access cues that they cannot hear. Thus, psychoacousticians must take great care when designing experiments to parse out the contributions of audibility and true binaural abilities.

Binaural Summation

In general, binaural summation is not greatly altered by sensorineural hearing loss. Hall and Harvey (1985) and Hawkins et al. (1987) found that binaural summation for loudness was not altered by sensorineural hearing loss, if the sounds presented to both ears were audible. However, Whilby et al. (2006) argued that binaural summation abilities vary greatly across listeners. They suggested that listeners with SNHL fell into two distinct groups: those who experienced much less binaural summation than listeners with normal hearing and those who experienced much more binaural summation than listeners with normal hearing. Some listeners with SNHL appeared to have typical binaural summation, but the majority of listeners experienced deficits in several other binaural arenas.

Localization and Lateralization

As a rule, listeners with sensorineural hearing loss experience deficits in their sound localization and lateralization abilities (Akeroyd, 2014). A particular hallmark of these studies is wide variability of performance by listeners with SNHL. As an example, a comprehensive study evaluated minimum audible angles (MAAs) in the free field and JNDs for ITDs and ILDs over headphones for 140 listeners (Häusler et al., 1983). Regarding the MAA measurements, some listeners with bilateral sensorineural hearing loss had MAAs within the range of normal variability, but other listeners, both those with bilateral hearing loss and those with asymmetrical hearing losses, had abnormally large MAAs. Most of the listeners with bilaterally symmetric hearing losses presented with JNDs for ITDs and ILDs within normal limits, although some demonstrated larger JNDs than typical. Other studies evaluating sensorineural hearing loss have come to similar conclusions. For example, Koehnke et al. (1995) found considerable variability across listeners with hearing loss in their ability to detect ITD and ILDs. Hawkins and Wightman (1980) also measured substantial deficits in some listeners' ability to detect ITDs.

The reasons for poor ITD and ILD perception in listeners with sensorineural hearing loss are still unknown, but may be related to the following factors:

- *Audibility and low sensation level.* Both ITD and ILD discrimination are poor at low sensation levels for listeners with normal hearing (Dietz et al., 2013). Even if sounds are audible, low sensation levels might account for poor performance in listeners with hearing loss on these tasks. The real-world environment also may exacerbate these issues, particularly for the ILD.

In natural auditory scenes, the head shadow can lead to some sounds being inaudible, detrimentally impacting the perception of the ILD. Consider an example in which a head shadow renders a sound inaudible in one ear but audible in the other. In this scenario, the representation of the ILD in the auditory system may be larger than that present in the environment, causing distortions to the perception of space. Also consider a listener with small, 5-dB asymmetry in hearing. For example, if their hearing is 5 dB better in the right ear than in the left ear, a sound presented to the left ear will be associated with an ILD that is 10 dB larger than when a sound is presented to the right ear. The auditory system may be unable to compensate for these distortions, leading to disruptions in the perception of space.

These scenarios, however, do not explain the experimental results of poor ILD perception in listeners with SNHL, as most studies take great care to control for audibility and ensure that the ear has access to the true acoustic ILD. Thus, poor ILD perception is also a consequence of altered auditory processing. Although ensuring appropriate audibility in both ears is critical to provide adequate access to interaural cues for listeners with SNHL, we cannot expect appropriate audibility to fully restore perception of either ILDs or ITDs.

- *Abnormal coding of temporal and intensity information.* Physiological changes have been demonstrated to occur at levels peripheral to the superior olive that alter the way binaural information is processed by that structure. Regarding temporal coding, Ruggero et al. (1992) noted small shifts in the delay of the traveling wave after cochlear death, and Heinz et al. (2010) demonstrated that cochlear damage can also distort the across-frequency representation of temporal fine structure in auditory nerve fibers. Such temporal distortions would not need to be large to disrupt the fine temporal synchronization necessary for representation by the MSO. Alterations in the amount of basilar membrane vibration with level (Ruggero & Rich, 1991) also will yield abnormal excitation and inhibition within the LSO.

Although hearing aids can compensate for issues related to audibility, they cannot address abnormal physiological coding. We see evidence that audibility is not the only driving factor of abnormal sound localization in listeners with sensorineural hearing loss, as hearing aids do not appear to restore sound localization for many listeners. In fact, in some cases, listeners wearing hearing aids make more localization errors than when they are not wearing hearing aids, a finding that is discussed in Chapter 9.

Release From Masking

In general, listeners with SNHL do not benefit from the binaural masking release abilities to the same degree as listeners with normal hearing. Deficits are present in the:

- *Better-ear advantage.* Similar to listeners with normal hearing, listeners with hearing loss can benefit from the better-ear effect. However, listeners with bilateral hearing loss will experience deficits simply because their better ear is largely susceptible to masking. Listeners with asymmetrical hearing loss with normal hearing in one ear will need to strategically move their head or body so that their ear with better thresholds is also the ear with the better SNR. Generally speaking, the better-ear effect will be determined by degree of hearing loss in the better ear, with more hearing loss being associated

with more masking and a poorer ability to understand speech in noise. Arsenault and Punch (1999) showed that, on average, listeners with SNHL did not benefit from the better-ear advantage to the same degree as listeners with normal hearing.

- *Binaural squelch.* The representations of ITD and ILD are important for binaural squelch. Those listeners who experience deficits in the ability to represent ITD and ILD will also experience deficits with binaural squelch. In Arsenault and Punch's evaluation, listeners with SNHL experienced only 1.7 dB of advantage due to binaural squelch, in contrast to a 4.9 dB advantage experienced by listeners with normal hearing.

- *Masking level difference.* Several studies have demonstrated that the masking level difference is reduced in listeners with sensorineural hearing loss (Durlach et al., 1981). The size of the MLD typically decreases as the severity of hearing loss increases. That is, listeners with more severe hearing losses receive less of a binaural release from masking by presenting a signal (but not a noise) in antiphase across the ears. Small asymmetries across the ears can also reduce the size of the MLD. Yet, small differences in hearing levels between the ears cannot fully account for the reductions in the size of the MLD. The poor coding of interaural timing cues in these listeners provides a better explanation for the reduced MLD associated with SNHL.

- *Precedence effect.* Listeners with SNHL also may experience deficits in the precedence effect and be more susceptible to reverberation. However, studies report wide variability across listeners. Roberts et al. (2002) measured echo thresholds for click stimuli in listeners with normal hearing and with SNHL. The echo threshold was defined as the just noticeable delay that determined whether the listeners heard one (the echo stimulus was fused with the leading stimulus) or two clicks. Roberts et al. found large variability across listeners, even when stimuli were presented at the same sensation level for the two groups. Many listeners with sensorineural hearing loss had higher echo thresholds than those with normal hearing, but not all. As we have seen repeatedly in this text, no correlation was observed between audiometric threshold and echo threshold. Other studies, however, did not find an effect of sensorineural hearing loss on the precedence effect (Roberts & Lister, 2004). Studies which have measured localization dominance also have demonstrated large variability across listeners with sensorineural hearing loss, with some listeners making errors in the perceived origin of a sound source (Cranford et al., 1993; Goverts et al., 2002).

Perceptual Consequences of Changes to Binaural Perception

Poor binaural abilities in listeners with sensorineural hearing loss have clear implications for the perception of sounds in noisy environments. Binaural release from masking (in terms of the MLD and binaural squelch) is degraded by SNHL. The consequence of these factors is straightforward: Listeners will experience more masking and more deterioration of speech perception in noisy environments. As we know, communicating in noisy environments can be particularly problematic for listeners with sensorineural hearing loss, and the loss of binaural mechanisms for noise reduction has been implicated in these difficulties (Humes et al., 2013). Listeners can still rely on the better-ear advantage, but listeners will not gain great benefits from binaural listening. Deficits in the precedence effect are also asso-

ciated with greater susceptibility to masking in reverberant environments.

Regarding sound localization, listeners with SNHL generally have deficits in their ability to represent the ITD and ILD. Consequently, these listeners will have more difficulty determining where a sound is coming from in the azimuthal plane. Whereas listeners with bilateral, symmetric hearing losses have difficulty localizing sounds, a unilateral loss can make sound localization almost impossible. Yet, data do suggest that the brain adapts to unilateral hearing losses, with greater plasticity observed for children than for adults, with the degree and duration of hearing loss being important factors (Kumpik & King, 2019). Lastly, due to reductions in audibility and loss of high-frequency hearing, many listeners do not have access to the pinna cues to help them localize sounds along the median plane.

Adding to the problem is that hearing aids, even when they provide linear amplification, can distort the natural relationships between ITD and ILD. Microphone placement (as in a behind-the-ear hearing aid) can entirely remove pinna effects, and even though most hearing aids have algorithms that compensate for the spectral changes imposed by the pinnae, they commonly do not amplify sounds above 6 kHz, where pinna cues are most available. Taken together, microphone location, signal bandwidth, and processing delays can all contribute to substantial deficits in sound localization for listeners wearing hearing aids.

Summary and Implication

It is evident from this review of literature that listeners with sensorineural hearing loss experience substantial deficits in their abilities to take advantage of binaural cues, but there is also wide variability across listeners. Listeners with symmetrical SNHL will experience poor sound localization as well as difficulty in using their binaural hearing to separate target sounds from background sounds. Listeners with asymmetric SNHL experience even greater difficulties. As a result, the ability of many listeners with sensorineural hearing loss to utilize their two ears can be severely compromised, and they cannot benefit from the multitude of abilities afforded by hearing with two ears. Amplification can provide access to binaural cues by restoring audibility but would not be expected to restore poor sound localization due to abnormal encoding of binaural information.

SUMMARY AND TAKE-HOME POINTS

To summarize, having two ears affords many individuals a multitude of auditory abilities. Binaural summation abilities are demonstrated with better detection and discrimination. Two ears also provide information about the location of sound in space, with the duplex theory of sound localization being an important theory describing the mechanisms responsible for sound localization. Two ears provide substantial reduction in the effects of masking. The precedence effect works in concert with binaural unmasking and reduces the impact that echoes have on perception. Listeners with SNHL can have deficits in any or all of these abilities, and substantial variability is present in this population.

The following points are key take-home messages of this chapter:

- Two ears provide binaural summation, or improvements in detection, discrimination, and identification for two ears compared with one.
- Two ears provide the ability to localize sound. The duplex theory of sound local-

ization describes the relationship between acoustic cues and perception, with ITDs driving localization for low-frequency sounds and ILDs driving localization for high-frequency sounds.

- Listening with two ears reduces the effect of masking in the following ways:
  - The better-ear effect—an acoustic effect that is measured perceptually, describes how well the auditory system can take advantage of the ear with the better SNR.
  - Binaural squelch and the masking level difference are true binaural auditory effects that can improve our perception in noise.
  - The precedence effect—a true binaural auditory effect, effectively suppresses perception of echoes generated in reverberant environments.
- SNHL alters sound localization abilities for many listeners, although there is considerable variability in performance. Some listeners have near-normal sound localization abilities, but many listeners experience deficits. Restoring audibility does not correct these sound localization problems, as the deficits are likely due to changes in neural coding.
- SNHL also degrades the ability to binaurally inhibit background noise, which, in turn contributes to difficulties understanding speech in noisy environments.

EXERCISES

1. Discuss the three primary advantages of having two ears and how each of these advantages facilitates listening in everyday environments.
2. Describe why ITDs are only useful for low-frequency sound localization and why ILDs are only useful for high-frequency sound localization.

3. Big Bird and Elmo use different cues for sound localization at different frequencies, and one reason for this is their different head sizes. Big Bird has a head that is 3 times the size of Elmo.

   a. If ILDs are available to Big Bird at frequencies above 750 Hz, at what frequencies would ILDs be available to Elmo? (Be specific here—this answer requires a number.)

   b. Describe why Elmo has ILDs available at different frequencies than Big Bird.

   c. What happens to the ITD processing of Big Bird compared with Elmo?

4. You have a patient with a conductive hearing loss in his left ear. If that conductive hearing loss attenuates sound by 40 dB at all frequencies, calculate his available ILD at 6000 Hz if a sound is presented to his left ear at 40 dB SPL or if that sound is presented at 80 dB SPL. Using your answer, discuss whether his sound localization will be better at the moderate or at the high stimulus level. Use Figure 7–2 to inform your answer.

5. Woodsy the owl has been having trouble with finding his prey. His vision is already poor (he is an owl after all!) and he really needs his hearing for hunting. He goes to the "owl"diologist and has his binaural hearing tested. The owldiologist discovers that Woodsy has normal ILD thresholds at all frequencies, but his ITD thresholds are abnormally high.

   a. Discuss whether making sounds louder (i.e., linear amplification) might help Woodsy.

   b. What are some other options for Woodsy to localize sounds better? Think outside of the box and what you might be able to do to help with his ITD issue.

6. Duane has a low-frequency hearing loss, and his wife Keisha has a high-frequency hearing loss. Who will be better at localizing sounds with different elevations? Discuss.

7. Describe the difference between the better-ear advantage and binaural squelch.

8. Many people with hearing loss have been shown to have smaller MLDs (masking level differences) than people with normal hearing. What are at least two possible explanations for this finding? Please explain these answers.

9. Listeners with sensorineural hearing loss have greater difficulty communicating in reverberant environments than listeners with normal hearing. Given your knowledge of the effects of hearing loss on binaural hearing, explain why this might occur.

10. Suvali spends a lot of time at home but her family visits frequently. She has presbycusis (age-related hearing loss) and struggles to hear her family, with particular difficulty localizing the voices of her grandchildren. She has asked that they speak more loudly so that she can more easily figure out where they are. Do you think that this will help her? Discuss.

11. Jerome receives a behind-the-ear hearing aid, in which the microphone is located at the top of the pinna. Discuss whether this microphone placement will affect Jerome's abilities to localize sounds in elevation and in azimuth.

12. Vikram has asymmetrical hearing loss and requires different amounts of amplification in both of his ears. Discuss whether Vikram has near-normal abilities to localize sounds without his hearing aids and whether his hearing aids are likely to assist him in sound localization.

13. As discussed in Chapter 5, ANSD is a disorder that primarily affects temporal processing. People with ANSD have good ILD perception but not ITD perception. Using your knowledge of the mechanisms for binaural hearing, describe why this would be the case.

Visit the companion website for lab exercises.

REFERENCES

Akeroyd, M. A. (2014). An overview of the major phenomena of the localization of sound sources by normal-hearing, hearing-impaired, and aided listeners. *Trends in Hearing*, *18*, 1–7.

Algom, D., Rubin, A., & Cohen-Raz, L. (1989). Binaural and temporal integration of the loudness of tones and noises. *Attention, Perception, and Psychophysics*, *46*(2), 155–166.

Arsenault, M. D., & Punch, J. L. (1999). Nonsense-syllable recognition in noise using monaural and binaural listening strategies. *Journal of the Acoustical Society of America*, *105*(3), 1821–1830.

Bronkhorst, A. W., & Plomp, R. (1988). The effect of head-induced interaural time and level differences on speech intelligibility in noise. *Journal of the Acoustical Society of America*, *83*(4), 1508–1516.

Brownell, W. E., Manis, P. B., & Ritz, L. A. (1979). Ipsilateral inhibitory responses in the cat lateral superior olive. *Brain Research*, *177*(1), 189–193.

Cranford, J. L., Andres, M. A., Piatz, K. K., & Reissig, L. (1993). Influences of age and hearing loss on the precedence effect in sound localization. *Journal of Speech, Language, and Hearing Research*, *36*(2), 437–441.

Dietz, M., Bernstein, L. R., Trahiotis, C., Ewert, S. D., & Hohmann, V. (2013). The effect of overall level on sensitivity to interaural differences of time and level at high frequencies. *Journal of the Acoustical Society of America*, *134*(1), 494–502.

Duquesnoy, A. (1983). The intelligibility of sentences in quiet and in noise in aged listeners. *Journal of the Acoustical Society of America*, *74*(4), 1136–1144.

Durlach, N. I. & Colburn, H. S. (1978). Binaural Phenomena. In E. Carterette & M. Friedman (Eds.), *Handbook of perception* (Vol. 4, pp. 365–466). Academic Press.

Durlach, N. I., Thompson, C. L., & Colburn, H. S. (1981). Binaural interaction in impaired listeners: A review of past research. *Audiology*, *20*(3), 181–211.

Feddersen, W. E., Sandel, T. T., Teas, D. C., & Jeffress, I. A. (1957). Localization of high-frequency tones. *Journal of the Acoustical Society of America*, *29*(9), 988–991.

Gardner, M. B., & Gardner, R. S. (1973). Problem of localization in the median plane: Effect of pinnae

cavity occlusion. *Journal of the Acoustical Society of America*, *53*(2), 400–408.

Goverts, S. T., Houtgast, T., & van Beek, H. H. (2002). The precedence effect for lateralization for the mild sensory neural hearing impaired. *Hearing Research*, *163*(1), 82–92.

Hall, J. W., & Harvey, A. D. (1985). Diotic loudness summation in normal and impaired hearing. *Journal of Speech and Hearing Research*, *28*(3), 445–448.

Häusler, R., Colburn, S., & Marr, E. (1983). Sound localization in subjects with impaired hearing: Spatial discrimination and interaural-discrimination tests. *Acta Oto-Laryngologica*, *96*(Suppl. 400), 1–62.

Hawkins, D. B., Prosek, R. A., Walden, B. E., & Montgomery, A. A. (1987). Binaural loudness summation in the hearing impaired. *Journal of Speech and Hearing Research*, *30*, 37–43.

Hawkins, D. B., & Wightman, F. L. (1980). Interaural time discrimination ability of listeners with sensorineural hearing loss. *Audiology*, *19*(6), 495–507.

Heinz, M. G., Swaminathan, J., Boley, J. D., & Kale, S. (2010). Across-fiber coding of temporal finestructure: Effects of noise-induced hearing loss on auditory-nerve responses. In E.A. Lopez-Poveda, A.R. Palmer, & R. Meddis (Eds.), *The Neurophysiological bases of auditory perception* (pp. 621–660). Springer.

Henning, B. (1980). Some observations on the lateralization of complex waveforms. *Journal of the Acoustical Society of America*, *68*(2), 446–454.

Hirsh, I. J. (1948). The influence of interaural phase on interaural summation and inhibition. *Journal of the Acoustical Society of America*, *20*(4), 536–544.

Humes, L. E., Kidd, G. R., & Lentz, J. J. (2013). Auditory and cognitive factors underlying individual differences in aided speech-understanding among older adults. *Frontiers in Systems Neuroscience*, *7*, 55.

Jeffress, L. A. (1948). A place theory of sound localization. *Journal of Comparative and Physiological Psychology*, *41*(1), 35.

Jesteadt, W., & Wier, C. C. (1977). Comparison of monaural and binaural discrimination of intensity and frequency. *Journal of the Acoustical Society of America*, *61*(6), 1599–1603.

Koehnke, J., Culotta, C. P., Hawley, M. L., & Colburn, S. (1995). Effects of reference interaural time and intensity differences on binaural performance in listeners with normal and impaired hearing. *Ear and Hearing*, *16*(4), 331–353.

Koenig, W. (1950). Subjective effects in binaural hearing. *Journal of the Acoustical Society of America*, *22*(1), 61–62.

Kumpik, D. P., & King, A. J. (2019). A review of the effects of unilateral hearing loss on spatial hearing. *Hearing Research*, *372*, 17—28.

Licklider, J. C. R. (1948). The influence of interaural phase relations upon the masking of speech by white noise. *Journal of the Acoustical Society of America, 20*(2), 150–159.

Marks, L. E. (1980). Binaural summation of loudness: Noise and two-tone complexes. *Perception and Psychophysics, 27*(6), 489–498.

Mills, A. W. (1958). On the minimum audible angle. *Journal of the Acoustical Society of America, 30*(4), 237–246.

Mills, A. W. (1972). Auditory localization (binaural acoustic field sampling, head movement and echo effect in auditory localization of sound sources position, distance and orientation). *Foundations of Modern Auditory Theory, 2*, 303–348.

Pollack, I. (1948). Monaural and binaural threshold sensitivity for tones and for white noise. *Journal of the Acoustical Society of America, 20*(1), 52–57.

Roberts, R. A., Besing, J., & Koehnke, J. (2002). Effects of hearing loss on echo thresholds. *Ear and Hearing, 23*(4), 349–357.

Roberts, R. A., & Lister, J. J. (2004). Effects of age and hearing loss on gap detection and the precedence effect: Broadband stimuli. *Journal of Speech, Language, and Hearing Research, 47*(5), 965–978.

Robinson, D. E., & Jeffress, L. A. (1963). Effect of varying the interaural noise correlation on the detectability of tonal signals. *Journal of the Acoustical Society of America, 35*(12), 1947–1952.

Ruggero, M. A., & Rich, N. C. (1991). Application of a commercially-manufactured Doppler-shift laser velocimeter to the measurement of basilar-membrane vibration. *Hearing Research, 51*(2), 215–230.

Ruggero, M. A., Rich, N. C., & Recio, A. (1992) Basilar membrane responses to clicks. In Y. Cazals, L. Demany, & K. Horner (Eds.), *Auditory physiology and perception* (pp. 85–91). Pergamon Press.

Shaw, W. A., Newman, E. B., & Hirsh, I. J. (1947). The difference between monaural and binaural thresholds. *Journal of the Acoustical Society of America, 19*(4), 734.

Simon, J. R. (1967). Ear preference in a simple reaction-time task. *Journal of Experimental Psychology, 75*(1), 49.

Stevens, S. S., & Newman, E. B. (1936). The localization of actual sources of sound. *American Journal of Psychology, 48*(2), 297–306.

Strutt, J. W. (Lord Rayleigh; 1877). *The theory of sound* (Vol. I). Macmillan.

Wallach, H., Newman, E. B., & Rosenzweig, M. R. (1949). A precedence effect in sound localization. *Journal of the Acoustical Society of America, 21*(4), 468.

Wenzel, E. M., Arruda, M., Kistler, D. J., & Wightman, F. L. (1993). Localization using nonindividualized head-related transfer functions. *Journal of the Acoustical Society of America, 94*(1), 111–123.

Whilby, S., Florentine, M., Wagner, E., & Marozeau, J. (2006). Monaural and binaural loudness of 5-and 200-ms tones in normal and impaired hearing. *Journal of the Acoustical Society of America, 119*(6), 3931–3939.

Yost, W. A. (1974). Discriminations of interaural phase differences. *Journal of the Acoustical Society of America, 55*(6), 1299–1303.

Yost, W. A., & Dye Jr., R. H. (1988). Discrimination of interaural differences of level as a function of frequency. *Journal of the Acoustical Society of America, 83*(5), 1846–1851.

Zwislocki, J., & Feldman, R. S. (1956). Just noticeable differences in dichotic phase. *Journal of the Acoustical Society of America, 28*(5), 860–864.

8

Psychoacoustics and Advanced Clinical Auditory Assessment

LEARNING OBJECTIVES

Upon completion of this chapter, students will be able to:

- Discover how dead regions in the cochlea may be identified using psychoacoustics tools
- Evaluate the role of psychoacoustics in behavioral tests of retrocochlear pathology from a primarily historical perspective
- Demonstrate the connection between psychoacoustics and the identification of nonorganic hearing loss
- Consider psychoacoustics principles in the measurement of tinnitus perception
- See how diagnosing auditory processing involves psychoacoustics

---

INTRODUCTION

The previous chapters of this book have reviewed psychoacoustic characteristics of the auditory system in both ears with normal hearing and ears with sensorineural hearing loss. In many cases, we observed that SNHL leads to changes to psychoacoustic abilities and that the degree of these changes can vary considerably for these listeners. We also observed that these abilities represent levels of perception that are not well captured by absolute thresholds. In fact, in many cases the amount of the elevated threshold does not provide a robust indicator of the degree of deficits experienced by an individual listener.

Given the wide range of variability in perceptual abilities of listeners with sensorineural hearing loss documented throughout this text and the importance of auditory perception for speech understanding, a cogent argument could be made for including additional psychoacoustic tests into an audiological assessment. Importantly, audiological assessment is rooted in the tools and developments of psychoacoustics—there are a variety of clinical tests based on psychoacoustics that are part of modern audiology. Measurement of absolute thresholds, as done for the audiogram, is a prime example of the use of psychoacoustics in audiology. Developments regarding measurement and interpretation of auditory detection and masking have been critical to the ability to appropriately diagnose sensorineural hearing loss. In addition to the audiometric measurements of threshold, the audiologist has on hand a variety of psychoacoustic tests that assist with diagnosis of auditory disorders, including but not limited to, sensorineural hearing loss, tinnitus, and auditory processing disorder. Although some of these psychoacoustical assessments are not commonly used today, they nonetheless should be accessible within an audiologist's toolbox. These tools can, in some cases, support the diagnosis or identification of multiple auditory disorders, can be used with complicated patients, and can inform treatment strategies.

We discuss advanced applications of psychoacoustics to diagnostic audiology, by touching on the following topics, starting with measurements based on detection and advancing to higher levels of perception:

- Dead regions
- Nonorganic hearing loss (pseudohypacusis)
- Retrocochlear assessment
- Tinnitus evaluation
- Auditory Processing Disorder

DEAD REGIONS

Dead regions are regions in the cochlea in which all inner hair cells (or auditory nerve fibers) are lost or not functioning. It is notably difficult to identify a dead region from the audiogram because elevated audiometric thresholds (e.g., >70 dB HL) may result from either malfunctioning inner hair cells or a dead region + off-frequency listening. The logic behind this is as follows: For an ear with intact inner hair cells, the hair cells that innervate the basilar membrane at the place of maximum vibration will be the ones that code that vibration (as illustrated in the top panel of Figure 8–1). If those inner hair cells are damaged (as reflected by the gray hair cells), the threshold will be

elevated. On the other hand, if there are no inner hair cells or auditory nerve fibers innervating that region (i.e., a dead region), then there is no mechanism for afferent activity in the auditory pathway. Increasing the tone level (as would be done in audiometric testing), however, causes an increase in the spread of excitation along the basilar membrane. Hair cells distant (i.e., "off frequency") from the place of maximum vibration can respond to that tone (as shown in the bottom panel of Figure 8–1). In this way, an individual with a dead region could have an elevated threshold at the test frequency, but the response is due to a response occurring at a cochlear location distant from the place of maximum vibration. Thus, the audiogram itself does not provide sufficient information to determine whether a response on the audiogram is due to functioning but damaged cells and fibers or due to off-frequency listening.

Although dead regions are not easily identified from the audiogram, the ***threshold equalization noise (TEN)*** test, available on some audiometers, can be used instead (Moore et al., 2000). This test uses the principles of masking and involves measuring a patient's threshold in a special noise, created based on the principles of masking and measurements of the auditory filter. The noise is designed so that if inner hair cells are intact, thresholds measured within this noise should be the same as the level of the TEN. When using the TEN test, thresholds are first measured in quiet. Then, thresholds are measured in the presence of the TEN set to either 50 dB HL or 10 dB above the patient's threshold, whichever is greater. For example, if a patient's threshold was 50 dB HL at 2000 Hz when tested in quiet, the audiologist would re-measure the threshold in the presence of a TEN presented at 60 dB HL. In this scenario, if the individual does not have dead region, the threshold is expected to be 60 dB HL in the TEN (the masked threshold), but an individual with a dead region would have a masked threshold at

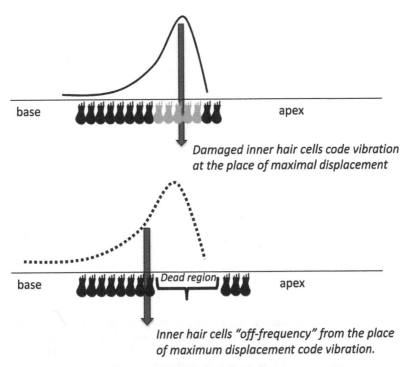

Damaged inner hair cells code vibration at the place of maximal displacement

Inner hair cells "off-frequency" from the place of maximum displacement code vibration.

FIGURE 8–1. Illustration of the hair cells responsible for coding vibration on the basilar membrane. The top panel illustrates excitation resulting from a pure tone for an ear with intact inner hair cells. The arrow indicates that the hair cells responsible for coding the excitation are located at the place of maximum vibration. The bottom panel illustrates excitation resulting from a pure tone for an ear with a dead region. The arrow indicates that the hair cells responsible for coding the excitation are located more basally than those at the place of maximum vibration.

least 10 dB greater than the level of the TEN (≥70 dB HL). For this individual with a dead region, off-frequency listening requires a more intense tone to overcome the threshold-equalizing noise because the region of the cochlea that corresponds to the detection is not the same location as the maximum vibration.

Figure 8–2 shows an audiogram without a dead region in the left panels, with thresholds measured in quiet (unfilled circles) and in the presence of the TEN (indicated with the "T"s). The level of the TEN is shown by the asterisks. Here, we see that the thresholds in the TEN overlap with the asterisks, indicating there is no dead region. The right panel of Figure 8–2 illustrates the same audiogram, but for an individual with a dead region. In this example, the individual has thresholds consistent with a dead region at frequencies of 2000 Hz and above. Thresholds are 10 dB or greater than the level of the TEN for these frequencies, evident in the gap between the asterisks and the "T"s.

Testing for dead regions is not terribly common in audiology, but some research suggests that there may be clinical value to establishing whether an individual has a dead region. This work has suggested that providing amplification to frequencies associated with dead regions may be disruptive to speech perception. For example, Vickers et al. (2001) evaluated speech perception in listeners with high-frequency dead regions and found that individuals with dead regions either did

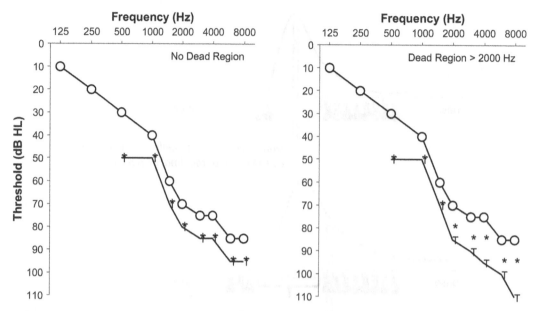

FIGURE 8–2. Illustration of two audiograms measured in quiet and in TEN noise. The left panel depicts thresholds for an individual without a dead region and the right panel shows thresholds for an individual with a dead region. Thresholds in quiet are plotted as circles; thresholds in the TEN noise are plotted as "T." The level of the TEN noise is indicated by the asterisks.

not benefit from amplification of frequencies within their dead region or experienced poorer speech perception when amplification was provided. Follow-up studies indicate that amplification may be more problematic for individuals with low-frequency dead regions. For example, Vinay et al. (2008) found that low-frequency amplification for individuals with a low-frequency dead region could be very disruptive to speech perception.

RETROCOCHLEAR ASSESSMENT

Before physiological tests and Magnetic Resonant Imaging (MRI) were developed, audiologists conducted behavioral assessments of **retrocochlear** auditory disorders, or disorders in the auditory system at a level above the cochlea in the auditory pathway. In many cases, a retrocochlear disorder is caused by a tumor of the auditory nerve or brainstem. A common finding in patients with acoustic tumors is an asymmetry in thresholds between the ears, with ≥15 dB HL or ≥20 dB HL considered *clinically significant*. Yet, audiometric asymmetry is a poor predictor of the presence of an acoustic tumor (present in less than ½ of patients who present with tumors), and other retrocochlear pathologies may also cause bilateral hearing loss, such aging, infection, neurological and vascular disorders, etc. As such, additional tests beyond the audiogram are almost always needed to facilitate the diagnosis of retrocochlear pathology. Physiological tests such as otoacoustic emissions (a test of cochlear function), immittance testing (a test of middle ear and brainstem function), auditory brainstem response (ABR; a brainstem evoked potential), and MRI are now used for a retrocochlear assessment. Audiologists no longer routinely conduct behavioral tests to determine whether a hearing loss is retrocochlear.

Psychoacoustic tests for retrocochlear assessment have reasonably good *test specificity* (ability to identify the non-retrocochlear ears), but their *test sensitivity* (the ability to correctly identify the ears with retrocochlear pathology) is relatively poor (Turner et al., 1984). However, there are patients for whom physiological tests are contraindicated, and there are some cases where retrocochlear assessment using behavioral techniques may still be needed. Some of these approaches with psychoacoustical roots are also described here for historical perspective.

Alternative Binaural Loudness Balancing (ABLB) Test

This test for retrocochlear hearing loss is based on the absence of *loudness recruitment,* a phenomenon associated with loss of outer hair cells. A listener with SNHL is expected to experience loudness recruitment, and this clinical method allows a quick assessment of recruitment, but only for people with unilateral hearing loss. In cases of suspected retrocochlear hearing loss and unilateral hearing loss, the tester can conduct the ***alternate binaural loudness balancing method*** (**ABLB;** Fowler,

1936) to determine if the ear with SNHL experiences recruitment or not

The ABLB is straightforward—a tone is presented at a specific dB HL to the patient's healthy ear. The audiologist presents a tone at the same frequency to the patient's poorer ear. The tones are always presented sequentially (e.g., alternating). In one approach, the patient hears the reference tone in the better ear and tells the audiologist to increase or decrease the level of the sound in his poorer ear until it is equally loud to the tone in his healthy ear. Another approach is to present the fixed tone to the poorer ear. Whatever the approach, the audiologist repeats the measurement multiple levels (usually in 10- or 20-dB steps, depending on the degree of hearing loss). The audiologist then plots a laddergram, in which one rung of the ladder plots the dB HL levels in the healthy ear and the other rung of the ladder shows the loudness-matched levels (in dB HL) in the other ear. Figure 8–3 illustrates that a laddergram from a patient with recruitment in the right ear will show nonparallel rungs (loudness will grow faster in the ear with SNHL than in the healthy one;

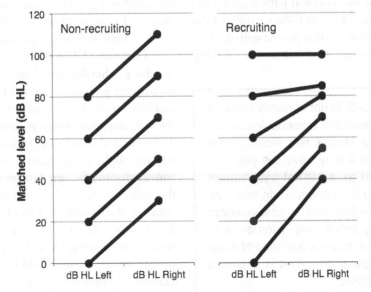

FIGURE 8–3. Laddergrams for a non-recruiting ear (*left panel*) and a recruiting ear (*right panel*).

see the right panel of Figure 8–3). An ear that does not exhibit recruitment will show parallel rungs (see the left panel of Figure 8–3). This type of laddergram might be indicative of retrocochlear pathology.

Short-Increment Sensitivity Index (SISI)

The *short-increment sensitivity index* (SISI; Jerger et al., 1959), a test based on *intensity discrimination*, was developed to determine whether a retrocochlear pathology was present At the time, the SISI test was promising, which was exciting for the audiology community, due to limited availability of tests to establish retrocochlear site-of-lesion. In the SISI test, a listener was presented with a continuous tone at 20 dB SL. Every 5 seconds, a 200- or 300-ms increment was imposed on that tone, with an increment level of either 5, 2, or 1 dB. The listener responded when a tone was heard, and only the 1 dB increments were counted. Early results suggested that listeners with normal hearing and retrocochlear pathology could only detect 0% to 20% of the increments. Those with cochlear pathology, on the other hand, could detect 60% to100% of the increments, or *more* than people with a retrocochlear pathology. At the time, the thinking

> While the SISI is not currently used for the assessment of retrocochlear disorders, Frank Musiek has recently suggested that it may have the potential to be used as a clinical assessment of intensity discrimination. In this way, it could be included in assessments of auditory processing disorder or in applications in which a source of auditory perceptual difficulties is unknown (Musiek, 2022).

was that loudness recruitment perhaps assisted with detection of these increments. However, Hirsh et al. (1954) demonstrated that differences in intensity discrimination were not present between listeners with and without recruitment (see Ch. 4), and further evaluations of the SISI have also shown it to be a poor indicator of retrocochlear pathology.

Performance-Intensity Function

Speech testing is also a common component of a standard audiometric assessment. Two types of speech tests are routine: the speech recognition threshold (SRT) and word recognition scores measured at a supra-threshold stimulus level. The SRT is a rapid assessment of speech understanding and is a measurement of the level at which 50% of a set of 2-syllable words (spondees) are correctly identified. The SRT is expected to closely approximate the pure-tone-average of 0.5, 1, and 2 kHz (PTA) of the audiogram, within about ±5 dB. Word recognition scores, on the other hand, provide an upper limit for a patient's ability to understand speech. Word recognition scores are generally measured using a set of single-syllable words, presented at an audible level. The percentage correct identification is reported.

Like the SRT, word recognition scores are also predictable based on the audiogram for patients with sensorineural hearing loss of cochlear origin. Yet, a patient with a retrocochlear hearing loss might present with poorer than expected word recognition scores. This finding might result from aging and other non-worrisome factors, but poor scores may also reflect retrocochlear pathology. Further evidence of retrocochlear pathology can be evident in word recognition measures as a function of the stimulus level. As with the *psychometric function*, there should be an increasing relationship between presentation level and word recognition scores. In some cases of retrocochlear disorder, however, word recognition may decrease with increasing intensity, a phenomenon called *rollover*. Figure 8–4 illustrates a *performance-intensity (PI) function*, a plot relating performance on a speech task (here, word recognition scores in percent correct). The PI function consistent with a cochlear site of lesion is plotted using solid symbols, and the PI function demonstrating rollover is plotted with unfilled symbols. Although the patient demonstrating rollover needs referral, these results also provide valuable information regarding rehabilitation. Large amounts of amplification would be contraindicated for this patient due to his poor word recognition scores at higher stimulus levels.

Békésy Audiometry

Békésy audiometry (Békésy, 1947) is an automatic method of measuring audiometric thresholds which can be used for audiometric screening, establishing cochlear versus retrocochlear hearing losses (Jerger, 1960), and identifying pseudohypacusis (discussed in the next section; Jerger & Herer, 1961). Descendent from the *method of adjustment*, Békésy audiometry initially involves presenting an audible tone to an individual, and the individual is instructed to press a button as long as they hear the tone. The tone's level decreases until the patient stops pressing the button, at which point, the level of the tone will increase. In this way, the patient controls the level of the tone, and the level of the tone oscillates between *just above* and *just below* the threshold. Thresholds can be obtained for different frequencies using either a frequency sweep or a fixed-frequency approach. Békésy audiometry generally results in a tracing of signal level versus time, and the reversal points between "just above" and "just below" the patient's threshold can (in some cases) be averaged together to determine the threshold.

Two conditions are needed to identify retrocochlear inolvement. In one condition,

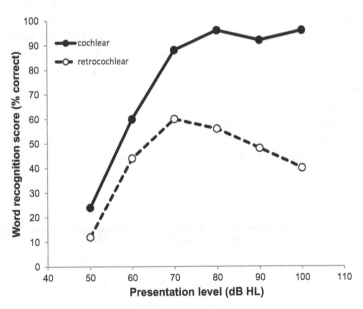

FIGURE 8–4. Performance-intensity functions for word recognition for a listener with a presumed cochlear site of lesion (*filled circles*) and a presumed retrocochlear site of lesion (*unfilled circles*).

the signal is periodically interrupted or pulsed, and in the other condition, the signal is continuous. By comparing the Békésy traces between the pulsed and continuous conditions, the site-of-lesion can potentially be established. Figure 8–5 illustrates the most common patterns that result from Békésy audiometry, when measured for a single frequency. The potential interpretations of these common patterns are as follows:

Type 1—Continuous and pulsed tracings overlap (inconclusive site-of-lesion)

Type 2—Continuous tracing yields thresholds that are slightly worse than the pulsed tracing (<20 dB, but usually about 3 to 5 dB; cochlear site-of-lesion)

Type 3—Continuous tracing *decays* to a much higher level than the pulsed tracing (retrocochlear site-of-lesion)

Type 4—Continuous tracing >20 dB worse than the pulsed tracing (inconclusive site-of-lesion, often considered retrocochlear)

Type 5—Pulsed tracing yields worse thresholds than the continuous tracing (nonorganic hearing loss).

The Type 3 pattern illustrates retrocochlear involvement, at it shows data from a listener who has difficulty maintaining their perception of a continuous sound; that is, their auditory system *adapts* to the sound.

The abnormal auditory adaptation requires the level of the continuous signal to be continually increased for this listener to hear it. This increased auditory adaptation is a characteristic of some retrocochlear pathologies. In contrast, when pulsed tones are tested in Békésy audiometry, the procedure converges on a threshold in the pulsed condition, which is not influenced by auditory adaptation.

> A procedure similar to continuous Békésy audiometry is the *tone decay test*, which is a test in which a listener raises their hand as long as they can perceive a sound, presented for one minute. Individuals with a retrocochlear pathology whose perception of sound decays over time would not be able to perceive the sound for the full minute.

As mentioned previously, Békésy audiometry is not widely used for the assessment of retrocochlear disorders. However, automated audiometric approaches that apply the method of adjustment, such as Békésy audiometry, can be extremely useful for identification of hearing loss. Such approaches have been demonstrated to be valid and to have the same test-retest reliability as manual audiometry for audiometric assessment for most adults when testing over earphones (i.e., air conduction; Mahomed et al., 2013). As a result, these

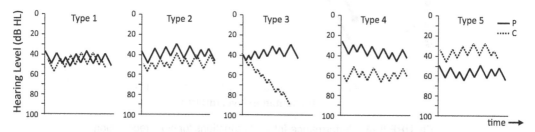

FIGURE 8–5. Common Békésy tracings (types 1–5). The level of the signal (in dB HL) is shown plotted as a function of time for pulsed (*solid lines*) and continuous (*dotted lines*) conditions.

approaches are excellent for auditory screenings and easy-to-test populations. That said, automated audiometry is not a substitute for a skilled audiologist obtaining an audiogram for difficult-to-test patients or children.

IDENTIFICATION OF NONORGANIC HEARING LOSS

Another common application of psychoacoustics to diagnostic audiology is the assessment of nonorganic hearing loss, commonly called *pseudohypacusis.* Nonorganic hearing loss may occur both consciously and unconsciously, and nonorganic losses manifest themselves in the form of an overly conservative criterion and lead to an overestimate of audiometric thresholds. That is, measured auditory thresholds are poorer/higher than the true threshold. Determining whether a patient has pseudohypacusis is not always easy and requires an attentive experimenter/ audiologist. There are numerous clues to pseudohypacusis, and although some may be identified during collection of an oral case history, those specific to the audiogram include:

- *Absence of a shadow curve.* An audiometric shadow curve should be present in patients with true unilateral hearing loss. The shadow curve is a false audiometric curve that occurs because a patient hears a sound in a nontest ear due to bone conduction from the sound presented in a test ear. The *interaural attenuation* is roughly 0 to 10 dB for bone conduction and 40 to 80 dB for air conduction. Patients with true, and large, unilateral hearing losses should present with a shadow curve during audiometric testing. The absence of a shadow curve when there should be one is clear evidence of a nonorganic hearing loss.
- *Disagreement among test results.* An audiometric assessment often includes measurement of the SRT, expected to closely approximate the PTA from the audiogram, within ±5 dB. Any SRT that is better than expected provides a sign of nonorganic hearing loss. Word recognition scores also provide clues, and scores that are better than predicted by absolute thresholds also suggest nonorganic hearing loss.
- *No false positives.* Patients following appropriate instructions are expected to provide some false positives during threshold testing. The complete absence of false positives can be indicative of false hearing loss.

Modifications to Standard Audiometric Procedures

Once pseudohypacusis is suspected, obtaining an accurate audiogram can be relatively difficult, and sometimes requires the support of physiological tests. However, in other cases a behavioral audiogram can be obtained without physiological assessment, and whereas it is easier to do so for a patient feigning a unilateral hearing loss, it is not impossible for bilateral hearing loss. Here, we discuss some of the strategies employed in audiology and how they are connected to psychoacoustic principles.

For patients with bilateral pseudohypacusis, the audiologist must make modifications to the audiometric procedures to determine true absolute thresholds. Standard audiometry applies procedures specifically designed to encourage patients to provide a neutral or slightly liberal criterion. However, in the cases of pseudohypacusis, these practices have not achieved that goal. Patients may adopt a loudness criterion by pressing the button for sounds above a specific, remembered loudness, or a patient may use knowledge of the 10-down, 5-up procedure and count steps to exaggerate their hearing loss. Both strategies can be disrupted by various procedural modifications rooted in the principles of Signal Detection Theory and thereby encourage the patient to adopt a more neutral criterion.

Consequently, the first step in audiometric testing for patients with suspected pseudohypacusis is to reinstruct the patient. This allows patients to be aware that the audiologist may be suspicious of the test results and gives the patient the opportunity to readjust their criterion, whether it is consciously or unconsciously overly conservative. In many cases, re-instruction is sufficient to obtain a true audiogram. During the audiometric threshold search, the audiologist may need to adjust the step size used in testing (often it is lowered to 2 dB or even varied across presentations to discourage a false criterion) or increase the variability of the timing of the presentation intervals. Another approach would be to use only ascending trials but start the threshold search at a level that is expected to be inaudible. In effect this approach removes familiarization but also removes an audible anchor for the patient. Ultimately, these practices effectively make it difficult for the patient to maintain an overly conservative criterion, but they also discourage specific strategies of feigning hearing loss, including counting and those based on remembered loudness.

The Stenger Test

For unilateral hearing losses, the audiologist can apply the *Stenger* test (Altshuler, 1970) to identify pseudohypacusis, which is based on the principles of lateralization The test relies on the psychoacoustic principle that a listener will lateralize a binaurally presented sound to the ear with the louder sound. When applying the Stenger test, the audiologist presents stimuli to both ears: The sound in the better ear is presented 10 dB above audiometric threshold (10 dB SL). The sound in the poorer (presumed pseudohypacusic) ear is presented

at 10 dB below the measured (but presumed false) threshold. The patient who is not feigning hearing loss will respond to this stimulus because the binaural sound will lateralize to his better ear, and he will hear it. In contrast, the patient with pseudohypacusis will not respond to this stimulus, as the sound will lateralize to the feigned ear because it is above his true audiometric threshold. This result provides evidence of pseudohypacusis because the tester knows that she can hear the sound in the healthy ear.

Once the Stenger test has identified the presence of pseudohypacusis, the *principle of contralateral interference* can be used when attempting to obtain true thresholds in the feigned ear. When applying this technique, the tester presents a stimulus at 10 dB SL in the better ear, and the sound level in the poorer starts at 0 dB HL is increased in 5- or 10-dB steps until the patient stops responding. This level is the contralateral interference level. The actual threshold is then inferred as being about 15 to 20 dB lower than the contralateral interference level.

Békésy Audiometry

As mentioned previously, Békésy audiometry can also be a useful tool for the assessment of pseudohypacusis by comparing tracings obtained between pulsed and continuously presented tones. A Type 5 Békésy pattern (illustrated in Figure 8–5), shows the pulsed tracing at a higher level (i.e., lower on the audiogram) than the continuous tracing. This pattern is indicative of pseudohypacusis. Rintelmann and Carhart (1964) suggested that this pattern occurs when an individual attempts to establish a false threshold by setting an internal loudness criterion (rather than a detection one). They argued that a pulsed stimulus is judged as softer than a continuous tone when presented at the same sensation level, causing an individual using a loudness criterion to require the pulsed tone to be presented at a higher level than the continuous tone to achieve the same loudness. Rintelmann and Harford (1967) found that a Type 5 Békésy tracing correctly identified pseudohypacusis about 75% of the time. Because no test of pseudohypacusis is 100% accurate, Békésy audiometry remains a useful tool, albeit not very common, for identification of nonorganic hearing loss in contemporary audiology.

TINNITUS EVALUATION

The prevalence of *tinnitus*, the perception of a sound in its absence, in the population is rising, along with a greater number of people presenting with sensorineural hearing loss. For the military, tinnitus is a long-standing issue, as it is currently the #1 service-connected disability. Unfortunately, there is no current diagnostic test for tinnitus, and diagnoses are based on self-report. Animal and human studies are currently under way that may ultimately lead to objective tests. However, diagnoses are currently made in conjunction with self-report, case history, and characterization of tinnitus.

Tinnitus assessment generally involves two separate evaluations: one which measures the reaction to the tinnitus (e.g., how bothersome or disruptive the tinnitus is), and one which measures the perception of the tinnitus (i.e., what the tinnitus sounds like to the patient). Reactions to tinnitus are exclusively measured through questionnaires, such as the Tinnitus Questionnaire (TQ; Hallam et al., 1988), the Tinnitus Handicap Inventory (THI; Newman et al., 1996), and the Tinnitus Functional Index (TFI; Meikle et al., 2012). These questionnaires are used to determine how disruptive tinnitus is to an individual's daily life and are critically important for establishing whether tinnitus treatment is necessary. On the other hand, characterization of tinnitus

perception is used to determine what the tinnitus sounds like (e.g., its loudness, quality or timbre, and pitch). Tinnitus perceptions are not necessarily related to the distress an individual experiences due to tinnitus. However, knowledge of the perception of tinnitus is informative to determine the need for medical referral and may be used to customize certain tinnitus treatments.

Tinnitus characterization, when conducted, generally establishes the quality first via questionnaire, in which an individual specifies the term that best describes their tinnitus (e.g., tonal, noisy, buzzing, hissing, etc.). Then, an audiologist usually conducts a brief measurement of tinnitus quality, which involves a patient listening to a tone and a narrow band noise and selecting which better matches their tinnitus. The next steps are loudness matching and pitch matching. Using the stimulus type selected by the patient (tone or noise), a tinnitus loudness match uses a loudness balancing procedure, which involves presenting stimuli at various sound levels to find the sound level that closely matches the perceived loudness of the tinnitus. In most instances, the sound level that best matches the tinnitus loudness is about 5 to 15 dB above the patient's audiometric threshold. There is no relationship between the tinnitus loudness and the annoyance of the tinnitus, and today, tinnitus loudness matches are not considered to be clinically useful unless used for counseling or to assess a treatment designed to reduce tinnitus loudness.

Obtaining a tinnitus pitch match uses a procedure similar to loudness balancing, but rather, the frequency that best matches the pitch of an individual's tinnitus is measured. In the clinical test, pitch matching is conducted using pure tones or narrow bands of noise (depending on the results of the quality test) presented at about 10 dB above the audiometric threshold at that frequency. Using a *bracketing procedure*, the audiologist presents pairs of stimuli with different frequencies to a patient, who then selects which of the two stimuli best match the pitch of their tinnitus. The audiologist chooses the next two frequencies to present to the patient based on the patient's selection. Figure 8–6 illustrates a schematic of a typical bracketing procedure, with an example of stimuli chosen by sample patient in bold italics. The audiologist continues presenting pairs of stimuli until the method converges on a single frequency; this is the tinnitus pitch match. In the example from Figure 8–6, the method would converge on a final pitch match of 3000 Hz. Individuals with tinnitus sometimes experience *octave* confusions, which are confusions between their tinnitus pitch and sounds one octave away from the pitch measurement. An audiologist also tests for these by presenting stimuli at octave multiples to finalize the pitch match.

Despite its use in clinical practice, the bracketing procedure is well-known to have very poor test-retest reliability for tinnitus pitch matching (Penner, 1983), and repeat estimates of tinnitus pitch are strongly recommended (McMillan et al., 2014). Further, numerous investigators have determined that even when tinnitus is described as tonal, individuals with tinnitus may rate many different frequencies as being similar to their tinnitus (Noreña et al., 2002; Roberts et al., 2008). In a test of over 100 participants, Roberts et al. used a pitch similarity rating method and showed that frequencies in the region of hearing loss were assigned high similarity to the tinnitus pitch. Given the results of these studies, methodologies that converge on a range of frequencies or use multiple estimates of the tinnitus pitch provide a better characterization of the perception of tinnitus than one bracketing procedure. Because certain tinnitus treatments may require an accurate tinnitus pitch match, it is important to verify the tinnitus pitch match with multiple measurements, particularly if the bracketing method is used.

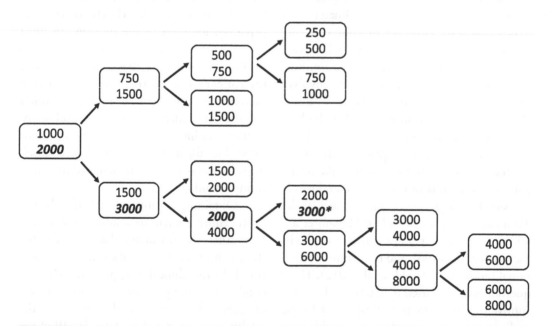

FIGURE 8–6. A sample bracketing procedure used for estimating tinnitus pitch. Frequencies shown in bold + italics represent example responses for a patient with a tinnitus pitch that matches a 3000-Hz tone.

In modern audiological assessment, the major useful diagnostic component of tinnitus assessment is that of tinnitus quality, although tinnitus quality is rarely measured using psychophysical techniques. Generally, tinnitus is characterized as being noisy, tonal, pulsatile, clicking, or hissing. Noisy, and more particularly, roaring tinnitus is a hallmark of Ménière's disease and can be informative from a diagnostic perspective. Pulsatile tinnitus can be indicative of high blood pressure, neurological pathologies, tumors, and so forth, and patients who characterize their tinnitus with similar terms should be referred for medical evaluation. Not all types of tinnitus are life threatening, as many forms of tinnitus are a consequence of aberrant neural activity within the central auditory system. Tinnitus can, however, be debilitating and can influence one's quality of life. Currently, no cure exists, and the goal of tinnitus treatment is tinnitus management. Some patients benefit substantially from ear-level sound therapies, noise maskers, and forms of cognitive therapy, all which help patients experience less distress from their tinnitus. In some debilitating cases, cochlear implants have successfully reduced the impact of tinnitus as well.

AUDITORY PROCESSING DISORDER

(Central) auditory processing disorder (APD) is defined as a single-locus disorder of the central auditory system (Moore, 2018). The British Society of Audiology identifies three types of APD: acquired APD, secondary APD, and developmental APD. Acquired APD is characterized by a known cause of the pathology (e.g., aging, trauma, or neurological event). Secondary APD is disruption to the central auditory pathway due to its association with a genetic cause or is secondary to peripheral hearing loss. Developmental APD presents in children with normal audiograms and has no known etiology. To date, it is generally accepted that acquired and secondary APD exist, but the evidence in support of the presence of developmental APD is limited, and as such, its existence is controversial (Moore, 2018)

Regardless of the source of the APD, diagnosis of the disorder can be challenging. The complexity of the auditory system, which includes bottom-up and top-down interactions among all levels of auditory processing (from peripheral to central), and the presence of speech-language, cognitive, and behavioral comorbidities among individuals who may present with APD, contribute to this difficulty. For those with acquired and secondary APD, we can link poor performance on specific auditory tests to a lesion or neurological change identified through some other mechanism (e.g., increased age, hearing loss identified on an audiogram, an associated pathology such as a stroke, etc.). But in the absence of some outside evidence of central auditory dysfunction, it can be difficult to determine why an individual may perform poorly on a set of psychoacoustical, speech, and/or language tests, as an auditory disorder is only one of many explanations.

Testing for APD requires a set of tests that attempt to establish central auditory function and behavior, separate from other neural processes (e.g., peripheral, cognitive, and speech/language). As such, a test protocol must include tests known to tap central auditory processes, such as temporal processing or binaural hearing tasks, and focus on nonspeech stimuli (Moore, 2006). Peripheral and cognitive assessments are also needed to rule out pathologies in those domains. What makes the diagnosis of APD so difficult is that auditory perception itself requires peripheral, central auditory, and cognitive processing. Auditory behavioral measurements require encoding of sounds by the peripheral auditory pathway and analysis of that information by the central auditory system. Cognition is also needed for an individual to make sense of and interpret the representations. Decision making, even at the lowest level of perception (detection), is required, as an individual must respond to the task requirements at hand. Consequently, no behavioral test taps into only central auditory function, and small changes to peripheral and cognitive function can influence results on a test designed to evaluate central auditory processing.

When tests for APD are conducted, behavioral assessments focus on temporal processing and binaural hearing. Temporal processing tests, such as gap detection and amplitude modulation detection, are not strongly influenced by peripheral factors, which make them good choices for an APD assessment. Binaural hearing tests are used because binaural interactions are represented at the level of the brainstem. As such, both types of tests can be helpful to determine whether APD is present. Individuals with APD are also expected to experience disruptions to speech perception when the speech is acoustically altered. Thus, an APD evaluation commonly includes tests of temporal processing, localization, lateralization, and dichotic listening. Speech tests generally include speech recognition in quiet, frequency-altered speech, time-compressed speech, and speech in competition. That said, tests of cognitive function are also necessary, as psychoacoustical and speech measures are negatively impacted by poor cognition (Lentz et al., 2022).

SUMMARY

Clearly, psychoacoustics has had a strong impact on diagnostic audiology. Even today, a variety of tests are conducted that rely on the principles of psychoacoustics from masking to the diagnosis of APD and the assessment of tinnitus. Although we rarely use behavioral

tests to identify retrocochlear disorders, there are cases where such tests are warranted, and an adept audiologist should be aware of the possibilities. There may come a time when additional psychoacoustic tests are adopted in the clinic to assess temporal, spectral, or binaural abilities in listeners. As we move toward precision medicine, it seems that using diagnoses of individual-specific disorders to influence treatment decisions may not be that far away.

The following points are key take-home messages of this chapter:

- Audiological assessment relies on several psychoacoustic principles, and behavioral testing is a core component in the diagnosis of auditory disorders.
- The principles of masking are important elements to the identification of dead regions.
- The ABLB and the SISI are techniques for retrocochlear assessment based on loudness recruitment, although they are not widely used in practice today.
- Békésy audiometry has been used in the past to facilitate diagnosis of both retrocochlear pathology and nonorganic hearing loss (pseudohypacusis). Although also not generally used for these purposes, automated methods based on Békésy audiometry for measuring hearing thresholds are both valid and reliable for many patients and experimental participants.
- Signal detection theory and lateralization are key principles applied in the evaluation of pseudohypacusis.
- Tinnitus evaluation relies on assessments of timbre, loudness, and pitch that are based on the techniques of loudness balancing and pitch matching.
- Temporal processing and binaural hearing measures are important pieces to identify APD.

EXERCISES

1. Explain how off-frequency listening could yield a threshold for a frequency associated with a dead region.

2. A patient's audiometric test results reveal a bilateral sensorineural hearing loss. The right ear has a PTA of about 20 dB HL, and the left ear has a PTA of 50 dB HL. Discuss why this patient should be assessed for retrocochlear involvement.

3. You decide to conduct a behavioral retrocochlear assessment for the patient in Exercise 2. Describe a test that would be appropriate and the results that would be expected if the patient had retrocochlear involvement to his hearing loss.

4. Provide two examples of cases when an audiologist may need to use behavioral techniques for retrocochlear assessment.

5. Behavioral tests of retrocochlear pathology typically have good specificity but poor sensitivity. Why is poor sensitivity a problem for a diagnostic test?

6. Using Erber's perceptual hierarchy, why is speech testing important for the diagnosis of retrocochlear disorders?

7. Consider the following situation: A patient presents with pseudohypacusis, and you, the audiologist, are attempting to obtain an accurate threshold. Nothing in the standard audiometric procedure seems to work. Given what you have learned in other chapters of this book, provide a methodological suggestion that might allow you to avoid problems with a conservative criterion. Discuss your reasoning.

8. Why can't we use the Stenger test for bilateral pseudohypacusis?

9. Discuss how tinnitus evaluation uses loudness balancing and pitch matching to discover the tinnitus perception.

10. Discuss how gap detection could be used in an assessment of central auditory function.

11. Discuss how measuring the masking level difference (MLD) could contribute to an assessment of central auditory function.

12. Explain why APD is difficult to diagnose using audiological testing.

REFERENCES

Altshuler, M. W. (1970). The stenger phenomenon. *Journal of Communication Disorders, 3*(2), 89–105.

Békésy, G. V. (1947). A new audiometer. *Acta Oto-Laryngologica, 35*(5–6), 411–422.

Fowler, E. P. (1936). A method for the early detection of otosclerosis: A study of sounds well above threshold. *Archives of Otolaryngology, 24*(6), 731–741.

Hallam, R.S., Jakes. S.C. & Hinchcliffe, R. (1988). Cognitive variables in tinnitus annoyance. *British Journal of Clinical Psychology. 27*, 213–222.

Hirsh, I. J., Palva, T., & Goodman, A. (1954). Difference limen and recruitment. *AMA Archives of Otolaryngology, 60*(5), 525–540.

Jerger, J. (1960). Békésy audiometry in analysis of auditory disorders. *Journal of Speech and Hearing Research, 3*(3), 275–287.

Jerger, J., & Herer, G. (1961). Unexpected dividend in Békésy audiometry. *Journal of Speech and Hearing Disorders, 26*(4), 390–391.

Jerger, J., Shedd, J. L., & Harford, E. (1959). On the detection of extremely small changes in sound intensity. *AMA Archives of Otolaryngology, 69*(2), 200–211.

Lentz, J. J., Humes, L. E., & Kidd, G. R. (2022). Differences in auditory perception between young and older adults when controlling for differences in hearing loss and cognition. *Trends in Hearing, 26*, 1–17.

Mahomed, F., Swanepoel, D. W., Eikelboom, R. H., & Soer, M. (2013). Validity of automated threshold audiometry: A systematic review and meta-analysis. *Ear and Hearing, 34*(6), 745–752.

McMillan, G. P., Thielman, E. J., Wypych, K., & Henry, J. A. (2014). A Bayesian perspective on tinnitus pitch matching. *Ear and Hearing, 35*(6), 687–694.

Meikle, M. B., Henry, J. A., Griest, S. E., Stewart, B. J., Abrams, H. B., McArdle, R., . . . Vernon, J. A. (2012). The tinnitus functional index: Development of a new clinical measure for chronic, intrusive tinnitus. *Ear and Hearing, 33*(2), 153–176.

Moore, B. C. J., Huss, M., Vickers, D. A., Glasberg, B. R., & Alcántara, J. I. (2000). A test for the diagnosis of dead regions in the cochlea. *British Journal of Audiology, 34*(4), 205–224.

Moore, D. R. (2006). Auditory processing disorder (APD): Definition, diagnosis, neural basis, and intervention. *Audiological Medicine, 4*(1), 4–11.

Moore, D. R. (2018). Auditory processing disorder (APD). *Ear and Hearing, 39*(4), 617–620.

Musiek, F. (2022). *The Short Increment Sensitivity Index (SISI): An auditory discrimination application?* https://hearinghealthmatters.org/pathways-society/2022/the-short-increment-sensitivity-index-sisi-an-auditory-discrimination-application/

Newman C. W., Jacobson G. P., & Spitzer J. B. (1996). Development of the Tinnitus Handicap Inventory. *Archives of Otolaryngology Head and Neck Surgery, 122*, 143–148.

Noreña, A., Micheyl, C., Chéry-Croze, S., & Collet, L. (2002). Psychoacoustic characterization of the tinnitus spectrum: Implications for the underlying mechanisms of tinnitus. *Audiology and Neurotology, 7*(6), 358–369.

Penner, M. J. (1983). Variability in matches to subjective tinnitus. *Journal of Speech, Language, and Hearing Research, 26*(2), 263–267.

Rintelmann, W. F., & Carhart, R. (1964). Loudness tracking by normal hearers via Békésy audiometer. *Journal of Speech and Hearing Research, 7*(1), 79–93.

Rintelmann, W. F., & Harford, E. R. (1967). Type V Békésy pattern: Interpretation and clinical utility. *Journal of Speech and Hearing Research, 10*(4), 733–744.

Roberts, L. E., Moffat, G., Baumann, M., Ward, L. M., & Bosnyak, D. J. (2008). Residual inhibition functions overlap tinnitus spectra and the region of auditory threshold shift. *Journal of the Association for Research in Otolaryngology, 9*(4), 417–435.

Turner, R. G., Shepard, N. T., & Frazer, G. J. (1984). Clinical performance of audiological and related diagnostic tests. *Ear and Hearing, 5*(4), 187–194.

Vickers D. A., Moore B. C. J., & Baer T. (2001). Effects of lowpass filtering on the intelligibility of speech in quiet for people with and without dead regions at high frequencies. *Journal of the Acoustical Society of America, 110*, 1164–1175.

Vinay, Baer, T., & Moore, B. C. J. (2008). Speech recognition in noise as a function of highpass-filter cutoff frequency for people with and without low-frequency cochlear dead regions. *Journal of the Acoustical Society of America, 123*(2), 606–609.

Vinay, & Moore, B. C. J. (2007). Speech recognition as a function of high-pass filter cutoff frequency for people with and without low-frequency cochlear dead regions. *Journal of the Acoustical Society of America, 122*(1), 542–553.

9

Improving Auditory Perception for Listeners With Hearing Loss

LEARNING OBJECTIVES

Upon completion of this chapter, students will be able to:

- Evaluate how nonlinear algorithms in conventional hearing aids influence various aspects of auditory perception
- Compare and contrast the effects of noise reduction algorithms and directional microphones on binaural hearing
- Explain the influence of cochlear implants on auditory perception

INTRODUCTION

Audiologists spend their time in the assessment and treatment of auditory disorders, and their ability to treat an individual's hearing loss is based on knowledge of both normal hearing and hearing loss. Much of an audiologist's profession is to provide rehabilitation options to individuals with a goal of improving their auditory and speech perception. Current assistive devices on the market do just that—they improve both auditory and speech perception for individuals who have hearing loss. Unfortunately, no assistive device can *cure* hearing loss, and the assistive devices on the market today focus on providing the ear better access to signals within the acoustic environment.

One approach to increasing auditory perception and speech understanding is to focus on technologies that improve perception in regard to the hierarchy of auditory perception. Hearing aids and cochlear implants were initially developed to provide a listener with more access to sounds; hearing aids through amplification and cochlear implants by direct stimulation of the auditory nerve. Both devices provide a listener with better detection, discrimination, identification, and comprehension than without the devices. Modern hearing aids and the speech processor of the cochlear implant reduce the noise present in the output signals by using directional microphones and digital noise reduction algorithms. As a result, both devices provide access to a more audible and potentially clearer signal, which is then processed by the neural mechanisms available to the listener. In this way, improvements to all levels of perception, including perception in noise, can occur. Both hearing aids and cochlear implants can be defined as successful and effective treatments for sensorineural hearing loss, if success is defined by better speech perception for almost all individuals who wear them.

In this chapter, we review common assistive devices: conventional hearing aids and cochlear implants. We also explore how these innovative assistive devices influence the acoustic representations of sound available to a listener and their effects on auditory perception.

We touch on the following topics:

- Impact of conventional hearing aids on the perception of sounds
- Amplification and compression
- Directional microphones and noise reduction
- Auditory perception by cochlear implant users

IMPACT OF CONVENTIONAL HEARING AIDS ON AUDITORY PERCEPTION

Modern hearing aids are an engineering marvel: They amplify sound in a frequency-specific manner, contain high-quality microphones and receivers, and have sophisticated software designed to modify sound that will ultimately assist the listener in a variety of acoustic environments. This is all done in a tiny device; many are smaller than an inch (2.5 cm). As we all know, hearing aids do not work like glasses, which correct for optical deficits in the eye. Sensorineural hearing loss is not an acoustic deficit; rather, it is a deficit in the sensory representation of acoustic stimuli. Consequently, hearing aids are limited in their ability to compensate for the distortions imposed by the ear, and so they alter the acoustics of input sounds in a way that supports speech perception.

Hearing aids can amplify sound, improve the signal-to-noise ratio through noise reduction or directional microphones, and even include specialized programs to assist with tinnitus tolerance or listening to music, and so forth. However, they cannot correct for many of the supra-threshold perceptual deficits experienced by listeners with SNHL.

Regardless, there is no doubt that hearing aids are beneficial to people with sensorineural hearing loss. Almost everyone who has a mild or greater hearing loss should wear them, and we could even argue that people with slight hearing losses (thresholds of 16 to 25 dB HL) may benefit from hearing aids. Primarily, hearing aids employ a sophisticated amplifier that increases the input level of sounds to the ear in a frequency-dependent manner, with the expectation that the auditory system will then decode the information present in the stimulus (with speech understanding being one of the goals). Consequently, hearing aids compensate for the most important auditory deficit, higher auditory thresholds, by amplifying sounds that fall below an individual's threshold. As a result, they improve speech perception.

Although hearing aids cannot directly alter supra-threshold deficits experienced by listeners with SNHL, the improved audibility provides access to higher levels of perception. Furthermore, technologies available in hearing aids may be able to help with these problems by manipulating the acoustics of the input sound. Many listeners with SNHL are expected to benefit from amplification and improvements to the signal-to-noise ratio, and although these technologies do not directly address the perceptual changes experienced by listeners, they can ameliorate some of the negative effects of those deficits by providing a cleaner, better signal. Modern hearing aids primarily work to compensate for three areas of perceptual deficits experienced by listeners with SNHL: reduced audibility through *amplification*, loudness recruitment through *compression*, and increased susceptibility to noise through *directional microphones* and *noise reduction*. Higher-level auditory perceptual deficits cannot be influenced directly by amplification, such as reduced frequency resolution, temporal processing, and pitch perception. And although hearing aids cannot restore binaural processing deficits, recent technological advances provide much better access to binaural information present in the environment. This section reviews how hearing aid algorithms improve, and sometimes degrade, the representation of information provided to listeners with sensorineural hearing loss.

Compression

Prior to the 1990s, most hearing aids employed *linear* (or constant gain) amplification, which meant that devices provided the same amount of gain for all input stimulus levels. For example, a linear hearing aid with 25 dB of gain would amplify a 30 dB SPL sound to 55 dB SPL, and a 75 dB SPL sound to 100 dB SPL. Linear hearing aids had multiple channels, which allowed for a different amount of gain in each channel, thereby accommodating hearing losses that varied across frequency. As a result, these hearing aids made sounds audible in a frequency-specific manner. Speech perception was improved by these hearing aids because of the amplification.

However, these hearing aids had some drawbacks. They included an output limiter, which set a maximum output sound level for each channel of the hearing aid. This output limiter prevented high-level sounds from becoming excessively loud due to the linear amplification. The output limiter distorted high-level sounds, and these devices provided too much gain to high-level sounds and not

enough gain to low-level sounds. Now, modern hearing aids all provide some form of non-linear amplification, which has contributed to better comfort for hearing aid wearers. ***Wide dynamic range compression (WDRC)*** is one of these popular non-linear amplification schemes. The pros and cons of using this type of algorithm are reasonably illustrative of other nonlinear forms of amplification, and so only WDRC is discussed here.

Fitting a modern nonlinear hearing aid generally starts with an audiometric assessment to determine the degree and type of hearing loss at various frequencies. The maximum amount of gain applied by the hearing aid is determined from the audiogram using a prescriptive rule and is set to somewhere between one-half and two-thirds of the amount of hearing loss. For nonlinear algorithms such as WDRC, the prescription determines the *maximum* gain, and the amount of gain applied varies depending on the level of the stimulus. Essentially, a simple form of WDRC works in the following way:

- *At low input levels, the hearing aid provides linear amplification.* That is, the gain provided by the hearing aid is constant regardless of the input level and is usually the maximum gain.
- *At moderate input levels, the hearing aid provides progressively less amplification.* The decibel level above which the algorithm switches from linear to compressive is called the *compression threshold* and can be dependent on frequency. A *compression ratio* is also required as part of the prescription, which specifies the reduction of the amount of gain after sound exceeds the compression threshold. For example, a 2:1 compression ratio indicates that for every 2-dB change in the input, a 1-dB change in output would occur. For example, a 50-dB SPL input sound might be amplified to 75-dB SPL,

and a 52-dB SPL input sound would be amplified to 76 dB SPL.

- *At high input levels, stimuli often receive minimal amplification.* This is related to the fact that many listeners with SNHL have similar LDLs to those with normal hearing. Hearing aids also offer a means for setting maximum output to avoid loudness discomfort and levels that could produce additional sensorineural hearing loss (overamplification).

Figure 9–1 illustrates this simple amplification scheme by plotting gain in dB versus input sound level. In this example, the maximum gain is 25 dB. Compression begins at the *compression threshold*, which here, is 40 dB SPL. The *compression ratio*, which in this example is 2:1, leads to a gradual decrease in the amount of gain with increasing level until, at 90 dB SPL and greater, the algorithm does not apply any gain.

The version of compression illustrated here is only an illustration, and many modern hearing aids employ expansion for very low-level sounds. Expansion is the opposite of compression—the amount of gain increases as the input level increases. Expansion reduces the audibility of low-level sounds, which ultimately prevents low levels of background noise from being amplified and reduces microphone noise in the hearing aid. A hearing aid with expansion would also have an expansion threshold that establishes the level below which expansion is adopted.

WDRC algorithms cannot act instantaneously, and so they also have a *compression speed,* which is a descriptor of the time it takes for a hearing aid to change the gain depending

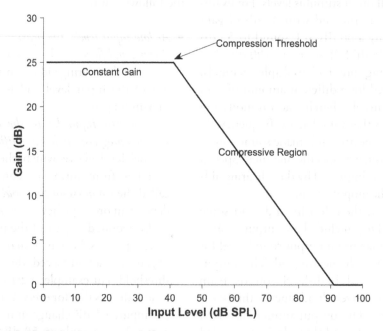

FIGURE 9–1. A schematic of the gain provided by a compression algorithm with a maximum gain of 25 dB, a 2:1 compression ratio, and a 40 dB SPL compression threshold.

on changes in the level of the stimulus. Compression speed is generally described as either being *fast* or *slow* (although other terms are also used). The compression speed influences the degree of temporal distortion imposed on a stimulus.

Compression algorithms provide perceptual benefits in several ways. Achieving audibility for speech signals is critically important for speech understanding, and compression algorithms do this in a way that achieves audibility without overly distorting signals at high levels. Compression algorithms accomplish a great deal in providing comfort for patients and restoring audibility. They have some negative consequences, however, and a patient's specific perceptual deficits might interact with the type of compression parameters used in amplification schemes.

Threshold and Loudness

Hearing aids all amplify sounds in the environment and, therefore, lead to improved thresholds. When WDRC is used, it increases the dynamic range available to a listener: Low-level sounds are amplified the most and high-level sounds are only slightly amplified. Consider a listener with sensorineural hearing loss who is fit with a hearing aid described in Figure 9–1 (maximum gain of 25 dB, compression threshold of 40 dB SPL, and a compression ratio of 2:1). For illustrative purposes, let us assume that this individual has an absolute threshold of 50 dB SPL. Without amplification, their dynamic range would be approximately 50 dB (or 50 dB SPL to 100 dB SPL). With amplification, however, all sounds between 25 and 50 dB SPL would become audible. Twenty-five dB of gain would be applied to sounds below 40 dB SPL and slightly less gain would be applied to sounds between 40 and 50 dB SPL. Because the hearing aid would not amplify high-level sounds, this individual's dynamic range becomes

75 dB (25 dB SPL to 100 dB SPL). The nonlinear amplification also influences loudness growth, by partially restoring loudness growth with intensity (Strelcyk et al., 2012).

Temporal Processing

Despite the benefits of WDRC in terms of improved audibility of low-level sounds and increased dynamic range, compression alters the natural fluctuations present in acoustic stimuli. Because low-level sounds are amplified more than high-level sounds, the acoustic waveform of a stimulus is less modulated after processing by a compression hearing aid. When the compression is fast acting, we may see improvements in temporal processing. For example, Moore et al. (2001) found that three listeners with SNHL had better gap detection in narrow bands of noise for compressed than for uncompressed stimuli. Brennan et al. (2015) showed that WDRC improved forward-masked thresholds and led to greater release of forward masking for nine listeners with SNHL. Lastly, Wiinberg et al. (2019) showed that listeners with normal hearing and SNHL both had better modulation detection thresholds when stimuli were processed by compression.

However, the distortions imposed by compression may also disrupt the waveform of speech and lead to poorer speech understanding. Hedrick and Rice (2000) evaluated stop consonants /t/ ("tip") and /p/ ("pip") and demonstrated that they were more confusable with one another after being processed by WDRC. That said, the temporal distortion imposed by WDRC likely has minimal influence on everyday listening because the WDRC algorithm provides substantial benefits by providing access to low-level speech sounds and, as discussed previously, assists with the encoding of temporal information in speech. Davies-Venn et al. (2009) found that whereas temporal distortion is a consequence of WDRC, the improvement in audibility outweighs the potential negative consequences of temporal distortion.

Spectral Contrast

Given that hearing aids include multiple channels to accommodate differing degrees of hearing loss across frequency, Plomp (1988) posited that the number of channels would interact with the compression imposed on those channels, with a consequence of smoothing the peaks and valleys in a sound spectrum. He argued that if one compression channel processed a spectral peak and another processed a spectral valley, the relationship between the output levels of the two channels would be altered from the original relationship. On the other hand, if the same channel processed the peak and valley, the peak and valley would undergo the same amount of amplification. This would preserve the spectral contrast in the stimulus.

To illustrate the effects of multichannel compression, consider a vowel, which is characterized by spectral peaks (the formants) and valleys, with a formant at 70 dB SPL and a valley that is at 45 dB SPL. The formant and the valley are processed by different channels but the same compression rule. If we apply a compression algorithm that applies 25 dB of gain below 50 dB SPL and has a 2:1 compression ratio above 50 dB SPL, the valley will be amplified by 25 dB and will have a level of 70 dB SPL at the output of the hearing aid. The peak, on the other hand, will also undergo compression but through a different channel. The peak will only be amplified by 10 dB (as it is in the region of compression), leading to an output of 80 dB SPL. In this way, processing the peak and valley through separate channels will reduce the 25 dB of spectral contrast to 10 dB.

Despite Plomp's hypothesis, a recent study by Kiliç and Kara (2022) showed no difference on a test of spectral resolution for stimuli processed through a channel free or a multichannel WDRC hearing aid. On the other hand, Bor et al. (2008) made acoustic and perceptual measurements and noted that the spectral contrast present in vowels decreased with increasing number of compression channels, and that perception of the vowels degraded as well. Listeners with sensorineural hearing loss made more vowel confusions as the number of channels increased. Performance was poorest for 16 channels, but relatively unchanged between 1 and 8 channels. The implications for these results are many, as vowel stimuli are not the only speech sounds that require the presence of spectral contrast. Yet, most studies on speech perception show that increasing the number of channels from one to eight improves speech perception, and that adding more channels does not drastically impact speech perception (Yund & Buckles, 1995). Such results suggest that our ability to perceive speech is very robust even in the presence of spectral distortion.

Binaural Perception

Providing amplification to a listener can provide a real benefit to a listener by providing access to binaural cues that may have been originally inaudible. Yet, a listener must wear two hearing aids to receive these benefits. There is clear evidence in support of bilateral compared to unilateral hearing aid fitting, as bilateral hearing aid wearers have better speech intelligibility in quiet and in noise and better sound localization than those wearing one hearing aid (Derleth et al., 2021). The ability of a listener to use binaural cues requires that they first be able to access, or hear, those cues. Hearing aids amplify the sound in the environment and, in part, restore interaural cues that may have been inaudible to the listener.

However, hearing aids do not provide full support for binaural hearing (see Zheng et al, 2022 for a review). Hearing aid microphones tend to amplify only up to 6000 Hz, and, therefore, do not provide access to binaural cues in high frequencies. Further, small differences in algorithmic fitting across the ears can negatively impact the binaural information available to the listener. Although binaural abilities of listeners with sensorineural tend to be substantially poorer than those with normal hearing, some listeners with SNHL do have spatial hearing, and many listeners experience binaural unmasking effects that require the representation of binaural cues. Unfortunately for these listeners, delays imposed by hearing aids may also impact the ITD representation and distort binaural perception. Compression algorithms that operate independently across the ears reduce the binaural cues available to a listener, with a significant impact on the ILD. Figure 9–2 illustrates how WDRC can impact the ILD.

In this example, a 3000 Hz tone at 70 dB SPL is presented to the listener's right ear. The top panel illustrates that head shadow of this individual produces an ILD of 15 dB. The middle panel illustrates how a compression algorithm might alter the ILD for an individual with a hearing loss of 50 dB HL. The bottom panel of Figure 9–2 shows that the right ear receives a sound level of 70 dB SPL that is amplified by 10 dB, and so the sound level at that ear is now 80 dB SPL. On the other hand, the left ear receives a sound at 55 dB SPL that is amplified by 17 dB, and the new sound level is 73 dB SPL. In this case, the ILD after hearing aid processing is 7 dB (80 dB SPL to 73 dB SPL), instead of 15 dB. In this way, the ILD is now reduced compared to the one present in the environment.

Multiple studies have demonstrated the detrimental effects of hearing aids on binaural hearing using sound localization tasks, as listeners with SNHL make substantially more localization errors while wearing their hearing aids compared to while unaided (for reviews

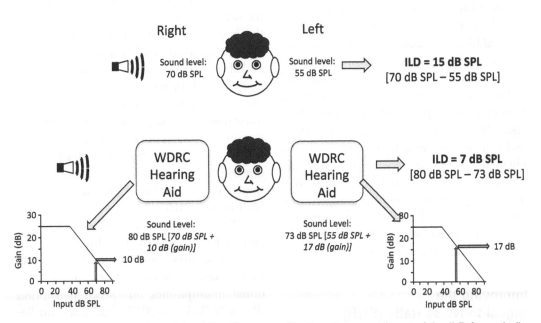

FIGURE 9–2. An illustration of the ILD without amplification (*top panel*) and of the ILD for an individual wearing a compression hearing aid (*bottom panel*) for a 2000-Hz sound presented at 70 dB SPL directly to the right of a listener. The top panel illustrates that the ILD is 15 dB. The bottom panel illustrates the impact of a compression hearing aid on the ILD for a listener with a threshold of 50 dB HL. For this listener, the hearing aid provides 10 dB of gain and 17 dB of gain to the right and left ears, respectively. Thus, the sound levels (at the output of the hearing aids) at the right and left ears are then 80 dB SPL and 73 dB SPL, respectively. In this case, the ILD becomes 7 dB in contrast to the original 15 dB.

see Akeroyd, 2014 and Zheng et al., 2022). We can conclude that bilateral hearing aids are not helpful for sound localization and often make localization worse compared to unaided conditions. However, binaural processing algorithms in paired hearing aids are likely to restore appropriate binaural acoustic cues. These algorithms have great potential to be beneficial to listeners experiencing binaural deficits associated with hearing aid processing and would allow listeners better access to the binaural cues in their environment. Such advancements may help listeners with spatial hearing and improved speech perception in noise due to better access of binaural unmasking cues.

Summary

Taken together, there is no doubt that nonlinear algorithms in hearing aids provide benefits to a listener with SNHL. These benefits include, but are not exclusive to, improving the audibility of sounds without exceeding uncomfortable loudness levels and expanding a listener's dynamic range. Listeners also tend to find these hearing aids more comfortable than their linear precursors. However, these algorithms include unintended side effects and can distort the temporal, spectral, and binaural cues. Improvements to hearing aid technology continue to reduce the amount of distortion provided by nonlinear algorithms, and in most cases, the positive effects of wearing a hearing aid far outweigh the negative consequences of the distortion.

Improving the Signal-to-Noise Ratio (SNR)

Improving the SNR is helpful to a listener—a better SNR allows a listener to apply their available auditory mechanisms without the detrimental effects of masking. Recall that under difficult listening conditions, a 1-dB improvement in the SNR can result in an

increase in intelligibility of between 7 and 19 percentage points. Due to the deficits associated with sensorineural hearing loss and the large potential benefits of a higher SNR, improving the SNR for listeners with sensorineural hearing loss has been a focus of modern hearing aids. A variety of techniques are used to improve the SNR, with common ones being directional microphones and noise reduction algorithms.

Directional Microphones

Directional microphones are a desirable feature in hearing aids and cochlear implants on the market today. In a nutshell, these microphones are more sensitive to sounds coming from a particular direction than to sounds coming from other directions. A common implementation of a directional microphone selectively represents sounds to the front of the listener more than sounds to the side or the back of the listener. Further, adaptive spatial algorithms are becoming increasingly available that do not always require the listener to look in the direction of the sound. For instance, a "speech-seeking" directional microphone would provide more amplification in the direction of algorithm-identified speech. Laboratory tests show advantages of directional microphones when listening to speech in noise, with improvements in the SNR of over 7 dB.

Perceptual research on directional microphones has been primarily directed toward speech perception and binaural hearing. Lab studies have demonstrated benefits of directional microphones on speech perception (Picou & Ricketts, 2017), but much smaller benefits are more commonly measured in real listening environments (Bentler, 2005). The reasons for this difference are many, and partly relate to vast differences in the acoustic setup used for laboratory and clinical tests in comparison to real-world acoustical environments. Traditional implementations of directional microphones also negatively alter the representation of environmental cues, particularly those involved in binaural hearing. Binaurally fitted devices that operate independently negatively impact sound localization and limit the ability of the auditory system to take advantage of binaural unmasking cues. Localization errors are common for listeners using directional technologies, as both ILD and ITD cues are distorted by the directionality (Picou et al., 2014).

New technologies designed to provide directionality may reduce the negative impacts on binaural cues. One approach is the development of algorithms that can retain the spatial cues present in the environment, such as an omnidirectional microphone that preserves the spatial information coupled with a directional microphone that attenuates the noise. Some manufacturers also have developed hearing aids that communicate with each other and can preserve the binaural cues present in the environment. These devices have great potential to provide access to binaural cues for those listeners with SNHL who have binaural hearing. In this way, better access to spatial cues would be provided to the hearing aid wearer and further allow that listener's auditory system to engage its binaural mechanisms such as binaural squelch and binaural unmasking and better support speech understanding in noise.

Noise Reduction Algorithms

Although not as effective as directional microphones, *digital noise reduction (DNR)* algorithms improve the SNR, but more notably offer improved listening comfort for assistive device wearers and reduce listening effort in difficult listening situations (Desjardins & Doherty, 2014). A common noise-reduction algorithm is based on the different spectrotemporal modulations present in speech compared to noise, and an algorithm generally evaluates the degree of modulation of the signal in each hearing aid channel. When the algorithm detects steady-state noise in specific channels, the gain is reduced in those channels. In this way, more gain can be applied to the channels that include speech only, thereby increasing the SNR. These algorithms may also reduce the gain in low frequency bands to decrease upward spread of masking. Algorithms such as these work rather well when the background noise has few fluctuations but are not as successful when the background noise is highly fluctuating (such as in an environment with one other person talking) because the algorithm identifies the fluctuations as speech.

However, DNR algorithms also have the potential to influence the availability of the psychoacoustic cues available in the environment. Given that these algorithms apply gain on a channel-by-channel basis, they alter the spectral shape of an input sound. Similar to the effects of WDRC, we might expect that disruptions to the spectral representation of a stimulus may impair abilities that require a faithful representation of the spectrum. Although the general spectral shape of a stimulus is not a critical parameter for speech understanding, music and timbre perception do rely on an adequate representation of spectral shape. DNR algorithms also distort binaural cues impacting sound localization abilities and sound segregation based on binaural cues, particularly the ILD. As noted previously, hearing aids that communicate with each other may also be helpful in resolving these situations, and algorithmic advances also promise to improve their distortions.

AUDITORY PERCEPTION BY COCHLEAR IMPLANT USERS

Cochlear implants (CIs) are prosthetic devices that are intended to provide access to sound for individuals who have sensorineural hearing losses and are (generally) not successful with hearing aids. To date, the cochlear implant remains the single most successful sensory implant, and many CI users who were implanted at a young age can achieve near-normal spoken language skills. Although many CI users can achieve fully intelligible speech production and strong speech perception skills in quiet, the CI does not provide *normal hearing*, as it delivers a significantly impoverished representation of sounds in the environment compared to that represented an ear with normal hearing. Speech perception in noise also remains a challenge for listeners with a CI, but the CI often provides an enormous improvement for perceiving spoken language for individuals with severe and profound sensorineural hearing losses.

General Principles of the CI

The CI is an extraordinary device that may allow individuals with moderate-to-profound sensorineural hearing loss to communicate through spoken language. The cochlear implant device consists of an external microphone and external speech processor, which converts useful environmental acoustic signals into electric signals. The electrical signal is then wirelessly transmitted through the scalp to an implanted electrode array in the cochlea. The speech processor codes the amplitude envelopes of speech by modulating digital pulses, delivered through the electrode array, which generally contains between 12 and 22 electrodes, depending on the manufacturer. These digital pulses stimulate the auditory nerve, activating the natural neural pathway for hearing. Whereas the CI provides access to sound for many, it also has numerous limitations that relate to auditory perception (Moore & Carlyon, 2005). Some of these limitations are as follows:

- *Electrode array depth:* The cochlea itself imposes some restrictions on the insertion depth of the electrode array, which can be a surgical and mechanical challenge to insert an electrode array down the full 2.5 turns of the cochlea. Some CI electrode arrays can be implanted to 2 to 2.25 turns of the cochlea, whereas others are shorter and penetrate to about 1.5. These shorter implants, therefore, do not usually provide access to low-frequency sounds.

- *Physiological degeneration:* Atrophy of the auditory nerve (occurring prior to implantation) can disrupt the ability to represent the signals generated by the CI.

- *Stimulation strategy:* Some CI stimulation strategies use a set of pulse trains that effectively *override* the natural phase-locking abilities of the auditory nerve. Some CI encoding strategies use the same rate of pulse trains for all electrodes, so any perceptual code based on phase-locking of the auditory nerve is unavailable to these CI users.

- *Number of channels:* A modern CI has about 12 to 22 electrodes, and current spread between the electrodes can lead to smearing of information between channels.

Auditory Perception

The role of the CI is to provide access to the acoustic environment via stimulation of the auditory nerve. We can measure how well a listener with a CI perceives this information by using psychoacoustic techniques. However, there are differences in the way perception is measured for CI users compared to those who have *acoustic hearing* (the typical mechanism of hearing). The mechanism of hearing for a CI user is commonly referred to *electric hearing*, due to the fact that the auditory system is stimulated by an electrical signal. A CI user may have access to both electric and acoustic hearing, depending on the type of implant and whether one or both ears are implanted with a CI. When testing electric hearing, scientists can present stimuli over loudspeakers or by connecting the CI to a computer interface. In this way, the experimenter may more closely simulate real-world experiences precisely control the signals by delivering them to the CI through a direct connection.

Threshold and Loudness

By providing electrical stimulation to the auditory nerve, the CI effectively bypasses the damaged cochlear structures that lead to elevated audiometric thresholds. Improvement to threshold (preimplantation measured via acoustic hearing vs. post-implantation measured via electrical hearing) can be significant. Prior to implantation, CI users typically have thresholds in the moderate-to-profound range for acoustic hearing. Post-implantation and activation, some CI users have thresholds better than 10 dB HL! But others may have thresholds in the range of 40 to 50 dB HL. Regardless, most achieve a vast improvement in auditory threshold when wearing the cochlear implant. However, recall that some CIs do not penetrate the entire length of the cochlea, and these CIs may not be able to stimulate frequency regions below 300 to 1000 Hz. CI users with good low-frequency hearing pre-implantation may be able to supplement the electrical stimulation provided by the CI with low-frequency acoustic hearing. For others, modern cochlear implant processing strategies can give some CI users access to low-frequency information, and neural reorganization may provide some additional access.

In comparison to listeners with normal hearing, the dynamic range of a CI is relatively small, but it can be anywhere from 3 and 80 dB. As such, loudness growth for CI users is generally more rapid than for listeners with normal hearing (Fu, 2005). Yet, comparing loudness growth between CI users and listeners with normal (acoustic) hearing is not straightforward. Compensation for rapid loudness growth can be implemented through the speech processing algorithm. This compensation can yield more typical loudness growth, which has been demonstrated to result in better speech perception for CI wearers (Fu & Shannon, 1998). Strikingly, CI users demonstrate JNDs for intensity that can be roughly half that of listeners with normal hearing (i.e., they have better intensity discrimination; Pfingst et al., 1983). As such, it appears that there are mechanisms by which a CI user can *compensate* for the reduced dynamic range.

Spectral Resolution

The spectral resolution, or frequency selectivity, of listeners with a cochlear implant is considerably poorer than for listeners with normal hearing. A modern CI typically has 12 to 22 electrodes and sometimes only a subset of these electrodes is activated for any individual CI user, further reducing the number of electrodes available. Increasing the number of physical electrodes is not presently advised, as current spread between adjacent electrodes has been shown to compromise spectral resolution and speech perception abilities. Other important factors likely contribute to the frequency selectivity of the CI user, such as the alignment between the acoustically stimulated electrodes and the cochlear location that normally processes that frequency range (Başkent & Shannon, 2005). Thus, there are numerous reasons why the spectral resolution of CI users is not robust.

Yet, good spectral resolution does not appear to be necessary to support speech perception in quiet, as illustrated by studies that have measured the speech perception abilities as a function of the number of active electrodes. Fishman et al. (1997) and Friesen et al. (2001) both showed that increasing the number of active electrodes leads to better speech perception, regardless of whether speech was measured in quiet or in noise. Figure 9–3 shows these effects for speech in quiet and speech presented at +5 dB SNR using sentences from the HINT (Hearing in Noise Test). For reference, data obtained from listeners with normal hearing, but processed by a cochlear implant simulation (a noise vocoder), are also shown. In all cases, increasing the number of electrodes (or channels, for the listeners with normal hearing) improved word identification up to a point. Approximately eight electrodes were sufficient to lead to good speech perception in quiet for CI users. More electrodes/channels supported better speech perception for both groups of listeners, but those wearing CIs did not achieve high levels of speech perception in noise.

Frequency selectivity can be measured more directly using the spectral ripple discrimination task (Henry & Turner, 2003). This task provides a rapid assessment of frequency selectivity by using a broadband stimulus (in contrast to the typical notched-noise method

discussed in Chapter 3). In this task, a listener discriminates between two broadband sounds, each with a spectral ripple. One stimulus has a positive spectral ripple (the standard), which is in essence, a rectified sine wave imposed on the spectrum, and the other stimulus is an *inverted* version of the spectral ripple, or a cosine wave. Figure 9–4 illustrates typical spectral ripple stimuli used in this kind of experiment. The ripple rate (which describes the spacing between the ripple peaks) is varied, and the fastest ripple rate that a listener can detect is a representation of the spectral resolution of an individual. Faster ripple thresholds align with better spectral resolution. The top panel of Figure 9–4 illustrates a stimulus that would be associated with a ripple threshold of 0.5 cycles/octave, or relatively poor spectral resolution, whereas the bottom panel illustrates a stimulus that would be associated with a better ripple threshold of 2 cycles/octave. When measured using this technique, CI users generally have spectral resolution that is about three

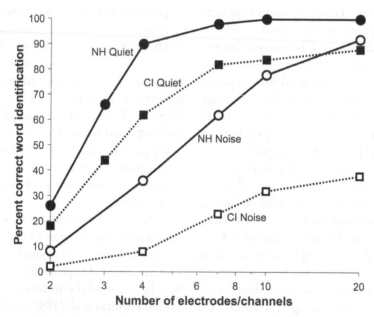

FIGURE 9–3. Effects of the number of electrodes on speech perception for listeners with normal hearing and CI users. Adapted from Friesen et al. (2001).

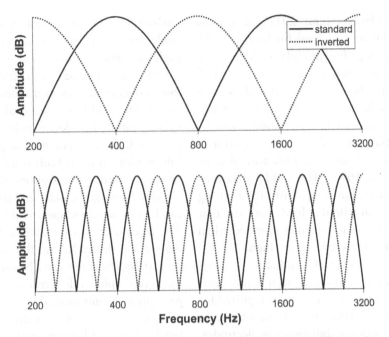

FIGURE 9–4. Sample stimulus spectra used for the spectral ripple test. The top and bottom panels illustrate amplitude spectra for spectral ripples of 0.5 and 2 cycles/octave, respectively. Solid lines indicate spectra for the standard stimulus and dotted lines indicate spectra for the inverted stimulus.

times worse than listeners with sensorineural hearing loss and eight times worse than listeners with normal hearing (Henry et al., 2005). There is wide variability in the spectral resolution of CI users, and better spectral-ripple discrimination thresholds are associated with better speech recognition thresholds (SRTs) in noise (Won et al., 2007).

Temporal Processing

Temporal processing is critical for speech perception of listeners with CIs, due to the limited spectral resolution available to these listeners. Measures of gap-detection and amplitude-modulation-detection have been widely used to assess the temporal processing abilities of CI users. Some CI users exhibit near-normal temporal processing abilities, but there is considerable variation across listeners (Garadat & Pfingst, 2011). As previously mentioned, it can be challenging to compare data between these two groups of listeners due to the exceptional differences between the mechanisms responsible for hearing and the differences in the ways in which perception must be measured. When a direct connection is used, the temporal change is imposed on the pulse train, but when stimuli are presented over loudspeakers, the experimenter has less control over the stimuli. Regardless of how temporal processing is measured, there is wide variability in the temporal processing abilities of CI users.

In some cases, particularly when electrodes are stimulated directly, many CI users exhibit temporal processing thresholds that are better than those measured for listeners with normal hearing. For gap detection, CI users report thresholds in the 1 to 2 ms range (Garadat & Pfingst, 2011), in contrast to thresholds of 2 to 3 ms for listeners with normal hearing. For modulation detection, the shape and cutoff frequency of the TMTF is very similar between CI users and listeners with normal hearing (Fraser & McKay, 2012). However, some CI listeners show modulation detection thresholds that are superior to that measured in listeners with normal hearing (Shannon, 1992). The TMTF measured in CI listeners, however, illustrates a strong dependence on stimulus level, with the best temporal processing measures reported when stimulus presentation levels are high.

One advantage of conducting experiments using a direct connection is that temporal processing measures can be reported for each electrode. There is wide variability in temporal processing abilities across electrodes, perhaps due to differences in the neural survival pattern across electrode locations for a single user and across CI users (Shader et al., 2020). Forward masking and temporal integration experiments also demonstrate wide variability across listeners. For forward masking, CI users show a 100 to 200 ms decay time window, very similar to that measured in listeners with normal hearing (Shannon, 1990). For temporal integration, the time window is also similar between CI users and those with normal hearing, but CI listeners benefit very little from the increased duration of stimuli (Donaldson et al., 1997).

Taken together, for high stimulus presentation levels, CI users generally have temporal processing abilities that are similar (or sometimes better) than listeners with normal hearing. Converging evidence also indicates a strong positive correlation between temporal processing abilities and speech perception (Fu, 2002).

Pitch

The electrode array of the cochlear implant represents the acoustic information in the environment in a tonotopic manner—electrodes nearer the base of the cochlea present high-frequency information whereas electrodes nearer the apex of the cochlea present low-frequency information about the acoustic signal. The cochlear implant also stimulates hearing through an electric pulse train. Therefore, the CI has the potential to provide pitch information through both place and temporal codes. Unlike when testing listeners with acoustic hearing, the place and temporal code can be evaluated independently in CI users. The place code can be assessed by stimulating specific electrodes and the temporal code by varying the pulse rate. Notably, CI users can perceive pitch information, but their pitch perception is substantially compromised in comparison to listeners with sensorineural hearing loss and listeners with normal hearing (Moore & Carlyon, 2005).

To establish whether pitch can be conveyed via place in listeners who wear a cochlear implant, a single electrode can be stimulated with the pulse train. In one study, Nelson et al. (1995) applied fixed-rate pulse trains sequentially to two different electrodes and asked listeners to determine which electrode evoked a higher pitch. Evidence of an active place code would be the perception of a higher pitch for the more basal electrode, due to tonotopic organization. The majority of participants reported higher pitch when the more basal electrodes were stimulated, indicating that CI listeners do have access to a place code. Some listeners were able to determine a pitch difference for adjacent electrodes (e.g., the 5th and 6th electrode) with 100% accuracy, but others required electrodes to be spaced very widely apart. These listeners did have access to a place code, but it did not provide a strong mechanism for pitch.

In the cochlear implant, pitch can also be conveyed through the temporal code by varying the stimulation rate. Zeng (2002) measured whether CI listeners could perceive differences in pitch by stimulating an individual electrode with pulse trains of different frequencies (50 to 500 Hz). By using stimuli like these, he was able to measure the frequency difference limen (FDL). His results indicated that frequency discrimination worsened with increasing stimulation frequency and was very poor for pulse rates greater than 300 Hz. His work demonstrated that these CI users had access to a temporal code for pitch perception, but only up to a point. There are substantial individual differences, however, and alternative stimulation strategies may provide better support for pitch perception (McKay et al., 1994; Müller et al., 2012).

Binaural Hearing

Listeners with two cochlear implants (and to some extent, individuals with combined acoustic and electric hearing) have the potential to experience binaural auditory perception, although binaural cues are not always well-preserved by the CI due to software and circuitry in the speech processor. There is fairly strong support for bilateral cochlear implantation when listeners meet the criteria for two CIs, as these individuals have better speech understanding and better sound localization than those who receive one cochlear implant. Evidence indicates that many listeners with bilateral CIs can utilize sound localization cues, although it may not be surprising that binaural auditory perception is poorer for CI users than for those with normal hearing.

Grantham et al. (2007) measured sound localization errors in CI users and noted that average localization error for a CI user was about 24°, whereas it was <8° for listeners with normal hearing. Thresholds for both ILD and ITD discrimination were also much higher for CI users compared to those with normal hearing, but CI listeners were better able to perceive the ILD than the ITD (Grantham et al., 2008). Although listeners with CIs benefit from spatial release from masking, not surprisingly, these benefits are not as striking as for listeners with normal hearing. CI users have access to binaural summation, better-ear effects, and binaural squelch with the better-ear effect being the dominant cue (Buss et al., 2008). Findings such as these support the practice of bilateral cochlear implantation (Litovsky et al., 2006), as many listeners with CIs do have access to binaural cues.

Summary

Psychoacoustics has been a primary driver in the development of cochlear implant technologies that can facilitate better speech perception for these listeners. CI users have far better perception than prior to receiving the implant, but the CI does not typically provide auditory perception that approaches that of listeners with normal hearing. The spectral resolution of the CI is relatively poor, but temporal processing skills of CI users are strong. Speech perception by CI users is correlated with temporal processing skills, and improving the spectral resolution of the cochlear implant is likely to lead to improvements in speech perception, particularly in noise. CI users also have access to pitch and binaural hearing, although these abilities do not rival that of listeners with normal hearing.

SUMMARY AND TAKE-HOME POINTS

The various devices designed to support auditory perception have a goal of improving perception of everyday sounds, primarily speech but also music and environmental sounds. None of these devices cure hearing loss, but they improve auditory thresholds so that the neural mechanisms responsible for higher level perception may engage for the tasks at hand. There is clear evidence that better auditory thresholds (provided by amplification or stimulation of the auditory nerve) lead to better speech perception. Amplification alone provides better access to necessary auditory perceptual cues, even though nonlinear algorithms within these devices, like directionality and noise reduction, may be somewhat detrimental. Collectively, however, those distortions have less of a negative impact on speech perception than the benefits provided by improved audibility.

The following points are key take-home messages of this chapter:

- The improved audibility provided by hearing aids is associated with improved performance on various psychoacoustic tasks.
- Psychoacoustics also reveals aspects of hearing aid technology that need improvement, as some of those technologies distort the acoustic cues provided to the wearer.
- Cochlear implants provide superior auditory perception for individuals who wear them, but most CI users are required to rely on temporal information for speech perception, as spectral information is substantially limited.

EXERCISES

1. Assume a situation in which a listener with sensorineural hearing loss receives linear amplification that ensures audibility but does not exceed uncomfortable levels. Discuss the effects of linear amplification (in this case, simply making the sound audible) on the following:
   a. masking of pure tones
   b. loudness perception
   c. temporal processing
   d. ILD processing
   e. ITD processing
   f. Pitch perception
2. Explain why digital noise reduction would provide little benefit to a listener

with sensorineural hearing loss unless she also received amplification.
3. Discuss why low-frequency amplification will exacerbate upward spread of masking experienced by a listener with SNHL.
4. Ling has a monaural hearing loss and wears a hearing aid in one ear that amplifies sound by 20 dB across all frequencies. Her hearing aid has an average time delay of about 4 ms, and the delay is greater at low frequencies than high. Considering the topics discussed in this text, how might these perceptual abilities be affected by this hearing aid?
   a. Absolute threshold in her aided ear
   b. Speech understanding in her aided ear
   c. Sound localization based on the ITD
   d. Sound localization based on the ILD
   e. Binaural release from masking
5. List the primary factors that limit frequency selectivity for a CI user.
6. Discuss why a CI user relies more on temporal cues than spectral cues for speech perception.
7. Do you think an individual who wears a CI on the deaf ear and has typical hearing in the other ear will be able to perceive the ITD or ILD? Provide your reasoning.
8. Pedro has a unilateral cochlear implant that preserved his good low-frequency hearing. He has good hearing in his other ear. After receiving the implant, the audiologist notes that he has good acoustic hearing at frequencies below about 500 Hz in the CI ear and that he relies on electric hearing for frequencies of 1000 Hz and above.
   a. Does Pedro have the potential to perceive the ILD and ITD?
   b. Does Pedro have the potential to achieve binaural release from masking, as with the MLD?
   c. Does Pedro have the potential to access better-ear effects and binaural squelch? Discuss.

REFERENCES

Akeroyd, M. A. (2014). An overview of the major phenomena of the localization of sound sources by normal-hearing, hearing-impaired, and aided listeners. *Trends in Hearing, 18,* 1–7.

Başkent, D., & Shannon, R. V. (2005). Interactions between cochlear implant electrode insertion depth and frequency-place mapping. *Journal of the Acoustical Society of America, 117*(3), 1405–1416.

Bentler, R. A. (2005). Effectiveness of directional microphones and noise reduction schemes in hearing aids: A systematic review of the evidence. *Journal of the American Academy of Audiology, 16*(07), 473–484.

Bor, S., Souza, P., & Wright, R. (2008). Multichannel compression: Effects of reduced spectral contrast on vowel identification. *Journal of Speech, Language, and Hearing Research,* 51(5), 1315–1327.

Brennan, M. A., McCreery, R. W., & Jesteadt, W. (2015). The influence of hearing-aid compression on forward-masked thresholds for adults with hearing loss. *Journal of the Acoustical Society of America, 138,* 2589–2597.

Davies-Venn, E., Souza, P., Brennan, M., & Stecker, G. C. (2009). Effects of audibility and multichannel wide dynamic range compression on consonant recognition for listeners with severe hearing loss. *Ear and Hearing, 30*(5), 494.

Derleth, P., Georganti, E., Latzel, M., Courtois, G., Hofbauer, M., Raether, J., & Kuehnel, V. (2021). Binaural signal processing in hearing aids. *Seminars in Hearing, 42*(3), 206–223.

Desjardins, J. L., & Doherty, K. A. (2014). The effect of hearing aid noise reduction on listening effort in hearing-impaired adults. *Ear and Hearing, 35*(6), 600–610.

Donaldson G. S., Viemeister, N. F., & Nelson, D. A. (1997). Psychometric functions and temporal integration in electric hearing. *Journal of the Acoustical Society of America, 101,* 3706–3721.

Fishman, K. E., Shannon, R. V., & Slattery, W. H. (1997). Speech recognition as a function of the number of electrodes used in the SPEAK cochlear implant speech processor. *Journal of Speech Language and Hearing Research, 40,* 1201–1215.

Fraser M., & McKay C. M. (2012). Temporal modulation transfer functions in cochlear implantees using a method that limits overall loudness cues. *Hearing Research, 283*(1–2), 59–69.

Friesen, L. M., Shannon, R. V., Başkent, D., & Wang, X. (2001). Speech recognition in noise as a function of the number of spectral channels: Comparison of acoustic hearing and cochlear implants. *Journal of the Acoustical Society of America, 110,* 1150–1163.

Fu, Q. J. (2002). Temporal processing and speech recognition in cochlear implant users. *NeuroReport, 13*(13), 1635–1639.

Fu, Q. J. (2005). Loudness growth in cochlear implants: effect of stimulus rate and electrode configuration. *Hearing Research, 202,* 55–62.

Fu, Q. J., & Shannon, R. V. (1998). Effects of amplitude nonlinearity on phoneme recognition by cochlear implant users and normal-hearing listeners. *Journal of the Acoustical Society of America, 104*(5), 2570–2577.

Garadat, S. N., & Pfingst, B. E. (2011). Relationship between gap detection thresholds and loudness in cochlear-implant users. *Hearing Research, 275*(1–2), 130–138.

Grantham, D. W., Ashmead, D. H., Ricketts, T. A., Labadie, R. F., & Haynes, D. S. (2007). Horizontal-plane localization of noise and speech signals by postlingually deafened adults fitted with bilateral cochlear implants. *Ear and Hearing, 28*(4), 524–541.

Grantham, D. W., Ashmead, D. H., Ricketts, T. A., Haynes, D. S., & Labadie, R. F. (2008). Interaural time and level difference thresholds for acoustically presented signals in post-lingually deafened adults fitted with bilateral cochlear implants using CIS+ processing. *Ear and Hearing, 29*(1), 33–44.

Hedrick, M. S., & Rice, T. (2000). Effect of a single channel-wide dynamic range compression circuit on perception of stop consonant place of articulation. *Journal of Speech, Language, and Hearing Research, 43*(5), 1174–1184.

Henry, B. A., & Turner, C. W. (2003). The resolution of complex spectral patterns in cochlear implant and normal hearing listeners. *Journal of the Acoustical Society of America, 113,* 2861–2873.

Henry, B. A., Turner, C. W., & Behrens, A. (2005). Spectral peak resolution and speech recognition in quiet: Normal hearing, hearing impaired, and cochlear implant listeners. *Journal of the Acoustical Society of America, 118*(2), 1111–1121.

Kiliç, M., & Kara, E. (2022). The effect of multichannel and channel-free hearing aids on spectral-temporal resolution and speech understanding in noise. *Journal of the American Academy of Audiology, 33*(5), 285–292.

Litovsky, R., Parkinson, A., Arcaroli, J., & Sammeth, C. (2006). Simultaneous bilateral cochlear implantation in adults: a multicenter clinical study. *Ear and Hearing, 27*(6), 714.

McKay C. M., McDermott H. J., & Clark G.M. (1994). Pitch percepts associated with amplitude-modulated current pulse trains in cochlear implantees. *Journal of the Acoustical Society of America, 96*(5 Pt 1), 2664–2673.

Moore, B. C. J. & Carolyn, R. P. (2005). Perception of pitch by people with cochlear hearing loss and by cochlear implant users. In C. J., Plack, A. J., Oxenham, R. R., Fay, & A. N. Popper (Eds.) *Pitch: Neural coding and perception* (pp. 234–277). Springer.

Moore, B. C., Glasberg, B. R., Alcántara, J. I., Launer, S., & Kuehnel, V. (2001). Effects of slow- and fast-acting compression on the detection of gaps in narrow bands of noise. *British Journal of Audiology, 35*(6), 365–374. .

Müller, J., Brill, S., Hagen, R., Moeltner, A., Brockmeier, S. J., Stark, T., . . . Anderson, I. (2012). Clinical trial results with the MED-EL fine structure processing coding strategy in experienced cochlear implant users. *ORL, Journal for Oto-rhino-laryngology and Its Related Specialties, 74*(4), 185–198.

Nelson, D. A., Van Tasell, D. J., Schroder, A. C., Soli, S., & Levine, S. (1995). Electrode ranking of "place pitch" and speech recognition in electrical hearing. *Journal of the Acoustical Society of America, 98*(4), 1987–1999.

Pfingst, B. E., Burnett, P. A., & Sutton, D. (1983). Intensity discrimination with cochlear implants. *Journal of the Acoustical Society of America, 73*(4), 1283–1292.

Picou, E. M., & Ricketts, T. A. (2017). How directional microphones affect speech recognition, listening effort and localisation for listeners with moderate-to-severe hearing loss. *International Journal of Audiology, 56*(12), 909–918.

Picou, E. M., Aspell, E., & Ricketts, T. A. (2014). Potential benefits and limitations of three types of directional processing in hearing aids. *Ear and Hearing, 35*(3), 339–352.

Plomp, R. (1988). The negative effect of amplitude compression in multichannel hearing aids in the light of the modulation-transfer function. *Journal of the Acoustical Society of America, 83*(6), 2322–2327.

Shader, M. J., Gordon-Salant, S., & Goupell, M. J. (2020). Impact of aging and the electrode-to-neural interface on temporal processing ability in cochlear-implant users: Amplitude-modulation detection thresholds. *Trends in Hearing, 24*, 1–14.

Shannon, R. V. (1990). Forward masking in patients with cochlear implants. *Journal of the Acoustical Society of America, 88*(2), 741–744.

Shannon, R. V. (1992). Temporal modulation transfer functions in patients with cochlear implants. *Journal of the Acoustical Society of America, 91*(4), 2156–2164.

Strelcyk, O., Nooraei, N., Kalluri, S., & Edwards, B. (2012). Restoration of loudness summation and differential loudness growth in hearing-impaired listeners. *Journal of the Acoustical Society of America, 132*, 2557–2568.

van den Bogaert, T., Doclo, S., Wouters, J., & Moonen, (2009). Speech enhancement with multichannel Wiener filter techniques in multimicrophone binaural hearing aids. *Journal of the Acoustical Society of America, 125*(1), 360–371.

Wiinberg, A., Jepsen, M. L., Epp, B., & Dau, T. (2019). Effects of hearing loss and fast-acting compression on amplitude modulation perception and speech intelligibility. *Ear and Hearing, 40*(1), 45–54.

Won, J. H., Drennan, W. R., & Rubinstein, J. T. (2007). Spectral-ripple resolution correlates with speech reception in noise in cochlear implant users. *Journal of the Association for Research in Otolaryngology, 8*(3), 384–392.

Yund, E. W., & Buckles, K. M. (1995). Multichannel compression hearing aids: Effect of number of channels on speech discrimination in noise. *Journal of the Acoustical Society of America, 97*(2), 1206–1223.

Zeng, F. G. (2002). Temporal pitch in electric hearing. *Hearing Research, 174*(1–2), 101–106.

Zheng, Y., Swanson, J., Koehnke, J., & Guan, J. (2022). Sound localization of listeners with normal hearing, impaired hearing, hearing aids, bone-anchored hearing instruments, and cochlear implants: A review. *American Journal of Audiology, 31*(3), 812–834.

Glossary

A

absolute threshold—the minimum detectable level of a sound in the absence of external noise.

adaptive staircase method—an adaptive method in which the signal levels are determined by a listener's previous responses.

alternate binaural loudness balancing method (ABLB)—an audiological method based on loudness matching between the ears. It is used to identify whether a listener with unilateral hearing loss experiences recruitment in the ear with poorer thresholds.

amplitude—the size of a stimulus.

amplitude modulation detection—an experimental paradigm in which a listener is asked to detect the presence of modulation on a sound. It measures the amplitude modulation detection threshold.

audiogram—a plot of absolute threshold in dB HL versus frequency.

auditory filters—a psychophysical model that describes the filtering process of the ear.

auditory nerve—the auditory portion of the vestibulocochlear nerve.

auditory neuropathy spectrum disorders (ANSD) —a rare auditory disorder that affects the typical synchronous activity in the auditory nerve.

auditory processing disorder (APD)—a condition that affects the way the brain processes auditory information.

auditory scene analysis—the process by which the auditory system organizes sound into meaningful elements.

autocorrelation—a process that determines the periodicities present in a stimulus.

B

bandwidth—the range of frequencies passed by a filter or contained within a stimulus.

Békésy audiometry—an automated form of audiometry that dates back to the 1940s. The level of a tone increases and decreases automatically, and a patient presses a button as long as he hears the tone.

best frequency—the frequency associated with the lowest threshold, used to characterize tuning curves.

better-ear advantage—an effect in which interactions between the head and a sound field cause one ear to have a better signal-to-noise ratio than the other.

better-ear effect—a quantification of the better-ear advantage. It characterizes the difference in speech in noise scores between the two ears.

binaural hearing—hearing with two ears

binaural masking level difference (BMLD or MLD)—an improvement in signal detection from binaural effects. It is characterized by a reduction in the masked threshold for a binaural signal presented with binaural noise when the signal (but not the masker) is presented out-of-phase at one of the ears.

binaural squelch—the ability to supplement the better ear advantage with binaural hearing and take advantage of the ear with the poorer signal-to-noise ratio.

binaural summation—improvements in auditory abilities from having two ears.

binaural unmasking—the ability of two ears to reduce the effects of masking noise.

bracketing procedure—a procedure in which a listener selects one of two sounds presented, and the tester presents two additional sounds based on that response. The process is repeated until the method converges.

C

carrier—(See "temporal fine structure.")

categorical loudness scaling—a procedure used to measure the loudness of sounds using categories ranging from very soft to uncomfortably loud.

center frequency—the frequency at the center of a filter's or a stimulus' frequency range.

central auditory processing disorder (CAPD)—(See "auditory processing disorder.")

cochlear implants—implantable devices that bypass the outer, middle, and inner ear, and stimulate the auditory nerve with electrical impulses.

complex tones—sounds that consist of multiple tones.

comprehension—the process by which sounds are assigned meaning.

compressive nonlinearity—the range of sound levels at which basilar membrane vibration grows more slowly than the input signal.

cone of confusion—a 3D conical surface extending out of each ear that represents the same ITD on the surface.

configuration of hearing loss—the shape of the audiogram.

contralateral interference—the process by which hearing a sound in one ear interferes with perception in the other.

count-the-dot audiogram—a visual way to predict speech intelligibility using the audiogram.

criterion—in relation to signal detection theory, the internal response above which a listener will say "yes, I hear a signal."

critical band—a measure of the effective bandwidth of the filtering provided by the ear. It is the range of frequencies within which one tone interferes with the perception of another.

critical duration—the duration beyond which thresholds no longer increase with increasing duration.

cross-modality scaling—listeners are given a set of terms ranging from "very soft" to "painfully loud."

cutoff frequencies—the highest or lowest frequencies before a filter attenuates sound.

D

dead regions—regions in the cochlea in which all inner hair cells (or auditory nerve fibers) are lost or not functioning.

decibel (hearing level, hearing loss; dB HL)—a decibel metric in which audiometric thresholds are referenced to normative data from adult listeners with normal hearing.

decibel (sensation level; dB SL)—a decibel metric in which sound levels are referenced to a listener's auditory threshold.

decibel (sound pressure level; dB SPL)—a decibel metric in which uses 20 μPa as the reference.

detection—the ability to perceive the presence of a stimulus.

dichotic—presenting different signals to both ears.

difference limen—(See the "just-noticeable difference.")

digital noise reduction (DNR)—an algorithm commonly used in hearing aids that adjusts the gain in each band with the goal of improving the SNR at the output of the hearing aid.

dip listening—the ability to take advantage of temporal waveform valleys that have a high Signal-to-Noise ratio to improve performance.

diotic—presenting identical signals to both ears.

diplacusis—the perception of hearing the same tone at a different pitch in each ear.

directional microphones—microphones that are more sensitive to sounds from particular locations compared to others. They are used in modern hearing aids to improve the SNR at the output of the hearing aid.

discrimination—the ability to hear that two sounds are different from each other.

duplex theory of sound localization—the theory that proposes two acoustic cues for sound localization: intensity differences across the ears for high frequencies and time differences across the ears for low frequencies.

dynamic range of hearing—the range of sound levels between absolute threshold and the threshold of discomfort or pain

E

effective masking level (EML)—the dB HL value to which threshold is shifted in the presence of a noise at that dB EML.

energy detector—a model of temporal integration that posits that the ear integrates the intensity over time up to the critical duration.

envelope—slow stimulus fluctuations in the waveform.

equal-loudness contour—a measure of sound pressure levels across frequency for which a listener perceives equal loudness.

excitation pattern—a psychoacoustic representation of the stimulus spectrum after auditory filtering.

existence region—frequency region over which the pitch does not change when harmonics are removed.

F

filter—a device that modifies sound.

filter (bandpass)—a filter that attenuates both high and low frequencies, while allowing a selected range through the filter.

filter (highpass)—a filter that attenuates low frequencies and allows high frequencies to pass through.

filter (lowpass)—a filter that attenuates high frequencies and allows low frequencies to pass through.

fluctuating masker benefit—an improvement in masked threshold provided by a fluctuating (modulated) stimulus.

forced-choice—an experimental paradigm in which more than observation intervals are presented, and the listener must determine which observation interval contained the signal.

forward masking—a process in which masking occurs when a masker precedes a stimulus in time.

Fourier analysis—a process by which complex sounds can be decomposed into sine waves.

frequency—the number of cycles a sound completes in a second.

frequency difference limen (FDL)—the just-noticeable difference in frequency.

frequency discrimination—an experimental paradigm that measures the ability to determine whether one sound has different frequency from another. It measures the JND for frequency.

frequency-gain functions—(See "transfer functions.")

frequency selectivity—the ability of the auditory system to represent one frequency as independent of another.

frequency specific—containing few frequencies.

fundamental frequency (f$_0$)—the lowest frequency of a complex tone. Other tones within the stimulus occur at integer multiples of the fundamental frequency.

fundamental frequency difference limen (F$_0$DL)—the just-noticeable difference in fundamental frequency.

G

gap detection—an experimental paradigm in which a listener is asked to determine whether a brief temporal gap is present in a sound. It measures the gap detection threshold.

H

harmonic sounds—complex tones containing frequencies that are related to each other by integer multiples.

harmonic template models—models that posit that the fundamental frequency of a sound is coded on the basilar membrane and can be derived from the location of the peaks of the traveling wave distributed along the length of the cochlea.

head-related transfer function (HRTF)—a three-dimensional function that codes for the spectral and phase changes that occur when sounds are presented at different locations with respect to the body.

head shadow—a reduction in intensity at the ear distant from the source.

hearing loss (conductive)—hearing loss associated with outer or middle ear disorders.

hearing loss (sensorineural)—hearing loss associated with cochlear damage.

hyperacusis—increased sensitivity to sounds.

I

identification—the level of auditory perception in which a sound is attached to an object or a label.

incomplete recruitment—(See "under recruitment.")

increment detection—(See "intensity discrimination.")

input-output (I-O) function—the relationship between the input of a system and its output.

intensity—the power in a sound, described as watts/m^2.

intensity discrimination—an experimental paradigm that measures the ability to determine whether one sound is more intense than another. It measures the JND for intensity.

interaural level difference (ILD)—the level difference (in dB) of a sound between the two ears.

interaural phase difference (IPD)—the phase difference of a sound between two ears.

interaural time difference (ITD)—the difference in arrival time of a sound between two ears.

J

just-noticeable difference (JND)—the smallest difference on some dimension between two sounds that is detectable or discriminable.

L

lateralization—localization of sounds that are perceived as being inside the head.

level per cycle (LPC)—(See "spectrum level.")

localization—the ability to locate the position of a sound in space.

long-term spectrum of speech (LTASS)—the spectral distribution of speech.

loudness—the attribute of auditory sensation by which sounds can be ordered on a scale ranging from soft to loud.

loudness balancing—a procedure in which level of a sound is adjusted so that its loudness matches that of a reference sound.

loudness discomfort level (LDL)—the level of sound in dB at which sound is uncomfortably loud.

loudness growth function—a function that relates the loudness of sounds to intensity.

loudness level—level of an equally loud 1000-Hz tone in dB SPL for a test sound, measured in phons.

loudness recruitment—an abnormally rapid growth of loudness. This is common in listeners with SNHL.

loudness summation—a perceptual phenomenon in which wider bandwidth sounds are perceived as narrower bandwidth sounds, even if they have the same dB level.

M

magnitude estimation—a procedure in which a listener estimates the relationship between the loudness of one sound with another at a different intensity.

magnitude production—a measurement technique in which a listener adjusts a sound to be a specified size. In a loudness experiment, a listener might adjust the level of a test sound to be a specified amount louder than a reference sound.

masker—a stimulus that raises the threshold of another stimulus.

masking—the process by which the presence of one sound interferes with the perception of another.

masking pattern—the amount of masking in dB for a single masker plotted as a function of the frequency of the signal being masked.

mel—the perceptual unit of pitch. One thousand mels is defined as the pitch associated with a 1000-Hz tone.

method of adjustment—a method to estimate threshold in which listener the adjusts the level of a stimulus to find threshold.

method of constant stimuli—method that involves stimulus presentations at randomly selected levels and a measurement of percentage detections (or discriminations).

method of limits—one of the three classical psychoacoustic procedures used to estimate threshold. The experimenter presents stimuli at a level below (or above) the threshold and increases (or decreases) the stimulus level until it is perceivable (or rendered inaudible) to the listener.

minimum audible angle (MAA)—the smallest angular separation at which two sounds are perceived as being in different locations.

minimum audible field (MAF) curve—a free-field, binaural measurement of the minimum detectable sound pressure level as a function of frequency.

minimum audible pressure (MAP) curve—a monaural measurement made over headphones of the minimum detectable sound pressure level as a function of frequency.

modified Hughson-Westlake method—a procedure used in clinical audiology to measure audiometric thresholds.

modulator—(See "envelope.")

monaural hearing—hearing with one ear.

monotic—presenting a stimulus to a single ear.

multiple looks hypothesis—a model of temporal integration, which states that increasing the duration of the stimulus provides more opportunities to detect the stimulus.

N

near miss to Weber's law—the JND for intensity, when expressed as a proportion of the intensity of the stimulus, decreases with increasing intensity across the audible range for tones.

noise—any unwanted sound. (See also "white noise" or "narrowband noise.")

noise (white)—random signal with a constant power spectral density.

noise (narrowband)—noise with a restricted frequency range.

notched-noise method—a technique used to estimate the size and shape of the auditory filter using a noise stimulus with a spectral notch.

O

observation interval—the interval of time during which a listener is expecting a stimulus.

organ of Corti—the sensory organ for hearing.

P

partial recruitment—(See "under recruitment.")

peak amplitude (pressure)—the maximum amplitude (pressure) value achieved.

performance-intensity (PI) function—a function relating performance on a speech recognition task to the intensity of the stimulus.

period—the time a sound takes to complete a single cycle.

phase locking—a characteristic of auditory nerve fibers in which they tend to fire at a particular phase of a low-frequency stimulus.

phon—the unit of loudness level equal in number to the decibel level of a 1000-Hz tone.

pitch—the perception on which sounds can be ordered from high to low.

pitch of the missing fundamental—(See "residue pitch.")

pitch strength—a characterization of the salience of the pitch of sounds, ranges from strong to weak.

place code for pitch—a spectral representation for pitch. The frequency of a sound is coded in

terms of the place of stimulation in the auditory pathway.

power law relationship—relationship between two variables that follows $y = x^p$.

power spectrum model of masking—a theory stating that masking is determined by the power at the output of a single auditory filter.

precedence effect—a binaural effect that describes the fusion of sound and its echo. Sound localization is based on the acoustic cues associated with the sound that arrives first at the ears.

profile analysis—an experimental paradigm that measures the ability to discriminate between sounds with different power spectra.

pseudohypacusis—false or feigned hearing loss.

psychoacoustics—the study of the relationship between the sound and its perception.

psychometric function—a function relating the percentage of sound detections or discriminations to a signal strength parameter.

psychophysical tuning curve (PTC)—(See "tuning curve [psychological].")

psychophysics—the study of the relationship between the physical stimuli and their perception.

pure tone—a sound with one frequency, characterized by a sinusoidal function.

R

rate-level function—a function relating a neuron's output firing rate to input stimulus level.

rating—(See "magnitude estimation.")

reaction time—the time it takes for a listener to react to a stimulus.

receiver operating characteristic (ROC)—a plot of hits versus false alarms.

recognition—(See "identification.")

release from masking (forward)—as a signal and forward masker become more separated in time, the masker has less of an effect on the signal detection threshold.

release from masking (general)—changes to the stimulus or the masker lead to less masking than for a tonal signal in a broadband noise masker.

residue pitch—pitch of a complex sound when the component associated with the fundamental frequency is removed.

resolved harmonics—harmonics that are represented independently in the excitation pattern.

response bias—(See "response proclivity.")

response interval—the interval of time during which a listener is expected to respond to a stimulus.

response proclivity—how the listener responds to the stimuli and associated biases.

retrocochlear—an auditory pathology that occurs beyond the cochlea.

root mean squared (rms) pressure—the square root of the average of the square of the pressure of the sound signal over a given duration.

S

scaling—(See "magnitude estimation.")

sensitivity (auditory)—the strength of the capacity to perceive a sound or a change in a sound.

sensitivity (test)—the ability of a test to correctly identify true positives (or patients with a pathology).

short-increment sensitivity index (SISI)—a psychoacoustical test in which a listener counts the number of small intensity increments imposed on a tone.

signal—a stimulus of interest.

Signal Detection Theory (SDT)—a framework to quantify the ability to discern between a signal and noise.

simultaneous masking—a paradigm in which maskers and signals are presented at the same time.

sinusoidally amplitude modulation (SAM)—a specific type of modulation in which the modulator is a sinusoid.

softness imperception—a theory that claims that the loudness of sounds at and near threshold may be higher for listeners with SNHL than for those with normal hearing.

sone—a unit of subjective loudness equal to the loudness of a 1000-Hz tone presented at 40 dB SPL.

sound—a pressure wave that results from oscillation of particles within a medium.

sound level—a general term describing the magnitude or amplitude of a sound.

specificity (test)—the ability of a test to correctly identify true negatives (or patients without a pathology).

spectral loudness summation—a phenomenon in which the loudness of a test stimulus increases as its bandwidth increases.

spectral splatter—refers to an unintended increase in the range of frequencies present in a stimulus, often caused by a rapid stimulus onset or offset or shortening the duration of a sound.

spectrum—a plot of amplitude versus frequency.

spectrum level—the amount of power in dB SPL within a sound contained within a 1-Hz band.

Speech Intelligibility Index (SII)—a measure that represents the intelligibility of speech under a variety of listening conditions.

speech recognition threshold (SRT)—the level in dB HL at which words can be identified 50% of the time.

staircase method—(See "adaptive staircase method.")

Stenger test—a test based on the principle of lateralization to identify the presence of pseudo-hypacusis.

Stevens' power law—a characterization of how loudness changes with intensity. Empirically, loudness grows in proportion to stimulus intensity raised to the power of 0.3.

T

temporal acuity—(See "temporal resolution.")

temporal code for pitch—a mechanism in which the pitch of a stimulus is based on the temporal patterns of neural impulses evoked by that stimulus.

temporal fine structure—rapid stimulus fluctuations in the waveform.

temporal integration—the ability of the ear to accumulate information over time to improve detection threshold.

temporal masking—(See "forward masking.")

temporal modulation transfer function (TMTF)—a plot relating amplitude modulation detection threshold to the modulation rate.

temporal processing—the general ability of the ear to represent stimulus changes over time.

temporal resolution—the ability to represent rapid changes in the envelope of sound.

temporal summation—(See "temporal integration.")

threshold equalizing noise (TEN) test—a test used to determine whether cochlear dead regions are present. In the absence of a dead region, thresholds measured in a TEN noise should be the same as the level of the noise.

time constant—the time frame over which temporal integration occurs.

time-frequency tradeoff—an acoustic principle in which short-duration sounds must have a spectrum with a wide bandwidth.

tinnitus—the perception of a sound in its absence.

tonotopic organization—different areas or cell populations of the brain respond to different frequencies. It begins at the basilar membrane and is maintained throughout the auditory system.

total power—the amount of power contained across all frequencies in a sound.

transfer function—a function that characterizes a system's frequency-gain characteristics.

traveling wave—a wave of basilar membrane vibration that travels through the basilar membrane until it reaches its place of maximum vibration.

trial—a sequence of the observation interval(s) plus the response interval.

tuning curve (physiological)—a plot relating the threshold sound level required to elicit a neural or basilar membrane response.

tuning curve (psychological)—a plot showing the level of a sound stimulus required to mask a fixed low-level signal.

two-tone suppression—a process in which one tone suppresses the neural activity produced by a second tone.

U

uncomfortable loudness level (UCL or ULL)—the level of sound in dB at which sound becomes uncomfortably loud.

under recruitment—a phenomenon in which the loudness of sounds, even at high levels, does not approach the loudness measured in listeners with normal hearing.

unresolved harmonics—harmonics that are not represented independently in the excitation pattern.

upward spread of masking—a phenomenon in which low-frequency sounds mask high-frequency sounds more than the reverse.

V

vestibulocochlear nerve—the VIIIth cranial nerve that is comprised of vestibular and auditory/cochlear fibers.

volley theory—a theory first proposed by Wever and Bray that individual fibers could be synchronized to a waveform, even if they did not fire on every cycle. A group of fibers could then code for the frequency of sound via their pooled response.

W

waveform—a plot of instantaneous amplitude versus time.

wavelength—the distance sound travels in a single cycle.

Weber fraction—the mathematical characterization of Weber's law: $\Delta S/S=k$, where S is the size of a stimulus and k is a constant.

Weber's law—the just-noticeable change in a stimulus is a constant ratio (or percentage) of the original stimulus.

white noise—a broad bandwidth stimulus that has a relatively flat power spectrum and randomly distributed instantaneous amplitude in the waveform.

wide dynamic range compression (WDRC)—a nonlinear hearing aid algorithm that makes low-level sounds audible and high-level sounds more comfortable.

Y

Y—an experimental task in which a stimulus is either present or absent, and a response is either *yes* or *no* to indicate whether a sound was heard.

Index

Note: Page numbers in **bold** reference non-text material.